NATURAL
HEALTH,
NATURAL
MEDICINE

NATURAL HEALTH, NATURAL MEDICINE

A COMPREHENSIVE
MANUAL FOR WELLNESS
AND SELF-CARE

ANDREW WEIL, M.D.

REVISED EDITION

HOUGHTON MIFFLIN COMPANY
Boston • New York

This book is not intended to be a total replacement for standard (allopathic) medicine, which has its place in the diagnosis and treatment of disease. Any unusual, persistent, or severe symptoms should be evaluated by a physician. The natural treatments suggested here, although generally safer than pharmaceutical drugs, can affect different people differently, occasionally producing adverse reactions. If a condition fails to respond to these treatments, you should consult a physician to see about another course of action.

For information about permission to reproduce selections from this book, write to Permissions, Houghton Mifflin Company, 215 Park Avenue South, New York, New York 10003.

Library of Congress Cataloging-in-Publication Data
Weil, Andrew.
Natural health, natural medicine : a comprehensive manual for wellness and self-care / Andrew Weil. — Rev. ed.
p.   cm.
Includes bibliographical references.
ISBN 0-395-73099-6 (pbk.)
1. Health.   2. Nutrition.   3. Naturopathy.
4. Medicine, Popular.   I. Title.
RA776.W417   1995   94-42040
613 — dc20   CIP

Printed in the United States of America

Book design by Robert Overholtzer

AGM 10 9 8 7 6 5 4 3 2

CONTENTS

PREFACE TO THE
REVISED EDITION

As I WORKED to update the text of this manual, our nation was noisily debating health care reform. I am happy to see the federal government addressing the issue at last, but I do not see discussion of questions that will make any real difference. The challenge is not to figure out who will pay for the present system, but to change the fundamental nature of medicine and people's expectations of it and to move society in the direction of greater self-reliance. To that end, people need more knowledge about how to prevent the diseases of lifestyle that are now widespread and how to handle common health problems on their own.

I wrote this book to help readers take greater charge of their health. It is filled with practical information about treatment and prevention, information that is now corrected and updated to incorporate what I have learned in the past five years. I have received hundreds of letters from readers who have used the book successfully to deal with a wide range of ailments. The methods recommended here work, and they are more effective, safer, and less expensive than many conventional treatments. Try them and you will see.

The focus of my present work is teaching doctors how to combine the best ideas and practices of conventional and alternative medicine into a new system, Integrative Medicine, that will be cost-effective and practical. One part of this effort is the development of standards for training physicians; another is the formulation of protocols for the treatment of common health problems by natural methods. I am also working on research projects that will document the cost-effectiveness of these methods, to convince insurance companies to reimburse the expense of many of the preventive and alternative interventions that most people now have to pay for themselves.

We are in the midst of a revolution in medicine that will continue whatever course the national debate on health care reform takes. This book gives you the basic information that will allow you to join that revolution and help bring about a healthier society.

Tucson, Arizona
December 1994

INTRODUCTION

THIS BOOK is a complete guide to preventive health maintenance plus suggestions for treating many common ailments on your own with methods that are safe, natural, effective, and not as expensive as standard medical treatments. If you are unfamiliar with the concept of preventive maintenance, I can summarize it for you in a few words: timely and appropriate investment of energy in your well-being will save a great deal of trouble, pain, and money down the road. Many people understand the value of preventive maintenance in caring for their cars. They get regular oil changes and tune-ups, and they pay attention when a warning light comes on. It is strange that more of us do not apply the same concept to our bodies, which are infinitely more valuable.

The most common reason for neglecting preventive maintenance is lack of information. I have always felt that the main work of doctors should be to educate, to give people the information they need to keep themselves healthy most of the time. Prevention of disease should be primary, treatment secondary. One of my main motivations in writing this book is to help you avoid the need for treatment.

In addition to teaching medical students, I have for some years practiced natural and preventive medicine in Tucson, Arizona, always encouraging well people to come in for preventive health checks and advice about diet, exercise, and stress reduction. I am in a small minority of physicians who practice this way, but there will be more of us in the future.

Mainstream medicine continues to be the same as it has been, but more so: more expensive, more reliant on technology, more focused on the physical body to the exclusion of mind and spirit. One trend of recent years has been the appearance of health maintenance organizations (HMOs) that offer prepaid medical care. As corporations interested in making a profit, HMOs want their staff doctors to see as many patients as possible during their time on duty, with the result that doctors have less time than ever to spend with patients. They cannot take detailed histories or get to know the people they treat. For their part, patients seem to feel that since they have paid in advance for care, they might as well take full advantage of it. They come in for every headache, sore throat, twinge, and pain, giving up more and more responsibility for their own well-being. It is discouraging to see in HMOs thick medical charts on men and women in their twenties and thirties. Most of these patients have no sense of their own health and their own power to affect it for good or ill. They also do not know how much better off they would be if they took care of common ailments on their own.

Blind faith in professional medicine is not healthy. In my book *Health and Healing* I explained the limitations and dangers of regular (allopathic) medicine and reviewed a number of kinds of alternative or complementary medicine. I urge you to read that book, both to inform yourself about the strengths and weaknesses of these systems and to get a sense of the philosophy of health and treatment that is the foundation of this book.

In short, allopathic medicine is very good at managing trauma, acute bacterial infections, medical and surgical emergencies, and other crises. It is very bad at managing viral infections, chronic degenerative disease, allergy and autoimmunity, many of the serious kinds of cancer, mental illness, "functional" illness (disturbances of function in the absence of major physical or chemical changes), and all those conditions in which the mind plays an active role in creating susceptibility to disease. It is not wise to go to an allopathic doctor with a disease that allopathic medicine cannot treat. It is also not wise to go to other sorts of practitioners with diseases that allopathic medicine can treat very well. For more detail on these points, please read *Health and Healing*.

I want you to know at the outset that I expect a lot of you as a reader. I expect you to want to be more responsible for your own health and wellness and more independent of professional medicine. I expect you to be willing to experiment and to make changes in your lifestyle. I expect that you will use good judgment and common sense in deciding when a problem is outside your limits of competence and should be taken to a doctor.

For example: if you develop fevers, night sweats, and enlarged lymph nodes, you should not ignore those symptoms or waste time trying to get help from alternative practitioners. You should go directly to an allopathic physician for a complete physical exam and blood tests. I would give the same advice to anyone who developed any alarming, dramatic, or persistent symptoms that might indicate infection, malignancy, or malfunction of a vital organ. The greatest failure you can make in trying to be your own doctor or in trying to rely on natural treatments is to miss the diagnosis of a condition that is fully and easily curable by standard allopathic medicine.

People often ask me, "How can I find a good doctor?" I have no simple answer to that question except to give you what I think are qualities you should look for when you shop around. First, a doctor should show interest in you as a person as well as a medical case. He or she should take the time to ask questions about you and answer your questions fully. My experience is that a thorough history is the best diagnostic instrument available; slighting it is bad medicine. One of the most common complaints I hear from patients who have had unsatisfactory experiences with allopathic medicine is that practitioners do not take the time to address their concerns and questions.

Next, a doctor should be a good teacher. You should emerge from a visit to your doctor better equipped to deal with problems in the future, with more knowledge and tools to help you practice preventive maintenance and wise self-care. The most effective way to teach is by example. A good doctor embodies and exemplifies good health. I could not tell patients to clean up their diets, start exercising, learn to breathe correctly, and meditate if I were not committed to those actions myself. In shopping for a physician to use in time of need, look for one who will inspire you to work at preventive maintenance by his or her own way of being.

I often teach medical students not to hesitate to say "I don't know" when they don't. To me that statement is a positive sign in a doctor. Yet another is openness to new ideas and willingness to try out new concepts and procedures. Ask prospective doctors what they think of vitamins, herbal remedies, acupuncture, manipulation, hypnotherapy. Are they willing to consider and learn, or do they dismiss everything unfamiliar as quackery?

Finally, and most difficult, I'm afraid, is finding a doctor whose philosophy of health and treatment is consistent with that presented here and in *Health and Healing*. A main point of this philosophy is that healing is the birthright of every human being. It does not have to be put into people or imposed on them from without but, rather, gently encouraged. Do not stay in treatment with doctors who discount the possibility of healing or who make you feel that you are incapable of experiencing it. Also, your physician should adhere to the famous injunction of Hippocrates: "First, do no harm!" All too often today doctors ignore that prescription and jump right in with drastic treatments before giving the body's own healing systems a chance. Awareness of and reverence for the healing power of nature — another principle of Hippocrates — has been a constant theme of my own research and practice, one that I will try to convey to you in these pages.

You can use this book in several ways. Part I gives you basic information about designing a healthy lifestyle. Read it through, try the suggestions, and see how you respond to them. You do not have to make all the changes at once. Go at your own pace and do not stick with any regimen that does not give you results after a reasonable trial.

Part II gives you very specific advice about reducing your risks of getting the diseases that kill most people prematurely in our society. As you will discover, heart attacks, strokes, and cancer are not simply the results of bad heredity and bad luck. They are often diseases of lifestyle, and lifestyle can be changed. Some of the recommendations will be easy to follow, others hard. You can decide for yourself how many of them you need to implement, based on your own sense of risk.

Part III gives you tools in the form of natural treatments you can use yourself. Here I want you to experiment in earnest. Keep notes on your experiences. See if you can make these simple measures, dietary supplements, and herbs work for you as they do for me and my patients.

Finally, Part IV gives detailed recommendations for the treatment of a large number of common ailments. I have not included in this list the kinds of medical disasters that ought to be dealt with by allopaths. Instead I have concentrated on the problems that people bring to me most frequently and that respond well to gentle, natural therapy and lifestyle modification. In these cases strong allopathic drugs and surgery should be used only as last resorts, after simple measures fail. This section is a reference work to consult in time of need, or you can browse or read it through all at once. You will find that much of the advice here echoes the general themes of earlier parts of the book. Following Part IV, in Appendixes A and B, I give the names and addresses of organizations and companies that can provide you with referrals to nonallopathic practitioners and with recommended materials.

Our ideas about how to maintain health and prevent disease change as we acquire more knowledge and experience. When you read the section on fats in Chapter 1 you will see examples of such a change. Not long ago we thought that olive oil was not good for the heart and that safflower oil was a healthy fat. Today we think very differently. The information in this book is the best available at the moment, consistent with the findings of scientific research, with clinical experience, and with my own personal experience. Doubtless we have more to learn, and doubtless we will change our minds on some issues that now seem so clear. For this reason I urge you again to be willing to experiment and to trust your own experience. You are ultimately the one responsible for your health. I have given you the best directions I know to help you on your journey to wellness. I leave it to you to put them into action and modify them according to your individual needs, guided by the experience you acquire.

PART I

PREVENTIVE
MAINTENANCE

1

WHAT SHOULD I EAT?

WHAT SHOULD I EAT? This simple question has no simple answer. Many people will try to persuade you that they know the right way to eat, but so much of the information is contradictory that the more theories you listen to, the more confused you will be. I have read convincing arguments against every category of food you can name: meat, fish, poultry, milk, cheese, butter, fruit, vegetables, vegetable oils, wheat, eggs, bread, yeast, sugar, spices, and so on. If all these arguments were right, we would starve in the midst of plenty, our minds finding endless causes to avoid everything our bodies craved.

I enjoy seeing how the rules of different dietary systems conflict totally. In yoga philosophy, foods are grouped in three categories, from highest (expressing the quality of balance) to lowest (expressing the quality of inertia). Fresh yogurt and white rice are in the top group; brown rice is at the bottom. In macrobiotics, a dietary system invented in Japan, brown rice is the best thing you can eat, milk products and white rice among the worst.

What should I eat? The first guideline I can give you is that there is no one right way. A particular diet may be right for you at this stage of your life, but it may not be right for me, and it may not be right for you a year from now. We are all different physically and biochemically, with different and changing dietary needs. Do not believe anyone who tells you he has discovered the one right way to eat. For any dietary system you name, I will show you examples of terrifically healthy people who violate all its rules. I read an interview recently with a Russian woman who had reached the age of 106 and was still vigorous. Her answer to the usual question about the secret of her success was "I never eat vegetables."

Some authorities say that human beings are meant to be vegetarians, others that we must eat animal products to be healthy. The fact is that human beings are omnivores, designed not only to survive but to do well on an astonishingly wide range of foods. Behind most of the rigid diets promoted in popular books and health food pamphlets is a most unhealthy assumption: that our bodies are inefficient and unresourceful, easily upset unless we consume exactly the right foods or combinations of foods. When you buy into these assumptions, you are underselling your body's natural resilience and capacity for adaptation. Do not accept this harmful belief.

Also do not believe anyone who tells you that all illness results from poor diet or that dietary change can cure any illness. It's not so. Diet is one factor shaping health — an important factor, but not the only one. Diet has the distinction of being the only major determinant of health that is completely under your control. You have the final say over what does and does not go into your mouth and stomach. You cannot always control the other determinants of health, such as the quality of the air you breathe, the noise you are subjected to, or the emotional climate of your surroundings, but you can control what you eat. It is a shame to squander such a good opportunity to influence your health.

Changing your eating habits in order to improve your life can be a way to activate the body's healing system. It is difficult to give up familiar foods and try new ones. To do so requires committing mental energy toward the goal of improved health. I have seen a number of cures of serious illnesses in people who decided to go on long-term fasts, macrobiotic diets, yoga vegetarian diets, and other regimens. My interpretation of these cases, consistent with the theory I presented in *Health and Healing,* is that part of the reason for success is the mental shift represented by the decision to follow a demanding nutritional program. That mental shift may be more important than the specifics of a program. I usually ask my patients to make changes in diet as one way of increasing their chances of natural healing. I never use dietary adjustment as the only means of treatment.

I do not place much stock in the advice of professional nutritionists and dietitians. Nutritional science is primitive. Research on food and diet is much distorted by cultural biases and values, and the researchers are seldom able to see these distortions. As an example of a cultural bias, consider the different reactions you would have to eating a lobster tail or a plate of fried grasshoppers. The biological reality of the two organisms is similar, but most people in our culture consider one delicious, the other revolting. There is no agreement from culture to culture on the answer to the most basic question of all: what is food, what is not? Food and eating have enormous symbolic importance, and that is why we surround them with taboos and rituals. Different dietary preferences divide nations, religions, and sometimes families. Trying to find truthful information in this area is as easy as dancing through a minefield.

Nutritional science gave us the Basic Four food groups, the concept responsible for much of our unhealthy obsession with protein (more on this in a moment). Registered dietitians are frequently witting or unwitting tools of the food industry, since the information they dispense often comes from industry rather than from disinterested sources. If you are tempted to follow their recommendations, remember that dietitians are the people responsible for the food served in schools and hospitals.

Having given all these warnings, I will now offer you nine basic suggestions about how to design a healthy diet.

1. Eat with Your Senses, Not with Your Intellect

Your senses of taste and smell are excellent guides to what is good for you. Trust them. Practice developing these senses and paying attention to them. If you eat what you think is good for you even if you don't like it, you are not listening to the wisdom of your body. Eating foods you don't like that someone else says are good for you is even further off base. Above all, the food you eat should appeal to your senses and agree with your body. Eating is one of life's great pleasures, and I assure you that a healthy diet does not require any sacrifice of enjoyment, even if you give up foods you now like.

2. Eat with Full Attention and with Gusto

Your digestive system mirrors your state of mind, which is why so many digestive disorders are stress-related. If you eat while angry, anxious, or distracted, your body will not process food well, no matter how good the food. If you always eat while listening to the news on television or while discussing business, you are not giving the act of eating the attention it deserves. How your body handles what you eat may be more important than what foods you eat. You will digest food most efficiently if you eat with full attention and full enjoyment of the experience.

Once, when Saint Theresa of Avila (1515–1582) visited a monastery, the abbot served her a special dinner with a main dish of roasted partridges instead of the usual plain fare. To the astonishment of her host, Saint Theresa tore into the meal with abandon. The abbot admonished her, saying he thought it unseemly for a woman whose life was devoted to prayer to show such enthusiasm for the pleasures of the table. Saint Theresa replied, "When it's prayer time, pray! When it's partridge time, partridge!"

3. Eat a Widely Varied Diet

By varying what you eat, you protect your health in two ways. First, you ensure that you get all the nutrients you need. If you eat the same foods day after day, you are more likely to shortchange yourself of needed vitamins, minerals, or other elements. We probably do not yet know all of the nutritional factors required for optimal health. Only recently did we discover the need for zinc, for example. You don't have to memorize the government's recommended daily allowances of carbohydrate, fat, protein, and vitamins — just go for variety.

The second reason to vary your diet is that it is the best way to avoid eating too much of anything that is *not* good for you. There are surprisingly many toxins in the food we eat, both natural and man-made. Celery, basil, the common cultivated white mushrooms *(Agaricus bisporus)*, chickpeas, and many other vegetables contain natural toxins; most, but not all, are destroyed by the heat of cooking, which is a strong argument against raw food diets. (You will find more information on this subject at the end of this chapter.) Alfalfa sprouts, so loved by health food enthusiasts, contain a natural toxin called canavanine, which is definitely not good for you. That doesn't mean you should never eat alfalfa sprouts. It does mean that it is better not to eat them every day. Peanuts and peanut butter are usually contaminated with traces of aflatoxin, a very potent natural carcinogen found in a mold that grows on peanuts and other seeds. Does that mean you should exclude peanut butter from your diet? No, but again, you would be better off not eating it all the time or in large quantities.

In addition to the natural toxins are all the unnatural ones, such as pesticides, fungicides, hormones, antibiotics, and others too numerous to list, that are added to the food we buy. These substances are a serious problem in my view, with strong political and economic components. I will give you advice on how to minimize your consumption of dangerous additives in the next chapter. For now, let me just repeat that the best general safeguard against taking in unhealthy doses of dietary toxins, natural or not, is to select the foods you eat from a widely varied menu rather than concentrating on a few items.

4. Eat Fresh Foods

Dried, canned, frozen, and prepared foods are more and more prominent in modern diets. Many of these foods contain too much fat, salt, sugar, and unhealthy additives, and rarely do they taste as good as fresh foods. If this has not been your experience, please work further to develop your sense perceptions. If you pay attention to the appearance, taste, and smell of what you eat, your senses will lead you away from packaged foods toward fresh ones.

5. Eat Less Rather Than More

Research shows that animals fed somewhat less than the "recommended" daily allowance of calories live longer and have fewer diseases than those put on standard diets or allowed to eat as much as they want. It may be that the recommended daily allowances of nutrients are too high, that eating these amounts creates a state of chronic overnutrition that stresses our bodies. In fact, some scientists now talk about "undernutrition" as a way of promoting health and longevity. Of course, it is easy to say we should eat less rather than more, but it is hard to put into practice. Eating, as I have noted, serves functions other than simply supplying the body with nutrients. It is a symbolic act, a social function, and a source of pleasure.

Our bodies evolved through long periods of scarcity, when food was simply not easily available or not available at all times of year. The surviving fittest — our ancestors — were those individuals who best developed the ability to seek out food and put it to maximal use. That genetic heritage can be a liability in a world where food is ever present, in unprecedented quantity and variety. It is no wonder that obesity is such a common problem, no wonder that we are obsessed with dieting and weight reduction, no wonder that the concept of "undernutrition" is unpopular. Nonetheless, the research findings are clear: less is better than more, and it is worth trying to apply this lesson as best we can. One possibility is to eat smaller meals more frequently. Another is to fast occasionally (see pp. 203– 204). Another is to learn how to reduce the calorie content of dishes we like.

6. Learn to Appreciate Simple Foods

Much contemporary cooking, particularly in restaurants, is designed to excite the senses more than to provide good nourishment. As much as anyone else, I like to try novel dishes and strong flavors, but I think there is a risk in losing the ability to delight in utterly simple food, simply prepared. Can you take pleasure in an ear of sweet corn, just picked, lightly cooked, and eaten plain without butter or salt? How about a perfect garden tomato, sliced and served as is. Or a crisp green salad with a little olive oil and fresh lemon juice, a warm slice of homemade bread with nothing on it, or a plate of lightly stir-fried fresh vegetables over a mound of rice. Or a slice of really fresh salmon, grilled, and served only with lemon wedges. Or a section of perfectly ripe melon. If you cannot imagine eating corn and bread without butter, salad and tomatoes without gobs of creamy dressing, a stir-fry without a spicy sauce, salmon without butter or hollandaise sauce, melon without prosciutto or ice cream, I suggest you try learning to appreciate the pure tastes of these and other plain foods.

I am not urging you to live on gruel and water. You can still have

Mexican and Italian and Szechuan food, if it is made from healthy ingredients. My concern is that if sensory novelty is the main appeal of food, you will move in dietary directions that are not necessarily best for your health. Learn to enjoy simple foods prepared quickly and properly without fancy adornments.

7. Eat a Balanced Diet

We've all been told so many times to eat a balanced diet that we don't want to hear it anymore, but just what is a balanced diet? A balanced meal is supposed to provide the proper proportions of the three basic categories of nutrients: carbohydrates, fats, and proteins. You need to know what these nutrients are and how the body uses them in order to make intelligent choices of food. Let me explain what I know about nutrients.

CARBOHYDRATES

Carbohydrates are the most basic foodstuffs, relatively simple compounds of carbon, hydrogen, and oxygen. Plants make them from carbon dioxide, water, and the energy of the sun. The simplest carbohydrates are familiar sugars: glucose (grape sugar), fructose (fruit sugar), dextrose (corn sugar), and sucrose (table sugar, from sugar cane and beets). Starches are complex carbohydrates, larger molecules made up of units of simple sugars linked in chains. Plants make the simplest sugars by photosynthesis, then convert them into other sugars and starches as storage foods.

When we eat carbohydrates, our bodies metabolize or "burn" them, releasing their stored energy and breaking them down again to water and carbon dioxide. For both plants and animals, carbohydrates are high-quality fuels, since it takes relatively little work to dismantle these compounds and release their energy. Because the end products of carbohydrate metabolism are carbon dioxide and water, these are clean-burning fuels as well as efficient ones.

Sugar is instant energy for us, and, as the first form of bound solar energy made by plants, it is also the foundation of the body's energy economy. All other foods are converted into sugar for distribution to our tissues and cells. Many of our cells prefer to run on sugar, and some, such as the highly specialized nerve cells of the brain, can run only on sugar; they have sacrificed the metabolic equipment needed to burn starch, fat, and protein.

Starch is almost instant energy. To release the energy from starch molecules, plants and animals convert them back to sugars. Sugars have not always been as readily available as they are today, but starches have been mainstays of our diets at least since the invention of agriculture. Indeed, they are the staples of most cultures; rice, wheat, corn, beans, potatoes and other starchy roots and tubers, bread, pasta, and so on, are the satisfying "peasant foods" that give us comfort as well as nourishment.

In this century carbohydrates acquired a bad name. Sugar is maligned in all quarters, accused of causing a long list of ailments from tooth decay to depression. Many people think of starches as low-quality, fattening foods; the image they see when they think of pasta is that of a fat Italian peasant. Many health practitioners parrot the statement that refined sugar and flour provide nothing more than "empty calories." The fact that carbohydrates are so inexpensive relative to fats and proteins seems to lend credence to these notions.

Very recently, a new and more accurate view of these foods has begun to emerge. In this view complex carbohydrates are seen, correctly, as premium foods. Starch is really the perfect food — satisfying, easily digested and assimilated, a clean, fast, and efficient source of energy. Starches are fattening under two conditions: if you mix them with fat or if you do not exercise. A box of linguini I just bought asks and answers the question: "Pasta . . . Why the Fattening Image? Where do you find satisfying eating without blowing your calorie budget? In pasta! That's right. Far from being fattening, pasta scores a moderate 210 calories per serving and has virtually no fat at all." One inch below this blurb is a recipe for "Pasta with Four Cheeses," calling for the pound of linguini in the box plus 6 tablespoons of butter, 3 ⅓ cups of half-and-half, and a pound of high-fat cheeses. Most of us have learned to like these starch-fat combinations. We put butter in and on our bread, butter and sour cream on potatoes, butter, cream, and oil on pasta, and so on. These dishes are very caloric and will certainly increase your weight if you eat them immoderately.

If you are an active person, and if you learn to eat starchy foods without a lot of added fat, you can eat quantities of carbohydrates without problems. Starch calories are easily burned through aerobic exercise. Complex carbohydrates ought to be a major part of the diet, accounting for 40 to 50 percent of total calories consumed. (Some sample recipes follow in the next chapter.)

Refined carbohydrates, like white flour and polished rice, are just as good energy sources as whole wheat flour and brown rice. The difference is that some of the grain's constituents have been lost: the bran, which is an important source of fiber, and the germ or embryo, which has vitamins and other nutrients. There is nothing wrong with eating some white bread if it is made from high-quality un-bleached flour, especially if you also eat whole-grain products. I like various kinds of brown rice, and I also like good white rice (like basmati rice from India or Texas, arborio rice from Italy, and Japanese-style steamed rice). I eat a lot of whole-grain breads, and I like good French and sourdough bread made from unbleached white flour. I eat ordinary pasta and some whole-wheat pasta. (The best kinds come from Japan and Italy.)

If starch is the perfect food, what about sugar? The concept of sugar as empty calories is meaningless. Calories are calories, and the calories of sugar are just as good as those of meat, milk, olive oil, and potatoes. Of course, if you try to live on sugar alone, you will eventually get sick, because the body needs a lot more than carbohydrate calories.

The main difference between sugar and starch is that the body tends to burn sugar immediately and may be unable to store its energy. Starches do not create this difficulty. The body easily stores starch calories, turning them into sugar when needed. Many people report problems from eating foods high in sugar. A common experience is a quick "rush" of energy followed later by a "crash" into lethargy and depression. Some people just feel the crash, saying sweets make them logy and sleepy. Others say that mood swings disappear when they stop eating sugar. Some parents are convinced that sugar makes their young children hyperactive, that behavior and attention problems are much less severe if sugar is restricted or removed.

Of course, everybody is different. Some of us can handle sugar, and some cannot. In those who cannot, the problem may be a mild version of what happens with alcohol. Alcohol is a drug (discussed in Chapter 7, "Habits") that is also a food. The body metabolizes alcohol as a carbohydrate but burns it immediately, releasing a flood of caloric energy into the system. Charlie Poole (1892–1931), a legendary banjo player, song writer, and whiskey drinker from North Carolina, used to call his drug of choice "heavy sugar"; he died of complications from alcoholism at the age of thirty-nine. It is fashionable today to talk about addiction to sweets, and some people would like me to call sugar a drug rather than a food. I prefer to call sugar a food that may have druglike effects in some individuals. Addiction to sugar does not look different from addiction to food in general, but I certainly agree that sugar is a powerful source of pleasure.

Aside from its effects on metabolism and energy cycles, sugar is certainly bad for our teeth. It is a favorite food of the bacteria that cause dental caries. Some forms of sugar are worse than others in this regard, honey being particularly bad because of its stickiness, chocolate being surprisingly benign because substances in it disrupt the "glue" that bacteria make to adhere to enamel. Diets high in sugar may also predispose some people, especially women, to yeast infections, may aggravate some kinds of arthritis and asthma, and may raise the level of blood fats (triglycerides).

If sugar can hurt us, why do we like it so much? I think the human sweet tooth made sense at one time. Our very distant ancestors encountered sugar only in the form of ripe fruit and an occasional honeycomb. Since sugar is instant energy, those individuals who had a taste for it would be more likely to survive — to outrun a saber-toothed tiger or win a fight — and so pass on their genes. Evolution could not have anticipated that the modern world would be filled with sugar. (I can usually locate some within a minute or two of entering a home, store, or office.) It is normal and natural to crave sugar, but it is wise not to give in to the craving every time you feel it.

Many people who consult me mention that they crave sweets or have problems controlling their intake of sweets. When I ask them exactly what they are eating, they tell me ice cream, candy, pastries, and the like. These are not simply sweets, but combinations of sugar and fat. Such foods are loaded with calories, very seductive, and major contributors to obesity. See if you can satisfy your sweet tooth with sugar alone: with dried fruit, hard candy, fruit ices (sorbets or water ices), or even (my favorite) bites of pure maple sugar. These are healthier treats because they are fat free. Try to use them consciously — as a way of rewarding yourself, for example, instead of just eating them for no reason.

Those who condemn sugar totally should note that in India, the native home of sugar cane, that plant is held in highest esteem, and its various products are recommended as foods and medicines in ancient, sacred writings. Eaten consciously and moderately (be sure to rinse the mouth afterward), sugar is a delightful addition to the diet.

In metabolic terms sugar is sugar no matter what form it comes in. I see no advantage to raw sugar, brown sugar, honey, molasses, or maple syrup except that they contain trace minerals as impurities and may have strong flavors that make it harder to eat them as immoderately and unconsciously as most people eat white sugar. Fructose (fruit sugar) has recently become available in refined form. It is sweeter than sucrose (table sugar), offering the benefit of fewer calories per unit of sweetness. Also it may be less likely to disturb blood sugar levels than sucrose and thus may affect energy cycles less.

Sugar is all mixed up with human psychology. From an early age we learn that sugar is our reward if we are good, if we eat our unpleasant vegetables. A great many processed foods contain large amounts of sugar to make them taste good. Many condiments — ketchup, relishes, pickles — are loaded with sugar, as are many soft drinks. The sugar industry likes to tell us that sucrose has only eighteen calories per teaspoon, but most recipes call for *cups* of sugar, and there are a *lot* of teaspoons in a cup. It is worth paying attention to your sugar intake, whether in fruit, fruit juice, desserts, snacks, or prepared foods.

If you have never stayed off sugar for more than a few days, you might try doing so to see just how strong the habit is. If you are prone to depression, mood swings, or fluctuating energy levels, this experiment will show you whether sugar is affecting the condition.

FATS

Like carbohydrates, fats are made up only of carbon, hydrogen, and oxygen, and they also burn clean. But the molecules that compose fats — fatty acids — require more energy to assemble and so release more energy when burned.

Fats are the most calorie-dense nutrients, with nine calories per gram, almost twice that of carbohydrates and proteins. Plants make fats from carbohydrates and use them for long-term storage of solar energy. They often store fats in seeds to provide the developing embryo with concentrated nourishment until it can begin to make sugar on its own by photosynthesis. Animals make their own fats from carbohydrates and from the fats of plants and other animals.

Humans tend to like fatty foods. Many of us have a "fat tooth" in addition to a sweet tooth, and again I think this is a legacy of evolution. Fat is concentrated energy and hence survival. For people living near starvation or through cycles of feast and famine, a craving for fat makes sense, especially if fat is available only on special occasions, as when a large game animal is killed. Today fat is an everyday item.

When we talk about "rich" food, we are usually responding to a high fat content, which gives a pleasurable feeling in the mouth besides adding flavor. Our craving for fat and the amount of it in our diet is killing us, no question about it. High-fat diets shorten life by predisposing us to heart disease, vascular disease, cancer, and other serious illnesses. They are also the major cause of obesity.

Not only is the amount of fat you eat an important determinant of health, so also is the kind of fat and the way it is prepared. In this area there is much misinformation. First you must learn which foods are naturally high in fat. These include seeds (sesame, sunflower, and corn), nuts (especially walnuts, pecans, Brazil, macadamia, and coconut), a few legumes (peanuts and soybeans), a few fruits (olives and avocados), many meats (beef, pork, lamb), poultry (goose, duck, and unskinned chicken), some fish (salmon, mackerel, sardines, bluefish, and herring), chocolate, butter, cream, and cheeses made from whole milk. Of course, many prepared foods are high in fat because they are made from these products or are cooked in or with fats. Many people get 40 to 50 percent of their total calories from fat. This is not healthy.

Fats differ greatly in their composition, depending on which fatty acids predominate. We have all heard of saturated and unsaturated fats. These terms refer to the chemistry of fatty acids — whether all available carbon bonds in the molecular chain are occupied, or saturated, with hydrogen atoms. You don't have to be a chemist to figure out where a fat falls in the spectrum of saturation/unsaturation. Just put a sample in the refrigerator, and you will quickly see. Saturated fats become hard and opaque in the cold, and the higher the temperature at which they stay hard, the more saturated they are. Animal fats are the major source of saturated fat in our diets. Just think of how bacon fat looks in the refrigerator. Some vegetable fats are saturated too, notably coconut and palm oils; coconut oil remains hard and white even at room temperature.

At the opposite end of the spectrum are the polyunsaturated fats, which include many vegetable oils. They stay transparent and free-flowing under refrigeration. Safflower oil is the most unsaturated of the food oils. Moving from that extreme we find sunflower, corn, soy, and cottonseed oils. In the middle of the spectrum are oils made up mostly of fatty acids that lack saturation only at one point in the molecular chain. They are called monounsaturated fats. Olive and canola oils contain more monounsaturated fats than other oils, with peanut oil trailing somewhat behind. Olive oil becomes thick and translucent in the refrigerator; you can sometimes get it out of the bottle in this state, but only with difficulty. Canola remains clear and pourable but becomes visibly thicker. Bear in mind that all fats are mixtures of fatty acids, so the terms "saturation" and "unsaturation" refer to the predominant components. Even beef fat and lard, which are saturated by definition, have a substantial percentage of unsaturated fatty acids, while olive oil, which is monounsaturated, contains 14 percent saturated fat.

Over the past half century evidence has steadily grown of the dangers of diets high in saturated fat. A major clue appeared during World War II, when the supply of meat, eggs, butter, and cheese declined sharply in the countries of Western Europe caught up in the war. As consumption of these foods dropped, so did deaths from coronary heart disease. After the war, when consumption rates returned to normal, deaths from coronary heart disease rose to their prewar levels. The theory that saturated fat promotes atherosclerosis, a condition in which cholesterol is deposited in arteries, is now established as medical fact. In the Western world this condition has been accepted as a normal characteristic of human life. It is not. Atherosclerosis is a disease of lifestyle, particularly related to the regular consumption of foods high in saturated fat: meats, whole milk and its products, and prepared foods made with butter, lard, beef fat, coconut oil, and palm oil. The best defense against early death from heart attacks is to eliminate these foods from the diet or eat them only infrequently. Arterial disease begins early in life in many people who eat "typical" diets. Autopsies of eighteen- and nineteen-year-old soldiers killed in Vietnam showed that most of them already had cholesterol deposits in their coronary arteries.

In response to the growing awareness of the harmful effects of saturated fats, doctors and nutritionists began recommending fats from the other end of the spectrum, with the result that the food industry began to promote products high in polyunsaturates. Safflower oil, once a little-known cooking fat, enjoyed a boom of popularity. Research showed that replacing saturated fat in the diet with polyunsaturated fat lowered blood cholesterol. Monounsaturated fats were considered neutral, neither raising nor lowering cholesterol levels and the risk of heart attack.

Unfortunately, polyunsaturated fats have dangers of their own, which are still not widely known. Points of unsaturation in fatty acid chains are unstable and vulnerable to attack by oxygen, especially if fats are heated in the presence of air or left standing exposed to air. The products resulting from these oxidation reactions are highly reactive molecules that can damage DNA and other vital components of cells. Diets high in polyunsaturated fats increase the risk of cancer, speed up aging and degeneration of tissues, and may aggravate inflammatory diseases and immune-system disorders.

When fats oxidize and the dangerous compounds build up, they become rancid, and our noses can detect the change. If you do not know the odor of rancid fat, I urge you to train your nose to recognize it. Do not eat anything that has even a hint of that smell about it. If you eat foods high in fat, such as nuts, chips, and crackers, smell them first before you start putting them in your mouth. In sealed bags of snack foods, the telltale odors are often concentrated and easy to detect upon first opening the container. The more unsaturated a fat, the faster it will become rancid on exposure to air. Linseed oil is so unsaturated that oxidation rapidly changes its chemical structure, causing it to turn dry and hard. (This is the reason for its use as a base for oil paints.) Safflower oil develops a rancid odor much more quickly than other oils; before its recent popularity as a cooking fat, it was classed as a "drying oil" along with linseed.

There is another danger in polyunsaturated fats that are heated or subjected to chemical treatment. The molecular structure of some of the fatty acids may change from a natural configuration with a curved shape (called *cis-*) to an unnatural one with a jointed shape (called *trans-*). *Trans*-fatty acids, or TFAs, are never found in nature, and we do not know what the body does with them. We know that the body needs *cis*-fatty acids to construct cell membranes and hormones, but we do not know how it handles TFAs. It is possible that diets containing TFAs cause derangements of cell structure and function, predisposing a person to disease, accelerated aging, and premature death. The major sources of TFAs are margarine, solid vegetable shortening, and all partially hydrogenated vegetable oils. All of these are artificially saturated fats, polyunsaturated oils that have been put through high-temperature chemical reactions to change their consistency.

If both saturated and unsaturated fats can harm us, what are we to do? First and foremost, we should try to reduce the total amount of any kind of fat in our diets. Some very restrictive diets with only 10 percent of total calories as fat do wonders for patients with cardiovascular disease, but most of us would find such diets hard to follow. If you can get your fat intake down to 20–30 percent, you will still enjoy what you eat while greatly lowering your risks of disease. This means cutting way down on fried foods, whole milk products, meats, nuts, high-fat condiments like mayonnaise and salad dressings, rich sauces, and desserts.

It also means paying attention to the fat content of foods you buy. Labels have recently become more user-friendly by law. They now list calories from fat in an easy-to-read format, whereas before they stated only the weight of fat in a serving of the product. In the old format, a package of a part-skim-milk, low-sodium cheese could describe its nutritional content in this way: "Serving size: 1 ounce, calories 100, protein 8 grams, fat 8 grams, carbohydrate less than 1 gram." That sounds not bad, but let's work out the percentage of fat by calories. One gram of fat has 9 calories, so a 1-ounce serving of this "lite" cheese has $8 \times 9 = 72$ calories. To get the percentage of fat by calories, you divide 72 by the number of calories per serving (100) and multiply by 100: result, 72 percent. A cheese that is 72 percent fat is not a food you can afford to eat very often if you are trying to keep the total calories you consume as fat below 30 percent.

Here is another example: a 15-ounce bag of gourmet, all-natural, cheese-flavored popcorn from a natural food store. The serving size is 1 ounce. (I could eat eight servings in no time.) Each serving has 160 calories and 12 grams of fat. Multiply 12×9, and you get 108 fat calories. Divide by 160 and multiply by 100 to get the percentage of calories that are fat; the result is a hefty 67.5 percent. You would do well to go easy on this kind of snack food, natural or not. Beware of products that use formulations like "96 percent fat free." Such a product is 4 percent fat by weight, which could turn out to be a hefty percentage of fat calories, depending on its composition. Cheese that is 4 percent fat by weight might be more than 60 percent fat by calories, for example.

You can learn to like good bread without a coat of butter, to prefer breads made without any shortening, to eat fish and skinned chicken broiled without added fat, to use dairy products made from skim milk, and to modify recipes by halving or quartering the amount of fat called for without sacrificing flavor. In fact, you can develop a taste for richness of flavor rather than for fat content. Once you begin to make these healthy changes in your eating habits, you will look with astonishment at how much fat most people eat and how much recipes tell you to use.

Here is a recipe from the back of a bottle of vanilla extract in my cupboard:

CANDY EGGS

Cream ¹/₂ cup butter until soft. Add 2 teaspoons heavy cream, ¹/₂ teaspoon lemon juice and 1 teaspoon vanilla extract. Gradually add 1 pound powdered sugar, mixing well after each addition. Shape into "eggs" about 2 inches long and 1 inch in diameter. Chill. Melt a 6-ounce package chocolate chips in double boiler with 1 tablespoon butter and 1 tablespoon water, stirring constantly. Roll eggs in chocolate. Place on wax paper and refrigerate until set. Makes 18 eggs.

These might better be called Artery Bombs. Or take this dish from the back of a ten-ounce box of vegetable macaroni I bought at a health food store:

MACARONI HEALTH SALAD

Cook macaroni as directed. Drain. Mix with 4 cups chopped raw vegetables (carrots, celery, radish, cabbage, bean sprouts, etc.). Add 2 cups mayonnaise and 1 cup olive oil. Season to taste with salt and pepper. Mix well, chill. Serve on lettuce leaves garnished with chopped almonds and parsley.

Please do not eat food like this. This is more a dish of fat than a salad and certainly not healthy.

The next rule, after cutting down on fat in general, is to avoid eating from either end of the saturated-unsaturated spectrum. Since animal foods are the major sources of saturated fat, the easiest way to cut consumption of it to a minimum is to follow a vegetarian or semivegetarian diet, but be sure also to read labels of prepared foods to avoid getting the unhealthy tropical oils: palm and coconut. Strictly avoid all hydrogenated and partially hydrogenated oils, including margarine and vegetable shortening (like Crisco). For most of its history, margarine's only virtue was its cheapness relative to butter, but in the 1950s, with fixing of blame for atherosclerosis on saturated fat, margarine took on new life as a healthy alternative to butter rather than a cheap substitute for it. To this day, I find margarine more often than butter in the refrigerators of my colleagues. Margarine and other artificially hydrogenated fats appear to be worse for hearts and arteries than naturally saturated fats. In addition, they contain TFAs, the unnatural *trans*-fatty acids that may undermine health in other ways. You are better off eating a small amount of butter than any amount of margarine. Also try to avoid completely any products made with partially hydrogenated oils of any type. That rule eliminates virtually all commercial baked goods: cookies, crackers, chips, pastries, the lot.

You should also minimize intake of polyunsaturated oils and products made from them. I do not eat safflower oil, and I recommend that you do not either. Safflower's history as a food plant in the Western world is very recent; mostly we have grown it as a natural dye. We do not eat safflower seeds as we do other oil sources. The plant is native to India, and ancient medical texts from that country warn against using the plant as food. Recently plant breeders have developed new forms of safflower with a healthier proportion of monounsaturated to polyunsaturated fatty acids. You will see the term "high oleic safflower oil" on some products. Oleic acid is the principal monounsaturate in olives. I would rather get it in olive oil, which tastes better and has a long tradition of use as a food.

If you do use polyunsaturated oils, save them for use in salad dressings or other cold food. Remember, heating them makes them susceptible to oxidation, with unhealthy results. Even if you buy your cookies, crackers, and chips in health food stores, you will find most of them cooked with safflower oil or other polyunsaturates. Better leave these products alone or learn to make them at home with safer ingredients.

Monounsaturated fats, those in the middle of the spectrum that were once thought to do us neither harm nor good, now look like the safest ones to use. In moderation they do not increase the risk of cardiovascular disease, nor do they oxidize rapidly to become carcinogenic. Replacing saturated fat in the diet with polyunsaturated fat lowers both "good" and "bad" cholesterol in the blood (see the section on cholesterol in the next chapter). Substituting monounsaturated fat lowers only the bad cholesterol and is therefore more protective. Olive oil, for example, has a high percentage of monounsaturated fat. It is a flavorful oil, much liked by most people. Cultures that use it as their main cooking fat have less cardiovascular disease than others. In fact, olive oil turns up as a consistent theme in research on healthy diets in the Western world, and it appears the body has an easier time processing oleic acid than any of the other common fatty acids. Buy extra virgin (first pressing) or virgin (second pressing) olive oil and enjoy its rich color and fruity odor and flavor. An advantage of a highly flavored oil is that you can use less, adding it as a seasoning to foods rather than a principal ingredient.

If you want an unflavored oil high in monounsaturated fat, I recommend canola, a new introduction in the United States. Obtained from the seeds of a plant in the cabbage family, this oil is a traditional cooking oil of India and southern China, where it is known as rapeseed or rape oil. Breeders have improved the plant considerably, so that modern canola has an excellent fatty acid composition. Buy only "expeller pressed" or "cold pressed" brands at health food stores, and make sure the label says they are "organic," since ordinary rapeseeds carry pesticide residues. Supermarket brands have been extracted with heat or solvents that change the chemical structure of the fatty acids in unhealthy ways.

You have to be careful not only about choosing the right fats but also about making sure they have been handled properly. Just as partially hydrogenating an oil makes it dangerous, so do heating it, treating it with chemicals, and leaving it exposed to air. Most oils in supermarkets, except for olive oil labeled "extra virgin" or "virgin," have been extracted with heat or chemical solvents or both.

Buy oils in small quantities, not the giant size. Keep them in the refrigerator after opening. Never reuse an oil that has been heated to high temperatures; throw it out. Never heat an oil to the point of smoking. Smoke from overheated oil is highly carcinogenic. Get out of any place — your kitchen, a restaurant, someone else's kitchen — that smells of burning grease. It is dangerous to breathe those vapors. Always smell oils before using them and discard if there is any hint of rancidity. Never eat anything deep-fried in a fast-food restaurant or, probably, in any restaurant. Economics dictates that restaurants will use oils over and over until the tastes of oxidized compounds build up to unacceptable levels. Have you ever looked at the fat in a restaurant fryer? If you are lucky it will be brown; often it is closer to black, a carcinogenic soup. A few years ago I lectured on this subject at a state university. A woman in the audience spoke to me afterward. She managed a dormitory on campus and said the fat in the large deep fryers in the dorm kitchen was changed *once a semester*. She said she would try to remedy the situation.

Here are some comments on specific oils, beginning with the most unsaturated and going to the most saturated:

Safflower: too unsaturated; avoid it.

Sunflower, corn, sesame: too high in unsaturated fat; use moderately and do not heat.

Sesame, roasted (dark): a highly flavored seasoning used in Oriental dishes. Add small amounts to soup and stir-fries after cooking. Use in salad dressings and marinades.

Nut oils (walnut, hazelnut): expensive, flavorful, polyunsaturated. Use moderately in salads, marinades, and cold dishes.

Soy: cheap, similar to corn in composition, mostly polyunsaturated. Use moderately, if at all, and do not heat.

Cottonseed: too high in saturated fat, too low in monounsaturated fat. Also, because cotton is not classed as a food crop, the oil may contain more pesticide residues than other oils. Avoid it.

Peanut: has a good percentage of monounsaturated fat but has more saturated fat than canola oil and more polyunsaturated fat than olive oil. Use it moderately.

Avocado: mostly monounsaturated but unflavored and expensive. (Try a little seasoned, puréed avocado on bread as a replacement for butter or margarine.)

Olive: provides more monounsaturated fat than any other oil. Buy only extra virgin or virgin oil and use in both hot and cold dishes.

Canola: is substantially monounsaturated and has less saturated fat than any other oil (less than half that of olive). Use it as a general purpose, unflavored oil.

Palm, palm kernel, coconut: too high in saturated fat; avoid them altogether.

Cocoa butter: the fat in chocolate appears saturated (hard at room temperature) but may not be bad for your heart and arteries, because the body converts its principal saturated fatty acid (stearic) to a monounsaturated one (oleic). Best eaten in moderation but can be applied liberally to the skin to soothe rough, dry areas.

Vegetable shortening (Crisco): a mixture of saturated and unsaturated fats, but the oils have been deformed by chemical processing. Avoid it.

Margarine: ditto.

Chicken fat, lard, beef fat: too saturated. Avoid them entirely or minimize consumption. Unlike vegetable fats, they contain cholesterol.

Butterfat: is the most saturated of all the animal fats and contains the most cholesterol (more than twice that of beef fat). Try to minimize consumption of butter, cream, ice cream, and whole milk products. Read labels for the percentage of fat in these products.

I have not mentioned fish oils up to now. You may have read about their possible value in preventing heart attacks. Studies of Eskimos and European fishermen seem to show that regular consumption of oily fish from cold northern waters offsets the risk of a diet high in

Comparison of Dietary Fats

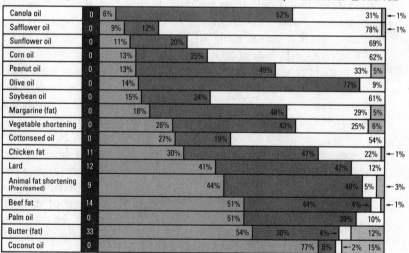

■ Cholesterol, mg/Tbsp.   ▨ Saturated Fat   ▧ Monounsaturated Fat   ☐ Polyunsaturated Fat   ▨ Other Fats

	Cholesterol	Saturated	Monounsaturated	Polyunsaturated	Other
Canola oil	0	6%	62%	31%	←1%
Safflower oil	0	9%	12%	78%	←1%
Sunflower oil	0	11%	20%	69%	
Corn oil	0	13%	25%	62%	
Peanut oil	0	13%	49%	33%	5%
Olive oil	0	14%	77%	9%	
Soybean oil	0	15%	24%	61%	
Margarine (fat)	0	18%	48%	29%	5%
Vegetable shortening	0	26%	43%	25%	6%
Cottonseed oil	0	27%	19%	54%	
Chicken fat	11	30%	47%	22%	←1%
Lard	12	41%	47%	12%	
Animal fat shortening (Precreamed)	9	44%	48%	5%	←3%
Beef fat	14	51%	44%	4%←	←1%
Palm oil	0	51%	39%	10%	
Butter (fat)	33	54%	30%	4%←	12%
Coconut oil	0	77%	6%	←2%	15%

*The values shown for saturated and polyunsaturated fats are based on Federal Regulations, Title 21, Sec. 101.25 (c)(2)(ii) (a,b), which state that: (a) saturated fat is the sum of lauric, myristic, palmitic, and stearic acids, and (b) polyunsaturated fat is cis, cis-methylene-interrupted polyunsaturated fatty acids. "Other Fats" include saturated and polyunsaturated fatty acids that are outside of these definitions.

Sources: Canola oil, animal fat shortening, vegetable shortening: data on file, Procter & Gamble. Margarine: H.T. Slover et al., "Lipids in Margarines and Margarine-like Foods," *Journal of the American Oil Chemists Society*, 62: 775–786 (1985). All others: J.B. Reeves and J.L. Weihrauch, *Composition of Foods*, Agriculture Handbook no. 8–4 (Washington: U.S. Department of Agriculture, 1979).

Reprinted by permission of Procter & Gamble. © 1989 P&G

saturated fats. The fat of salmon, sardines, mackerel, herring, and some other species contains unusual fatty acids, called omega-3's, that are present in only tiny amounts in most other animal and vegetable fats. The omega-3's may reduce the clotting tendency of blood (and thereby lower risk of heart attacks), may inhibit inflammation (the opposite effect of polyunsaturated vegetable oils), and have other beneficial effects. There are problems with fish as a food source (see below under "Protein"), and I do not recommend taking fish oil capsules as supplements (see the section on omega-3 fatty acids in Chapter 14). Eating some oily fish two or three times a week is a healthful addition to an otherwise mostly vegetarian diet.

For those who do not want to eat fish, soy and canola oils both provide small amounts of omega-3 fatty acids, the latter more than the former. A much richer source is linseed oil, also known as flax-seed oil. Not usually thought of as a food, linseed oil has a history of use as a dietary supplement and is available in most health food stores. It is so unsaturated that it must be specially protected from oxidation. Buy it only from reputable sources, in small, light-proof containers, packed under nitrogen. Keep it in the refrigerator and always smell it before using to make sure it is not going rancid. When very fresh, linseed oil is nutty and pleasant, but many samples I've tasted are not delicious. Some Mediterranean peoples get their omega-3's from purslane, a green vegetable *(Portulaca oleracea)* that is easily cultivated in home gardens. Other sources are hemp oil and hop seed oil, which are slowly becoming available.

I have devoted a lot of words to the subject of fat, but I cannot overemphasize the importance of knowing the role of dietary fat in health and disease, and I find constantly that people are unaware of the facts I have just presented. Let me conclude this section with a brief story. When I was discussing fats with a group of medical students and mentioned solid vegetable shortenings, one student asked, "Why do they call it shortening? What does it shorten?" Before I could respond, another student answered, "Your life."

PROTEIN

The chemistry of proteins is much more complex than that of carbohydrates and fats, and proteins are important to living organisms in more ways than as sources of energy. They compose many tissues of the body, such as muscle, skin, and bone; make up the delicate internal machinery of cells; and regulate many life functions. Protein molecules begin as long chains of amino acids, relatively simple compounds containing nitrogen. Amino acids are like the letters of an alphabet. We can make endless numbers of words from only twenty-six letters, and the body can make endless numbers of proteins from twenty amino acids. It can manufacture all of these building blocks on its own except for eight of them, the *essential* amino acids that we must get in our diet.

Once protein chains are assembled, they assume complex three-dimensional shapes by folding up in ways determined by their amino-acid sequences. The meaning of a protein "word" is as much in its contour as in its "letters." Because protein chemistry offers so many possibilities for distinctive sequences and shapes, proteins, more than any other components, differentiate organisms. The carbohydrates and fats in me are not that different from the carbohydrates and fats in you or in my dogs or in the plants in my garden, but my proteins are very different from the proteins of plants and other animals and even from your proteins.

Instructions for building cells and tissues and organs are encoded in DNA, the basic molecule of life that makes up genes. Information in the DNA genetic code (which is the same for all organisms) is expressed through the manufacture of specific proteins. Some of the most important proteins in all organisms are enzymes that catalyze or speed up biological reactions. As genes turn on or off, thereby starting or stopping the synthesis of particular enzymes, the machinery of cells is directed to build up the tissues that become you or a dog or a plant and then to regulate the functions of the finished organism.

You must have dietary protein to build new tissue and to repair damaged tissue. If you are a growing child you need to eat plenty of protein. If you are recovering from serious illness or injury, you need extra protein. If you are a nursing mother, your protein needs are higher than normal. But if you are not in these categories, your protein needs as a normal, healthy adult are not great, even if you are pregnant or engage in strenuous physical activity.

As little as two ounces (sixty grams) of a protein-rich food may be enough to prevent protein deficiency in most of us; four ounces will certainly do it. That means a four-ounce serving of meat *or* chicken *or* fish *or* cheese *or* tofu. Most people eat more than four ounces of protein at every meal. A breakfast of bacon and eggs with milk and cereal is already a protein overload at the start of the day.

If you eat more protein than your body needs for growth, repair, and maintenance of tissue, what becomes of it? It is burned as a fuel, just as carbohydrate and fat are, but protein is not nearly so efficient a fuel.

Because of the complexity of protein molecules, the body has to work harder to dismantle them and release their energy. The ratio of energy gained to energy expended is not as favorable as for carbohydrate and fat. High-protein diets impose a considerable workload on the digestive system and may contribute to feelings of fatigue and lack of energy. A frequent complaint of patients who consult me is lack of energy. If I can convince them to cut down on the amount of protein they eat, increase their intake of starch and vegetables, and do more aerobic exercise, most of them find that they feel better and have more energy.

The second problem with protein as a fuel is that it does not burn clean. Because of its nitrogen content, protein leaves "ashes" when it burns, toxic nitrogen wastes that must be eliminated from the system. After a high-protein meal, amino acids flood into the bloodstream. The liver has to work hard to metabolize them to a simple compound, urea, which is poisonous and must be removed by the kidneys. For this to happen, large amounts of water have to be excreted to flush the urea from the blood. In addition to the general workload on the entire digestive system, protein metabolism especially taxes the liver and kidneys.

Although doctors know that patients with serious liver or kidney disease must be maintained on very low protein diets, they often fail to warn patients with mild disorders about the dangers of eating too much protein. One way to keep liver and kidney ailments from getting serious is to spare these organs the extra work of processing the residues of protein metabolism.

The rapid weight loss that occurs with the ever-popular high-protein, no-carbohydrate diets promoted in books, magazines, and tabloids is mostly the result of diuresis — loss of water from the body into the urinary tract. You *can* lose ten pounds in a week of eating nothing but steak and grapefruit, but most of the weight is water, the consequence of the kidneys' efforts to get rid of urea. The chance of gaining it all back when you resume a normal diet is 100 percent. I have never met anyone who kept weight off by following this sort of regimen. It is also a terrible stress on the system.

The diuretic effect of high protein intake leaches minerals out of the body, including calcium. Loss of calcium from bones can produce osteoporosis, a condition that results eventually in skeletal deformity and fractures, especially of hips. In recent years osteoporosis has become a well-known disease feared by women, who, because of hormonal changes at menopause, become susceptible to it at younger ages than men. Many women today take hormone and calcium supplements to protect their bones, but they continue to eat protein-rich diets that neutralize the protection. Osteoporosis is not caused by calcium deficiency in the diet, nor can it be corrected by taking calcium supplements once it develops. It is caused by heredity (slender, light-boned women being most susceptible), lack of proper exercise (weight-bearing activities such as running, aerobics, and weight lifting increase the uptake of calcium by bones), low levels of sex hormones (as in women after menopause and men in their eighties), and diet. Although biochemists have known for many years that high-protein diets cause bones to lose calcium, this information seems not to get the attention of doctors and patients, most of whom would rather use pills once osteoporosis has developed than try to prevent it by modifying patterns of eating and exercise early in life.

I believe that high-protein diets can irritate the immune system in some people, aggravating allergies and autoimmune diseases (such as rheumatoid arthritis and lupus, in which the immune system mistakenly attacks the body's own tissues). Because proteins are the components that make an organism unique, the immune system reads them to decide whether materials in the body are self or foreign. When the immune system is overactive, as in allergy and autoimmunity, flooding the body with animal and plant protein may confuse it further and make resolution of these conditions less likely. I find that very low protein diets often contribute to improvement in patients with immune-system problems.

If too much protein is not good for us, why do we put such emphasis on it in thinking about food and in planning meals? Most people worry about not getting enough protein; almost no one thinks about getting too much. "Where are you getting your protein?" is a common question in our culture, asked often of people who move in the direction of vegetarianism. How many times have you been asked "Where are you getting your fat?" or "Where are you getting your starch?" Most meals revolve around centerpieces of protein-dense foods. Many cooks would not know what to put on the table for dinner if they were told to omit meat, poultry, fish, and cheese. Everyone would be looking around for the main course.

Our love of protein has a simple historical explanation, I think. Our ancestors came from agricultural societies in which poor people ate starch and rich people put meat on the table. Eating meat was a sign of affluence, resonating with subconscious associations to much more distant times when the ultimate success was success at the hunt. The hunter with the most status was the one who could provide meat most often. These cultural and economic prejudices operate very strongly today, bolstered by horrible visual images of protein-deficient children in famine-struck areas of the Third World. In fact, it would be hard to become deficient in protein in our country even if you tried. There is enough protein in green vegetables to supply the needs of a normal adult who eats large portions of them. I have put many patients on very low protein diets and have never seen problems result. The signs of deficiency are clear enough. If you are not getting enough protein, your hair and nails stop growing and wounds do not heal. If you do not have those symptoms, you would do better to worry about getting too much protein than too little.

Our culturally warped view of the value of protein foods naturally is reflected in our nutritional science. At the beginning of this chapter I referred to the Basic Four food groups, that most holy icon of nutritionists. All of us have seen the charts telling us we must select foods from each of the groups every day. Three of the four are protein foods: (1) dairy products; (2) meat, fish, poultry, eggs, and legumes; and (3) breads and cereals, which have significant protein in addition to their carbohydrate content. One average serving from group 1 or group 2 would provide more than enough protein for an entire day. I just received in the mail the current Australian version of this scheme. It creates a fifth basic food group consisting only of butter and margarine — have some extra fat with your excess protein!

Although different protein foods may be better or worse for our health, in considering total intake, protein is protein, whether it comes from animals or vegetables, whether it is beef or tofu. The only advantage of vegetable proteins is that they are less dense, often diluted by carbohydrate and fiber, so you can eat more of them before exceeding your protein needs. Vegetable proteins also differ from animal proteins in their amino acid content. In particular, they are usually low in one or more of the eight essential amino acids, which is why some nutritionists call them "incomplete." Animal products, being more closely related to human tissue, provide all of the amino acids in the right proportions.

If you are a vegetarian, you can compensate for the difference by combining foods in ways that complete their amino acid profiles, by eating grains and beans together, for instance. You have probably heard about "complementary proteins" or "protein combining," an idea that became very popular in recent years as more people became interested in vegetarian diets to improve both their personal health and the ecology of the planet. Although it may be desirable to combine proteins, it is certainly not necessary to do so. The body makes complete proteins from incomplete ones; it gets the missing amino acids from the large numbers of microorganisms in the intestinal tract and from recycled cells of the lining of that tract. Writers who popularized the concept of protein complementarity left many of us feeling that we could not safely be vegetarians unless we had calculators in our hands at all times. They also reinforced our cultural obsession with protein as the crucial nutrient, the one element of our diet we had to worry about. My advice is not to worry about protein at all and to eat less of it, whether from animal or vegetable sources.

Still, there are advantages and disadvantages to different kinds of protein foods. Let's review the major ones to see how they compare.

Red meat (beef, lamb, venison, etc.) is the choicest, most expensive source of protein in our culture. It provides complete protein, similar in composition to our own, in dense form, relatively undiluted by carbohydrate and fiber. Of course, this is a disadvantage if you are alert to the reality of protein excess, since it is easier to exceed your protein needs with smaller quantities of red meat. A major drawback is its high content of saturated fat and cholesterol. Much of the fat in beef, lamb, and pork is distributed through the muscle tissue and cannot be trimmed off; in fact, we tend to consider meat tastier and more desirable if it contains more of this sort of fat. People who cannot imagine a meal without a main dish of meat are at much higher risk of cardiovascular disease than people who follow a meatless diet.

When we eat animals raised for meat, we live near the top of the earth's food chain — the sequence of organisms in which those above feed on those below. Animals that eat other animals accumulate and concentrate many environmental toxins passed along this chain. That is one reason to eat mainly plants; they are at the bottom of the food chain and are generally less contaminated. In addition, current methods of raising animals make use of large amounts of drugs, hormones, and toxic chemicals to increase the weight and market value of animals destined for the table. These hazards of high-meat diets are less obvious and less well studied than the risk of cardiovascular disease but may be equally unhealthy. The drugs and hormones in meat may increase our chances of developing cancer, degenerative illnesses, and damage to the immune system. Finally, meat cooked rare may transmit certain viruses suspected of playing a role in causing cancer. Thorough cooking eliminates that danger but does not get rid of toxins and contaminants.

Also, our cultural love of meat is not sound for humanity as a whole, because raising grain to feed to animals is an inefficient and wasteful use of agricultural resources. The caloric energy in grain would go much further if it were fed directly to people. In addition, the ecological consequences of farming and ranching are dreadful. Herd animals have devastated the landscape in much of the world, and their wastes are a major contributor to groundwater pollution and to the heat-retaining capacity of the atmosphere (greenhouse effect).

More and more of my patients tell me they no longer eat red meat or eat it very seldom. This represents a major change in eating habits in our society, and as a believer in preventive medicine, I welcome it.

"White meat" refers to veal and pork. Some of those who tell me they have given up red meat continue to eat veal and pork, thinking that the switch is a big step toward a healthier diet. I do not see why. Veal has less fat than beef, but it is the most inhumanely raised of all the meats. (Veal calves are made anemic and prevented from moving in order to keep their muscles underdeveloped.) Pig farming has done less damage to our environment than cattle ranching, but I do not consider pork any lighter or healthier than beef, as the pork industry would have us believe. It is another major contributor to the excesses in our diets: of protein, saturated fat, and cholesterol. In short, white meat is not significantly different from red.

Poultry, particularly chicken and turkey, is an extremely popular and versatile animal food that offers one big plus over meat: its fat is mostly external to muscle and can be largely removed by skinning. Skinned chicken broiled or baked without added fat is a healthier source of animal protein than beef, veal, lamb, or pork in terms of cardiovascular risks. Of course, you lose this advantage if you cook your chicken with its skin, eat it fried, or douse it with butter or mayonnaise. Some kinds of domestic poultry — duck and goose, specifically — are much higher in fat than chicken or turkey. The fat of all these fowl is highly saturated and contains cholesterol. You should avoid eating it.

Another problem with poultry in general is chemical contamination. We raise domestic fowl in even worse ways than cows and pigs, confining them in unnatural conditions and plying them with drugs. If you have access to free-range chickens and turkeys that are guaranteed to be free of drugs and hormones, you can eat them in moderation as an alternative to meat. Otherwise be cautious about eating poultry frequently.

Eggs are part of many breakfasts, and they are ingredients in a wide variety of prepared foods, such as breads, cakes, cookies, ice cream, and pasta. The white of the egg is the protein source, and it is good-quality protein. The trouble is that most people eat whole eggs, not just whites, and egg yolk is a rich source of dietary cholesterol. If we just ate eggs by themselves occasionally, that would not be too bad, but many favorite dishes combine whole eggs with butter, cream, milk, and cheese, mixtures that are very dangerous for our hearts and arteries. Usually it is possible to modify recipes by leaving out eggs altogether or using just the whites. You can make excellent muffins, cookies, cakes, and pancakes without any eggs at all, you can buy pasta made only from flour and water, and you can read the labels of prepared foods to be aware of your consumption of egg yolks and whole eggs.

I see no advantage in eating fertile eggs instead of the usual unfertilized ones, but if you can get eggs from free-range chickens raised without drugs and hormones, it is worth the small extra trouble and expense to reduce your intake of chemicals that can harm you. Because of recent increases in the incidence of bacterial (especially salmonella) contamination of eggs, it is wise to cook them thoroughly.

Fish was once an excellent source of high-quality protein, low in fat compared to meat. In today's world it is less desirable as a food source because it is likely to be contaminated by the toxins we have dumped into rivers, lakes, and oceans. In general, ocean fish is safer than freshwater fish, but in both salt and fresh water, fish are often at the top of the food chain, where they concentrate all the toxins that accumulate in the bodies of smaller organisms. The least safe fish are therefore the large, carnivorous ones, as well as those that spend a lot of time in coastal waters, where pollutants are heaviest. I strongly recommend against eating swordfish, marlin, and other big ocean fish. Small fish that feed mainly on tiny marine organisms and live offshore, such as sardines and herring, are much safer; they also supply the omega-3 fatty acids that protect against heart attacks.

Other oily fish are salmon, mackerel, bluefish, and, to a lesser extent, albacore tuna. Bluefish often concentrates toxic amounts of mercury and should be eaten with caution if at all. Because tuna is a large fish, it is best eaten in moderation. Mackerel is a good source of omega-3 fatty acids but is available only seasonally. Salmon from clean northern waters is available most of the year and is usually of good quality. Alaskan salmon is wild; Norwegian salmon is farm-raised. Drugs are often used in fish farming to control diseases that result from crowding. These diseases may threaten the health — and eventually the existence — of wild populations of salmon. Farmed salmon may contain residues of these drugs and generally has less omega-3's than wild salmon.

Fish spoils quickly and should be eaten as fresh as possible, both for taste and nutritional value. In many areas of the country it is difficult and expensive to get really fresh fish. Raw fish, a traditional Japanese delicacy, has become very popular recently in the West. Japanese insist on using only the freshest fish for sushi; most sushi bars in North America cannot provide that quality. There is a small but real risk of getting parasitic worms from eating raw ocean fish. To my taste, fish is best when it is properly and lightly cooked. Like other protein foods, fish is more easily digested after cooking.

Shellfish are of two types, mollusks (clams, oysters, scallops, snails, mussels) and crustaceans (shrimp, lobster, crab). The feeding habits of these creatures and their preference for coastal waters make them riskier than most scale fish — they are likely to have picked up toxins and pollutants. Be careful about eating raw mollusks, which can transmit a variety of diseases, including hepatitis. Shrimp and lobster contain significant amounts of cholesterol, but since they are also very low in saturated fat, they are much healthier protein foods than meat, if they are not fried or prepared in butter and cream sauces. Shrimp should always be deveined before eating, since the "vein" is the digestive tube and may have higher concentrations of unwanted elements than the flesh.

Milk and milk products (cheese, yogurt) are popular protein sources, eaten in quantity by most people. The dairy industry would like us to believe that we never outgrow our need for milk and that milk is nature's most perfect food, but there are reasons to think otherwise. In fact, all of the nutritive factors in milk can cause problems.

Many people cannot digest milk sugar, or lactose. If you are not of northern European origin and if you stopped drinking milk after infancy, you have probably lost the ability to make lactase, the enzyme needed to metabolize lactose. Without the enzyme, lactose in the digestive system will result in bloating, flatulence, and general intestinal distress. Lactose-intolerant individuals can eat cultured milk products like yogurt, buttermilk, and cheese, in which the lactose has been broken down by bacterial action, or can add commercial enzyme preparations to milk before drinking it.

As noted in the section on fat, the fat in milk — butterfat — is the most dangerous of all animal fats for the health of our hearts and arteries. It gives us a whopping dose of saturated fatty acids and cholesterol and is a principal culprit in the development of atherosclerosis. When milk is made into cheese, the protein is concentrated, and so is the butterfat. Many cheeses range from 50 to 70 percent fat by calories, making them sources of fat more than of protein. Some of the high-fat cheeses are obvious: cream cheese, Brie, and Camembert, for example. Others, like Swiss and cheddar, are not so obvious. The great disadvantage of most dairy products as protein foods is the amount of unhealthy fat they provide. I recommend using only low-fat cheeses, and low-fat or nonfat yogurt. Part-skim mozzarella is available in all supermarkets, and you can purchase flavorful low-fat cheeses at most cheese stores. Read labels to determine the fat content of the dairy products you use, and remember to convert this information to percentage of calories that are fat.

Milk protein, or casein, can also cause trouble. It increases the production of mucus in most people and so aggravates such conditions as asthma, bronchitis, and sinusitis. Moreover, it acts as an irritant of the immune system in many cases of overactive immunity (allergies and autoimmune diseases). Even if skin tests do not demonstrate a true allergy to milk, removing it from the diet often leads to improvement in allergic conditions like asthma and eczema and in autoimmune diseases like rheumatoid arthritis and lupus. Eating nonfat milk products does not help, because they have the same amount of milk protein, and it is the protein that causes these unwelcome effects. Be aware that nondairy cheese substitutes made from soybeans and almonds may still contain casein to give them a more authentic texture. If you are trying to avoid milk protein, read labels of these products carefully.

Most commercial milk contains residues of the drugs, hormones, and chemicals used in abundance on modern dairy farms. Raw (unpasteurized, unhomogenized) milk may taste better than the ordinary variety, but unless it comes from a reputable, certified dairy, it may transmit serious infectious diseases. Even pasteurized milk can transmit a common virus (papillomavirus) that may be involved in a number of human cancers. Goat's milk may be easier for some bodies to digest than cow's milk. Depending on how it is produced, it can be pleasant or nasty in taste.

People of European origin are in a minority of the world's population in their liking for dairy products. Most human beings regard drinking milk in adulthood as outlandish if not disgusting. Milk probably is nature's most perfect food for baby cows, but not for human beings. Many people in our society could improve their health by reducing their consumption of milk and all products made from it.

Legumes (beans, peas, lentils, peanuts, soy products) are important protein sources for vegetarians, especially those who do not eat milk or eggs. The standard fare in many traditional cultures is a serving of legumes and grain, such as the tortillas and beans of many New World Indians. This combination provides all the essential amino acids with little fat. Except for soybeans and peanuts, legumes are very low in fat and high in complex carbohydrates as well as protein. Because the protein is diluted, you can eat more of these foods without overloading your system.

Some of the carbohydrates in beans are too complex for humans to digest. The bacteria that live in our intestines can break these carbohydrates down, but in doing so they produce a lot of methane gas as a by-product. This accounts for the flatulence many people experience when they eat beans. The usual suggestions offered to reduce the problem, like discarding the soaking water and adding fresh water before cooking, are not effective. The best solution is to select varieties of beans that have fewer of the indigestible elements (black beans, Anasazi beans) rather than more (pink beans, soybeans). Unprocessed soybeans, as well as products made from soy flour and grits, are so flatulent as to be unacceptable to many.

Many legumes contain toxins, which in most cases are destroyed by cooking, especially cooking in water. It is not a good idea to eat raw legumes, including peanuts and peas, all of which have an unpleasant raw bean taste that disappears with cooking. Raw chickpeas (garbanzos) contain a toxin that injures the immune system, producing a disease (called lathyrism) that resembles lupus. In India, where flour is commonly made from dry-roasted chickpeas, outbreaks of the disease have been so frequent that many states have banned their sale. The toxin disappears when chickpeas are boiled in water. Sprouts of legume seeds contain these same toxins and should never be eaten raw. In the case of alfalfa sprouts, this probably means not eating them at all, since cooking turns them to mush. Alfalfa sprouts contain canavanine, a well-known toxin that harms the immune system. Other common legume sprouts are lentils, mung beans, and chickpeas.

A common problem with bean dishes is insufficient cooking. When beans are cooked long and slowly until they begin to melt into the liquid, they become most delicious and most digestible.

For centuries the peoples of Asia have turned soybeans into an amazing variety of foods that are both digestible and delicious, including soy milk, tofu (the "cheese" made from soy milk), and products that are very like meat in appearance, taste, and texture. This soy magic reached its highest expression in the vegetarian cuisine of Buddhist temples. Western manufacturers in this century have tried to make fake hot dogs, cutlets, and bacon out of soy protein, but until recently their efforts were far inferior to the temple foods of China and Japan. Today, some of the Oriental soy products are becoming known in the West, and new ones are being developed here. For example, tempeh, a staple Indonesian food, can be found frozen in many natural food stores. A fermented soy product, it has a pleasing taste and meatlike texture that make it very acceptable to Western palates, especially when made into burgers or kebabs, or used in dishes that normally call for ground beef. It is also nonflatulent. Tempeh is so good, in fact, that I am surprised no one has yet created a chain of fast-food restaurants based on burgers made from it. If you have been turned off by tofu, try tempeh.

Grains are not as rich in protein as legumes but are important sources of both starch and protein in many vegetarian diets. Except for corn, grains are low in fat. Eat grains frequently, not just in the form of bread and pasta, but also in soups and main dishes. Try some of the less familiar ones: millet, buckwheat, wild rice, quinoa.

Nuts and seeds are protein-rich, and most of them are also very high in fat. Do not rely on them as major components of the diet.

In summary, most of us can benefit from reducing the amount of protein we eat by cutting down on animal foods, by diluting protein-dense foods with starches and vegetables, as in stir-fries and pasta dishes, and by unlearning our cultural preference for meals organized around centerpieces of meat, poultry, or fish.

Probably you have forgotten by now that all of this information on protein, fat, and carbohydrate came as amplification of the suggestion to eat a balanced diet. A balanced diet will be high in complex carbohydrates, low to moderate in protein, and low in fat. It will minimize both saturated and polyunsaturated fat and will include far fewer foods of animal origin than the standard diet.

To continue with suggestions for a healthy diet:

8. Eat Your Vegetables

Vegetables add variety to the diet and are excellent sources of potassium and other minerals, vitamins, and fiber. Most of them are very low in fat and calories, and some, like potatoes, sweet potatoes, and winter squash, are high in starch. In our society many people shun vegetables as boring or consider them too much trouble to prepare. I find that women like vegetables more than men do. Some men are strictly meat-and-potato eaters, except for occasional salads covered with high-fat dressings. A woman patient, recently widowed, told me her husband had died of colon cancer after a lifetime of meat-and-potato eating. "The only green thing I ever saw him eat," she told me, "was the olive he put in his martini."

Why do so many people not like vegetables? It can't be that vegetables taste bad, because all babies, both male and female, love puréed vegetables as baby foods. Dislike for vegetables develops later, perhaps when solid foods and unfamiliar textures are introduced, and I suspect that a lot of it is learned. Early on, children pick up the ideas that eating vegetables is a chore and that you get desserts as a reward. On top of this comes the hideous reality of badly cooked vegetables: the trays of limp broccoli, gray brussels sprouts, canned peas, and candied parsnips that have come out of home and institutional kitchens for decades. For vegetables to taste really good, they have to be fresh and properly prepared. That takes some knowledge and more time and effort than many people care to spend.

I've never met a vegetable I didn't like, although it took me a long time to make friends with some that I had bad experiences with as a child. Some people learn to like vegetables by using them as vehicles for butter or cream sauces or by dipping them in batter and deep-frying them, but these preparations do not promote health. Yoga practitioners say that we should eat at least one serving of lightly cooked greens each day: spinach, beet greens, chard, kale, collards, or mustard greens. I find this to be a good prescription, because for those on vegetarian diets, cooked greens are an important source of iron. They can be made very delicious with minimal effort and fat. Both raw and cooked vegetables should be in the diet, but you have to know which are good to eat raw and which are not. As I mentioned earlier, always avoid raw legumes and legume sprouts, including alfalfa sprouts. On the other hand, onions and garlic lose some of their virtues when cooked. They are still good to eat, but if you want to take advantage of the ability of onions to lower cholesterol or that of garlic to fight germs, eat them raw. A salad of different kinds of lettuce, radishes, carrots, cucumbers, onions, and tomatoes is a good way to get some raw vegetables in your diet. In the next chapter I give some sample recipes for easy, healthy, fresh-vegetable dishes I think you will like. Give them a try and be inspired to invent your own.

As mentioned earlier, many vegetables contain natural toxins. The sprouts and green skins of potatoes are poisonous and should always be removed before cooking. Celery, especially when affected by a very common fungus disease called pink rot, contains natural toxins that sensitize us to sunlight and may damage our immune systems. Pink rot is responsible for the brownish patches that discolor many celery stalks. Avoid these.

Most of the natural toxins in vegetables are heat-labile; that is, they are easily destroyed by the heat of cooking. All cruciferous vegetables (the cabbage family), for example, contain such toxins. Small amounts of raw cabbage and cauliflower will not hurt you, but they (and brussels sprouts, kale, collards, mustard greens, and broccoli) are better for you when lightly cooked. They may then offer some protection against colon cancer by affecting the chemical environment of the colon in a favorable way. Raw spinach, chard, and beet greens contain oxalic acid, which removes calcium and iron from the body; light cooking breaks down this compound. Raw cultivated white mushrooms contain three natural carcinogens. Two of them are destroyed by heat, but the third (agaritine) is not and is enough of a worry that I urge you to be cautious about including these mushrooms in the diet at all. In addition to the natural toxins in vegetables is the problem of residues of pesticides and fungicides used on commercial produce. I discuss this subject and give advice on protecting yourself in the next chapter.

Here are some guidelines about how to eat vegetables:

Never eat raw: peas, beans, alfalfa sprouts, lentil sprouts, mung bean sprouts, mushrooms.

Best when cooked a long time: beans, lentils, chickpeas, eggplant.

Better cooked than raw: beets and beet greens, chard, spinach, cabbage, broccoli, cauliflower, kale, brussels sprouts, collards, mustard greens, winter squash, green beans. Do not overcook green vegetables.

Good both raw and cooked: carrots, celery, onions, garlic, chives, scallions, summer squash, turnips, endive, asparagus, sunflower sprouts, tomatoes, peppers.

Better raw: lettuce, other salad greens (arugula, radicchio, watercress), cucumbers, radishes, buckwheat sprouts.

9. Experiment with Your Diet

The only way you will find out what you should eat for optimal well-being is by experimenting. Be willing to change your diet. Try new foods and new combinations of foods, leave others out. Note how your interest in and enjoyment of food varies as you make these changes. Use the suggestions I have presented here as general guidelines, but use your own experience as your best guide. If you read or hear of a dietary system that appears to be sound, give it a try, but do not hestitate to drop it if it fails to deliver any benefits or takes away from the enjoyment of preparing and eating food.

2

ANSWERS TO
COMMON QUESTIONS
ABOUT DIET AND HEALTH

THROUGHOUT THIS BOOK you will find information about nutrition and health, particularly regarding ways of preventing and treating specific diseases by changing your dietary habits. In this chapter I will answer some of the general questions I am asked most frequently.

I hear so much about fiber in the diet these days. How much do I really need and where do I get it?

Fiber is simply a term for the indigestible components of the plants we eat. It used to be called "roughage" and not so long ago was considered unimportant in the diet because it did not provide the body with energy. Fiber consists of carbohydrates that are too complex for our digestive system to break down. Vegetarians get a lot of fiber; those who eat mainly meat, potatoes, and white bread do not. Our present fascination with fiber is a nutritional fad. I think most people can benefit by increasing the amount of fiber in their diets, but we lack hard scientific evidence to support some of the claims made by promoters of high-fiber diets.

It is obvious that people who eat a lot of fiber have better-functioning intestinal systems than those who eat little. Fiber increases the bulk and frequency of bowel movements, and its lack is a common cause of constipation. The way to increase dietary fiber is to eat more fruits, vegetables, and whole grains.

Actually, there are five types of fiber, which differ in chemical structure and their degree of solubility in water. All of them contribute to our health, but they fall into two groups with different bene-fits. In the first group are the three types that are most helpful to our bowels and that may reduce the risk of diseases of the colon, including colon and rectal cancer. These are the insoluble fibers: cellulose and lignin, found especially in wheat bran and other whole grains, and hemicellulose, which is only partially soluble in water. Hemicellulose occurs in whole grains, nuts, seeds, fruits, and vegetables. Psyllium seed, a good source of hemicellulose, is the main ingredient in Metamucil and other "bulk laxatives" that make stools softer, larger, and easier to pass.

We do not know just how insoluble fiber works. One theory is that by speeding up the time that food takes to pass through the colon, insoluble fiber minimizes contact of potentially carcinogenic substances with intestinal cells. Carcinogens occur as breakdown products of bile acids and of protein metabolism. Cancer of the colon is not caused by lack of fiber — it may have a genetic basis — but in susceptible individuals, adequate amounts of insoluble fiber in the diet may offer significant protection. This kind of fiber also helps in cases of irritable bowel syndrome and diverticulitis.

Gums and pectins are the two kinds of water-soluble fiber. Gums from trees and legumes are added to many manufactured foods to improve their texture. Others occur in familiar seeds, including oats and sesame seeds. Pectins are present in fruits, vegetables, and seeds. These types of fiber bind bile acids and also bind cholesterol, preventing its absorption into the blood. The reason oat bran has become so popular is that its action in the intestines can lower blood cholesterol.

You should be eating forty grams of fiber daily, which is about twice what most people consume. You can easily increase your fiber intake by eating cereals containing bran, but you must read labels, since many products proclaiming themselves to be rich in bran are not. To be worthwhile, a cereal should give you at least four and preferably five grams of bran per one-ounce serving. Of course, you can simply buy straight bran and add it to your favorite cereal or other dishes. Cooked beans are also an excellent source of fiber; many varieties (for example, pinto, navy, and kidney beans) give you four grams of fiber in each half-cup serving.

One problem that results from increasing your fiber intake is flatulence, for the same reason that beans are gas-producing; when bacteria in the gut attack and digest these complex carbohydrate molecules, methane gas is released. Individuals differ greatly in their tolerance to this effect. If bran gives you gas, eat less of it, take smaller amounts more frequently, or concentrate instead on eating more fruits, vegetables, and whole-grain products. Taking bran as a supplement may cause two other problems. It may interfere with the absorption of minerals from foods, and it may impede bowel movements if you do not drink large amounts of water with it. Therefore I do not usually recommend the use of fiber supplements in the form of pills, powders, or straight wheat bran. I do suggest that constipated people try powdered psyllium seed husks with lots of water.

For most people the best advice concerning fiber is simply to eat more fresh vegetables and fruits as well as products made from whole grains. White flour is a very poor source of fiber. You would have to eat fifty loaves of white bread to get your daily allowance of forty grams from this source alone. If you eat fewer products made from white flour and more whole-grain foods of all sorts along with your vegetables and fruits, you will not have to worry about getting enough fiber in your diet.

How about diet and cholesterol? I hear a lot about oat bran. What else can I take to lower my cholesterol?

Controlling cholesterol has more to do with what you *don't* eat than with what you do. As I explained in Chapter 1, the amount of saturated fat you consume is the most direct dietary influence on how much cholesterol circulates in your blood. The most important preventive measure you can take is to reduce the percentage of saturated fat in your diet by cutting way down on meat, eggs, butter, whole milk and whole-milk products, and processed foods made with animal fats and tropical oils (palm and coconut).

Diet is only one factor affecting serum cholesterol — others are heredity, stress, smoking, caffeine, and exercise — and cholesterol is only one factor affecting the risk of coronary heart disease (see Chapter 9, "How Not to Get a Heart Attack"), but since you can change your eating habits more easily than some of these other variables, it is worth making some changes.

Because cholestrol has become a buzz word in our culture, food manufacturers now try to sell products by labeling them as low in or free of cholesterol. This is often misleading. For example, I have in front of me an "Italian Garlic-Herb Loaf" purchased at a nearby supermarket. It is half a large loaf of Italian white bread, spread with a very thick coating of fat mixed with spices and herbs, and meant to be heated in the oven. A main ingredient is "partially hydrogenated vegetable oil (soy and/or cottonseed)." Stuck on the plastic wrapping is a prominent red seal bearing the words "No Cholesterol!" This is truthful but deceptive. No vegetable oil contains cholesterol, but the large amount of saturated fat in that unhealthy topping will certainly make for plenty of cholesterol in your arteries. Do not be misled by "No Cholesterol" labels on containers of peanut butter, vegetable oils, shortenings, margarine, and other fats. There never has been cholesterol in these products, but they can cause your body to produce excessive amounts of it.

Actually, dietary cholesterol is less important than dietary fat, because our livers make cholesterol independently and are much more influenced by saturated fat in foods than by cholesterol. Most foods high in cholesterol are unhealthy, but that is because they are all of animal origin and with few exceptions are the major sources of saturated fat. It is the fat in meat, butter, and cheese, more than the cholesterol, that is bad for you. Shrimp is one of the exceptions to the rule; it contains significant cholesterol but very little fat. Therefore shrimp cooked without added fat is better for your arteries than meat. Egg yolks have a great deal of cholesterol and are much higher in fat. For people eating typical high-fat diets with a lot of meat and dairy products, eggs may not be a major contributor to high levels of serum cholesterol. For people who shift to a low-fat, mostly vegetarian diet, eggs become more significant. If you make the dietary changes I recommend, you will want to be careful about eggs. Even one meal of them can raise the blood level of cholesterol noticeably.

To emphasize the fact that people are biochemically unique, I must point out that very low fat, high-carbohydrate diets do not automatically improve lipid (fat) metabolism in all people. In some people such diets result in high levels of serum cholesterol and tri-glycerides. These individuals do better eating more protein and moderate amounts of carbohydrate and fat. Whenever you make a major dietary change to lower cardiovascular risk, you must monitor blood levels of cholesterol and triglycerides to be sure the changes are in the direction you want. Get a blood test called a "lipid profile," which includes all of these values, one month after starting a dietary regimen and again at three months.

Besides oat bran, which binds cholesterol in the gut and blocks its reabsorption, other foods can be helpful. Many fruits and vegetables have been shown to lower cholesterol, probably because they also contain water-soluble fiber. Onions and garlic — especially raw — lower cholesterol for unknown reasons not having to do with fiber, since they provide little of it.

Shiitake mushrooms, the meaty and flavorful black mushrooms of Chinese and Japanese cuisine, contain a substance (eritadenine) that encourages the uptake of cholesterol by body tissue, thus lowering the amount in circulating blood. One Japanese experiment showed that feeding human volunteers ninety grams (a little over three ounces) of fresh shiitake a day lowered serum cholesterol 12 percent in a week and also counteracted rises caused by adding butter to the diet. Dried shiitake, available at all Oriental groceries, are also effective, and fresh ones are becoming available in many markets as domestic cultivation of this delicious mushroom becomes more common. (By the way, shiitake are free of the natural carcinogens found in the common white cultivated mushroom.)

Chili peppers lower cholesterol, too, though we do not yet know how. They may suppress production of cholesterol in the liver. It is the hot compound in red pepper, capsaicin, that is responsible for this effect. Capsaicin is a powerful local anesthetic and may be good for our hearts and blood vessels in general. The hotter the pepper, the more capsaicin it contains. Another unusual source of cholesterol-lowering activity is Japanese green tea, which also appears to protect against cancer.

Moderate consumption of alcohol raises the level of "good cholesterol" in the blood. (See pp. 46–47 for a discussion of good and bad cholesterol.) Since alcohol is a strong drug with many adverse effects on health (see Chapter 7), I do not recommend it to people who do not already drink. I do recommend adding omega-3 fatty acids to the diet in the form of two to three servings per week of oily fish or linseed oil. You can find canned Norwegian sardines packed in sild sardine oil without salt. (Ordinary canned sardines have a very high sodium load.) Drain off as much oil as you can (you will get rid of 200 calories this way), and prepare the fish however you want. Fish oils protect against heart disease in several ways; they may help lower the total amount of cholesterol in the blood and in particular the level of the most dangerous fraction.

Many people attempt to reduce their cholesterol by taking high doses of niacin, vitamin B-3. I discuss this in Chapter 14, "Vitamins and Supplements." In the doses that are effective, niacin acts as a drug rather than a vitamin and can be risky.

In summary, the dietary adjustments that will allow most people to get their cholesterol down to the safe range are to: (1) eat less fat of all kinds; (2) eat less saturated fat in particular (replacing it with monounsaturated fat); (3) eat more fruits, vegetables, and whole grains; (4) add some oat bran to the diet; (5) eat more onions and garlic, some of them raw; (6) eat some oily fish or linseed oil; (7) eat shiitake mushrooms; (8) eat chili peppers in some form; and (8) cut out coffee, tea, cola, and other sources of caffeine, except for green tea. (See Chapters 7 and 9 for information on the effects of this drug.)

I'm confused by the terms "good" and "bad" cholesterol. What do they mean? And what about cholesterol-lowering drugs?

Cholesterol travels around the body in complicated ways controlled by the liver, which can remove it from the blood and secrete it in bile. Bile squirts into the small intestine to aid digestion of fats. Cholesterol in bile can be reabsorbed from the intestine and again enter the bloodstream. In the blood, cholesterol circulates in protein packages called lipoproteins. (The prefix *lipo-* means "fat.") One type of circulating cholesterol, the low-density lipoproteins, or LDL, is often called "bad cholesterol" because it damages arterial walls. High-density lipoproteins, or HDL, are the "good cholesterol." Some of them seem to protect arteries from damage.

In addition to knowing your total cholesterol, you should know how it breaks down into LDL and HDL. Total cholesterol should be under 180 (milligrams per deciliter of serum), but higher levels may be all right if the ratio of HDL to LDL is high. If you get your total cholesterol low enough — under 140, say — you may not need to worry about the HDL/LDL ratio. If the level of total cholesterol circulating in the blood is low enough, arterial damage will not occur even if the protective fraction is low.

A few individuals inherit a tendency to make large amounts of cholesterol no matter what they eat. They may require drug treatment to bring their cholesterol down to the normal range. For most of us diet *is* a major influence on the amount of fat and cholesterol in our blood. If you look through a microscope at a blood sample from someone who has just eaten a high-fat meal, you will actually see globules of fat mixed in with blood cells. Even a week of eating according to the guidelines in the last chapter will produce a measurable lowering of serum cholesterol in most people.

A few people are lucky enough to inherit efficient liver systems for clearing fat and cholesterol from the blood. They are the ones who can eat lots of meat, eggs, butter, and cheese all their lives and have low serum cholesterol and no arterial disease. Most of us cannot get away with that behavior. The ill effects may not be apparent in early life, but as we age, the results of arterial damage due to high levels of circulating cholesterol make themselves known. The sooner you change the dietary patterns that produce the problem, the sooner you begin to reverse the damage and decrease your risk of trouble.

I never prescribe cholesterol-lowering drugs. They are expensive and can be toxic to the liver. An herbal alternative is guggulipid, an extract of an Indian plant *(Commiphora mukul)* that is used traditionally in Ayurvedic medicine to treat obesity. Contemporary research shows that it lowers cholesterol in a manner similar to the pharmaceutical drugs, but with much less risk. Guggulipid is available in health food stores. Keep in mind that scientific research does not support the theory that artificially lowering cholesterol with drugs will lower the risk of dying from heart attacks. There *is* evidence that you can improve the health of your coronary arteries by a conscientious program of lifestyle modification that includes dietary change as one component.

Do I need to worry about additives in the foods I buy?

Yes, you do, and about some additives more than others. We are fortunate that today food manufacturers are required to list the ingredients in their products, mostly because pressure from consumer groups led to laws demanding this information. Only a few products, such as alcoholic beverages, are exempted from labeling requirements. I cannot urge you too strongly to read labels on the foods you buy.

A dangerous class of additives and one of the easiest to avoid are dyes. Chemicals that create color by reflecting light are energetic molecules, many of which are capable of interacting with and damaging DNA. Anything that damages DNA can injure our immune systems, speed up aging, and push us in the direction of cancer. I advise you not to eat foods made with artificial colors. Watch out for labels that use any of the following terms: "artificial color added," "U.S. certified color added," "FD & C red no. 3" (or green or blue or yellow followed by any number; these are food, drug, and cosmetic dyes approved for use by the Food and Drug Administration), or simply "color added" with no explanation.

Many synthetic food dyes that were considered safe for years have turned out to be carcinogenic. Some dyes approved for use in Europe are considered unsafe here and vice versa. Dyes are added to foods for the convenience of the manufacturer, not for the health of the consumer. You do not add dyes to food you make at home (at least I hope you don't), and you should not eat them in foods you buy. Try to convey to your children that garishly colored snack foods are weird and unhealthy rather than attractive. Simply stated: do not buy or eat foods with artificial colors. This is an easy rule to follow.

Some foods contain natural colors obtained from plants; I have no objection to these. The commonest is annatto, from the reddish seed of a tropical tree. Widely used in Latin American cooking to make yellow rice and breads, annatto is universally added to cheese to make it orange and butter to make it yellow. A red pigment obtained from beets, a green one from chlorella (freshwater algae), caramel and carotene from carrots are also safe.

Another class of additives is preservatives. You *can* make a case for using preservatives in food. They are natural or synthetic chemicals that block oxidation reactions, slowing down the development of rancidity in fats and interfering with the metabolism of bacteria and molds that also want to eat our food. I prefer to eat foods without preservatives, but if I had to choose between a rancid food and one with preservatives, I would take the latter without hesitation. Here are comments on some of the more commonly used preservatives.

Citric acid and ascorbic acid (vitamin C) are two natural antioxidants added to a number of foods. Both are completely safe. The synthetic preservatives BHA and BHT, which you will find on the labels of many prepared foods, may not be as safe. They may promote carcinogenic changes in cells caused by other substances.

Alum, an aluminum compound, is used in many brands of pickles to increase crispness. Aluminum has no place in human nutrition and may be harmful to us. Many brands of antacids contain aluminum salts as their active ingredients, and people who take them get much higher doses of this metal than comes from eating pickles or cooking in aluminum pots. (See p. 56 for more on cookware.) You should definitely stay away from these antacids, and you should look for brands of pickles made without alum. Baking powder is another source of aluminum; you can find brands in health food stores that do not contain it.

Nitrites, added to many cured meats, are not themselves carcinogenic, but they easily react with protein breakdown products in the digestive tract to form highly carcinogenic substances called nitrosamines. This reaction is blocked by vitamin C. If you eat any foods containing nitrites, take some vitamin C along with them (see pp. 186–187 for information on dosage). It is best to avoid hot dogs, sausages, lunch meats, and other products containing sodium nitrite or other nitrites — these foods are also high in saturated fat, dense animal protein, and salt. These chemicals are also found in smoked fish. Nitrates, which are usually added along with nitrites, do not form nitrosamines but may be converted to nitrites in the body.

More worrisome than preservatives are artificial sweeteners. Saccharin, a known carcinogen, should be avoided. Cyclamates, banned some years ago for suspected carcinogenicity, are now being reconsidered for use in food. They taste better than saccharin but cause diarrhea in some people. Avoid them too. Recently aspartame

(NutraSweet) has become enormously popular. The manufacturer portrays it as a gift from nature, but, although the two component amino acids occur in nature, aspartame itself does not. Like all artificial sweeteners, aspartame has a peculiar taste. Because I have seen a number of patients, mostly women, who report headaches from this substance, I don't regard it as free from toxicity. Women also find that aspartame aggravates PMS (premenstrual syndrome). I think you are better off using moderate amounts of sugar than consuming any artificial sweeteners on a regular basis.

A natural sweetener that may cause some people problems is sorbitol, originally derived from the berries of the mountain ash tree. Sorbitol tastes sweet but is not easily absorbed from the gastrointestinal tract and is not easily metabolized. It is a common ingredient of sugarless chewing gums and candies. If you eat a lot of it, you will probably get diarrhea. People with irritable bowel syndrome or ulcerative colitis should avoid sorbitol.

Monosodium glutamate (MSG), a natural product long used in Oriental cooking, is added to many manufactured foods as a "flavor enhancer." It is an unnecessary source of additional sodium in the diet and causes many allergic reactions, from stuffy noses to headaches to full-blown "Chinese restaurant syndrome" with flushing, sweating, racing heartbeat, throbbing headache, and other alarming symptoms. Omit MSG from recipes, do not buy products containing it, and when eating out in Chinese restaurants, request that food be prepared without it.

It is difficult to understand labels that list a lot of long chemical names. A good general rule is simply to avoid products whose chemical ingredients outnumber the familiar ones. Some chemicals are quite harmless, of course. For example, many commercial baked goods list ammonium bicarbonate on their labels. This is a form of baking powder that breaks down to ammonia and carbon dioxide, both gases that are driven off in the cooking process. Some other additives you need not worry about are malic acid, fumaric acid, lactic acid, lecithin, xanthan and guar gums, calcium chloride, monocalcium phosphate, and monopotassium phosphate.

As people become more concerned about toxins in their food, manufacturers respond by cleaning up their products. More and more labels assure you that products contain "no artificial preservatives" or "no artificial anything." This is all to the good. If you can't understand a label, however, or if the manufacturer can barely fit all of the chemical ingredients on it, better leave the product on the shelf.

You're telling me to eat more fruits and vegetables. But what about pesticide residues? Should I be worried?

In a word, yes. Recently, when I visited a friend on a farm in southern Minnesota, I stopped at the local farmers' co-op store to pick up some supplies that my hosts had ordered. Most of the products sold there were drugs, pesticides, and other poisons. There is a long and bitter debate raging over the safety of the many agricultural chemicals in common use today; however, the bottom line is that they can't possibly be good for us. The only question is just how bad they are.

One way to reduce consumption of these poisons is to grow some or most of your own food. You can grow a surprising amount of food in little space, and by gardening in containers, even people in apartments can produce some vegetables for the table. I find gardening to be a healthy enterprise on many levels. It is a physical and mental challenge, a wonderful way to dissipate emotional tension, and a source of great satisfaction when you pick the fruits of your labor. I recommend gardening to many people who consult me for medical problems.

If you can't grow your own food, you can buy from sources that promise it to be free of pesticides. The term "organic produce" may or may not have meaning, depending on local laws. In California, Oregon, and some other states, produce cannot be labeled "organic" unless it meets strict criteria. Quite recently some supermarkets have begun offering produce guaranteed to be low in or free of pesticide residues. Again this is in response to consumer demands. (See Appendix B for information on sources of organic produce.)

Since it takes extra effort and money to get pesticide-free fruits and vegetables, it is worth knowing which crops are most likely to be contaminated. The ones that worry me most are apples, peaches, celery, potatoes, grapes (and raisins), oranges, carrots, green beans, strawberries, the common white cultivated mushrooms, lettuce, peanuts, and wheat flour. If you eat these frequently it is worth finding pesticide-free sources. Otherwise, try to reduce your consumption of them. Whenever possible, peel fruits and vegetables before using them. Never cook or bake with orange, lemon, or lime rind unless you get it from pesticide-free fruit. Remove and discard the outer leaves of cabbage, lettuce, and other greens. Always wash your produce well, too, although I am not convinced that washing does a great deal, even if you use soap. Some pesticides are applied as "systemic preparations," which are taken up by the roots of plants and spread through all their tissues. Peeling and washing will not rid your food of these chemicals.

The wax used to coat some fruits and vegetables (apples, cucumbers, peppers) often contains fungicides, and no labeling is required to warn us of this. These chemicals are toxic and cannot be removed except by peeling, which doesn't work for peppers if you like to eat them raw. To prevent sprouting, potatoes are sprayed with a chemical that may be hazardous.

For years growers have maintained that they cannot produce good crops without reliance on these toxic chemicals, that organic farming may work for home gardens but is impractical on the commercial scale. Now, as a result of repeated scares over particular pesticides, the growing anger and concern among consumers, the obvious expansion of markets for pesticide-free fruits and vegetables, and grudging admission that widespread use of pesticides has moved us into worse battles with many species of insects, growers are discovering that natural farming methods do work. You can support this early trend by joining consumer action groups and making your demands for safe produce known. It is also worth working for laws requiring full disclosure of the chemicals used on the foods we buy.

What about food irradiation?

Food irradiation is a new method of preserving food by bombarding it with high-energy rays that disrupt DNA and kill organisms responsible for spoilage. Irradiation also causes chemical changes in foods, and these changes may or may not be harmful. Irradiation may be less dangerous than some chemical methods of preservation, but I do not like the way it is being pushed on the public without adequate investigation of possible risks. At the very least, irradiated food should be labeled as such, not with an innocent-looking flower symbol or the deceptive phrase "picowaved for your protection," but with a clear statement like "This product has been irradiated to preserve it from spoilage." If you are concerned about the growing use of irradiation in the food industry, join consumer action groups that are pressing for more research on its effects, for restrictions on its use, and for full disclosure of its use on product labels.

I'm beginning to feel it's unsafe to venture out of my house. Do I have to stop eating in restaurants? What do I do when I'm invited to eat at other people's houses?

Restaurant food usually provides too many calories, too much fat, too much saturated fat, too much salt, and too much protein. Since I like to eat out as much as anyone else, I have tried to find ways of minimizing the impact of restaurant meals on my dietary program. This is getting easier because more and more restaurants offer healthy dishes on their menus. Some advertise "heart healthy" entrées or note that some dishes meet American Heart Association standards for low content of fat, saturated fat, and cholesterol. Most fine restaurants, given advance notice, will be happy to accommodate your dietary needs with special dishes.

You will find it easier to get acceptable food in certain kinds of restaurants. For example, you can usually get fish, grilled or broiled without butter or oil, at seafood restaurants. You can always get pasta with tomato sauce and a salad with oil and vinegar at an Italian restaurant. Greek and Middle Eastern kitchens offer a number of good vegetarian appetizers and salads. At steak houses you can usually get a baked potato and salad. Chinese restaurants can always make stir-fried vegetables or vegetarian noodle dishes, even if these are not listed on the menu. Salad bars are fine if you stick to vegetables, avoid choices made with mayonnaise, and don't smother your salad in heavy, creamy dressing. Of course, you can find vegetarian and natural food restaurants in most cities, but there is no guarantee that you can order low-fat dishes at them.

Whatever kind of restaurant you go to, you can take some actions to protect yourself:

Do not eat a great deal of white bread.

Do not use butter on your bread.

Avoid cream-based soups.

Order salad dressings on the side. Use oil and vinegar dressing sparingly, if available.

Order simple entrées, such as chicken and fish, broiled or baked if
possible (request that chicken be skinned before cooking).

Request that food be prepared without butter or oil.

Request that rich sauces and toppings be served on the side.

Avoid fried foods.

Avoid high-fat desserts.

Do not hesitate to ask waiters for help in ordering or to ask whether
the kitchen can prepare special dishes to meet your needs.

This is not to take away all the fun of eating out. An occasional
splurge in a restaurant is not going to hurt you, but if you eat
out frequently, you will want to develop some skills at selecting
restaurants and foods that will not be harmful. I assure you that if
you begin to change your diet in the ways suggested in the last
chapter, you will gradually lose your taste for many popular restaurant foods, and when you do eat out, you will look around in
amazement at what most people are consuming.

When you go to other people's houses for dinner, it is perfectly
reasonable to let your hosts know in advance what you do and do
not eat. You can also use some of the same measures suggested
above for restaurant eating, particularly regarding butter, sauces,
salad dressings, and desserts.

What should I do when I travel?

Use the same kind of caution when you travel. Take food with
you if you can, select restaurants wisely, order carefully, and do not
be afraid to ask for the kind of food you like.

Airline food is bad and has been getting worse. Take your own
food on planes if you can. Most airlines offer special meals if you
order in advance, such as fresh fruit plates (often good), vegetarian
dinners (rarely good), and low-cholesterol meals.

Many hotels that cater to business travelers have restaurants with
some healthy selections on the menu. Search out good Italian and

fish restaurants. Inquire at local health food stores about vegetarian and natural food restaurants in the area.

What will I feed my children? They are going to demand all the foods you're telling me to give up.

Remember that healthy foods can also be delicious and appealing to the eye, nose, and palate. Eating habits develop at an early age. If you grow up in a family where hamburgers, hot dogs, French fries, chips, and milkshakes are treats, you will have a hard time changing your associations to those foods later in life.

If you think it's going to be a struggle to get your children to eat better food, it probably will be. Try to avoid the trap of using dessert as a bribe: eat your vegetables or you don't get your ice cream. One way to get children to eat the healthy dishes you prepare is to make it clear that nothing else will be served. If the choice is between good, healthy food and nothing, children will soon learn to eat what you put on the table and come to enjoy it.

As you learn to change your tastes and appreciate healthy food, you can be effective in helping others do the same. A good place to start is with your family. At the end of this chapter are suggestions for further reading, including several cookbooks that are useful. Also I hope you will try my sample recipes to convince yourself that you can make wonderful food without relying on unhealthy ingredients.

What are the advantages and disadvantages of different cooking methods, including microwaving?

Most professional cooks favor gas ranges because the temperature can be quickly adjusted. The disadvantage of cooking with gas is that it is a significant source of indoor pollution, so gas should be avoided by people with environmental sensitivities and respiratory problems. Gas ovens and stoves with pilot lights waste a lot of fuel; units with electric sparkers are much better. Electric stoves are much cleaner than gas but definitely slower. Cooking on them requires more attention and skill to compensate for their slow response to an adjustment of temperature.

Microwave ovens are very convenient for thawing and heating

and for making simple, individual servings. For many foods they do not give the same good results as conventional methods, no matter what their promoters say. Microwave radiation is not ionizing radiation; that is, it is not the sort that knocks electrons out of atomic orbits, creating charged particles that can damage DNA and thereby injure our immune systems and turn cells malignant. High doses of this radiation can cook human tissues that are exposed to it, and low doses may disrupt delicate control systems in our bodies. We know that cellular growth and development are regulated by small electric currents and electromagnetic fields. Microwaves may affect growth and development adversely.

One danger of microwave ovens, therefore, is leakage of this energy into the room. You can buy inexpensive microwave detectors to check for leakage, but they are not reliable. You can also hold a fluorescent light bulb in your hand and move it around the front of the oven while it is on. If the bulb lights or flickers, microwaves are leaking out. In general, microwave ovens do not leak unless they have suffered some physical damage. If you suspect leakage, have your oven tested by a professional. Do not use a leaky oven. Have it repaired or replace it.

Another consideration is what microwaving does to the chemical composition of foods. There is some evidence that microwaving proteins for ten minutes creates new, unnatural species of proteins that may be harmful. Given this possibility, I think it is prudent to use microwave ovens for heating and defrosting foods rather than for cooking main dishes.

People are usually unaware of a more immediate danger. If you microwave food in plastic containers or plastic wrapping, some of the plastic molecules will be driven into the food by the energy of the radiation. Never put food into a microwave oven in anything other than a glass or ceramic container, and never cover it with plastic wrap.

I can also give you some thoughts on cookware and ways of using it. I recommend against using aluminum pots because aluminum reacts with acid foods and is absorbed into your body. The iron in iron pots also does this, but iron is a needed nutrient while aluminum is not. Most men and most menopausal women do not require supplemental iron, but female vegetarians may, since meat is the principal source of iron in the typical diet. If you are a vegetarian or semivegetarian, you can do some, but not all, of your cooking in iron pots. It is possible to get too much iron, and that can have serious health consequences (see Chapter 14, "Vitamins and Supplements").

A reasonable choice for cookware that is safe, efficient, and reasonably priced is stainless steel with copper or aluminum bottoms to improve conductivity of heat. (Stainless steel by itself is a relatively poor conductor.) The bottom metals are not in contact with the food. Be aware, however, that stainless steel contains nickel, a toxic metal and common allergen. If you react to nickel-containing metal jewelry, you should not use stainless steel for long cooking of acidic foods, like tomato sauce. Probably the safest and most inert material for pots and pans is glass. High-quality nonstick pans are also good to have in the kitchen; they make it possible to sauté with little or no fat, and the coating does not react with food.

I strongly recommend against deep-frying. This cooking technique produces foods with excessive fat and, as explained in the previous chapter, is likely to result in unhealthy chemical changes in fats. You should try to phase out most fried foods, whether deep-fried or shallow-fried. Stir-frying is acceptable if you use minimal oil. A technique I like is steam-frying: put a tiny amount of flavorful oil in a hot skillet, add food, such as sliced or chopped vegetables, toss quickly, then add seasonings and some water or both and cover tightly. Cook just until vegetables are crunchy-tender, then remove the lid and cook off as much of the remaining liquid as you want.

Plain steaming is an excellent method of cooking that uses little energy and does the least damage to nutrients. It can be used for many foods, including breads, vegetables, and fish.

Boiling is a rapid method of cooking that may be preferable to steaming for less delicate vegetables, such as corn on the cob, potatoes, and beets. If you boil tender vegetables (peas, zucchini, or green beans, for example) and discard the water, you will lose some of their nutrients.

Broiling and baking use a lot of energy but produce tasty results. They are healthy methods of cooking if you observe a few cautions. The first is not to add extra fat to foods you bake and broil. The second is to avoid browning foods excessively, because foods become carcinogenic when they are cooked brown or black. Some experts feel so strongly about this danger that they recommend even cutting off dark crusts of bread. A third caution is not to inhale smoke from high-temperature cooking of foods containing fat and protein. It is also carcinogenic.

Charcoal grilling presents the same hazards. It produces carcinogenic smoke and unhealthy chemical changes in the outer layers of foods, especially flesh foods, cooked until dark. If you eat charcoal-grilled foods, get in the habit of cutting away the outermost layer. Never use charcoal-lighting fluid or self-lighting packages of charcoal, all of which put residues of toxic chemicals into the food. Buy a "chimney lighter" that uses a small amount of newspaper to turn pieces of charcoal into glowing coals. By the way, grilled vegetables are delicious and, because they are low in protein, much healthier than grilled flesh foods.

How harmful is salt?

It is very harmful for some people and probably not harmful for most of us. The culprit in salt is sodium, specifically the sodium ion, which the body uses to regulate many functions, including conduction of nerve impulses, the beating of the heart, and the control of fluid volume in the circulatory system. We do not need much salt to supply our sodium requirement. As little as a gram a day, a quarter teaspoon, may be enough, yet most of us eat many, many times that amount.

Carnivores get their sodium from the blood and tissues of the animals they eat. Herbivorous animals like deer and cows crave salt and will travel long distances to find salt licks and salt springs. The human craving for salt may go back only to the beginning of agriculture. Some traditional peoples who live mainly on wild game do not know salt and do not seek it out.

Once humans began to add salt to their food, they quickly came to like it and, in a sense, became addicted to it. Salt became a precious commodity, often thought of as a magical gift from the earth or sea. The economic importance of salt in human history is suggested by our word *salary,* originally meaning payment to buy salt.

Salt has gone in and out of favor with the medical community in this century. Currently it stands accused of causing or worsening high blood pressure (hypertension) and resultant strokes, congestive heart failure, kidney disease, fluid retention (edema, bloating), and headaches. Doctors often put heart, kidney, and hypertension patients on salt-restricted diets; health spas serve low-salt dishes; unsalted chips and crackers have appeared in supermarkets; and many products use the words "low in sodium" as an enticement to health-conscious consumers. It may be that some of our concern is a modern version of humanity's long-term fascination with salt as a special, magical, and powerful substance.

Some of us, perhaps as many as 20 percent of the population, are salt-sensitive to one degree or another. Salt can cause these people to retain more fluid, increasing circulatory volume and thereby adding to the workload of the heart and kidneys. Fluid retention can result in headaches and obvious swelling of the body, especially in women. People with congestive heart failure and kidney disease can reduce some of this workload by restricting their intake of sodium.

In Japan, where sodium consumption is very high, cerebral hemorrhage is a leading cause of death. Japanese people may get some protection from their addictive love of salt by their equal passion for soaking themselves in extremely hot water. The body can get rid of excess sodium in sweat as well as urine, and hot tubs encourage sweating. Despite the association of salt and cerebal hemorrhage in Japan, I do not think it is valid to say that salt causes high blood pressure, stroke, or heart and kidney disease. In most people with these problems, salt is not the cause, and by itself restricting sodium may not result in much improvement.

The ratio of sodium to potassium in the diet may be more important than the amount of sodium consumed (see Chapter 14); also, a deficiency of calcium may make some people more susceptible to problems from eating a lot of sodium. In any case, it is an oversimplification to say that eating salt is harmful. Nonetheless, I advise eating less salt, especially if you have a family history of hypertension, heart disease, or stroke or are salt-sensitive.

Not long ago, when salt was in better favor, doctors encouraged us to take salt tablets in hot weather, especially if we sweated a lot or were physically active. Today that prescription is very much out of fashion. In fact, it is rarely necessary to take supplemental salt, because the body is very efficient at retaining sodium and not losing too much in sweat and urine. Nevertheless, if you insist on playing tennis or running in the middle of the day during hot summer weather, you might want to take a little salt, especially if you develop muscle weakness.

Because a liking for salty food is a learned taste, you can unlearn it. Changing your sense of how much sodium tastes right is much easier than changing the attraction to fat and sugar. Begin by excluding foods with visible salt: pretzels, potato and corn chips, salted nuts, and the like. Make a rule never to add salt to food at the table. Then start to cut down on the amount of salt you use in cooking and moderate your use of salty products like olives, pickles, canned and smoked fish, and many cheeses.

As you unlearn your cultural preference for salt, you will be surprised to discover that foods you ate before now seem much too salty. This change will help steer you away from many processed and restaurant foods that are unhealthy for reasons other than their high sodium content. In time the food you prepare will be undersalted for some of your guests. Let them add salt or soy sauce at the table to suit their taste.

Reduced-sodium soy sauces are available at health food stores and some supermarkets. You can also buy "lite" salts that are half sodium chloride and half potassium chloride. By using the same amount as you would of regular salt, you cut your sodium intake in half. Read labels! Often these products are full of additives, including undesirable aluminum compounds that prevent caking. You can make your own additive-free lite salt by buying pure potassium chloride from a drug store or chemical supply house and grinding together equal weights of it and pure salt.

Finding pure salt is not that easy these days. Read labels to make sure you are not buying more than sodium chloride. I do not recommend iodized salt. Some people prefer sea salt to earth salt, but unless it has been well washed, sea salt may contain pollutants. I have in front of me an expensive French brand of sea salt that says it is from "the clear blue Mediterranean, evaporated to a sparkling white by sun and sea breezes, then washed in more clear Mediterranean sea water." The Mediterranean may have been clear and blue in the past, but today it is gray and polluted. You can find pure salt in health food stores and other stores. Just read labels to find out what you are getting.

How do you feel about drinking with meals?
I assume you mean drinking water, not alcohol or caffeine (tea, coffee, cola). Those substances are drugs, not just beverages, and are discussed in Chapter 7, "Habits." I don't consider fruit juices and most sodas simple drinks, because they are such concentrated sources of sugar. Simple drinks are water, mineral water, noncaffeinated herb teas, and mineral waters flavored with essences or small amounts of fruit juice.

I often hear and read advice to avoid drinking with meals because the water will dilute digestive juices. There is no truth to this. Water can pass freely in and out of the stomach, while food and digestive enzymes are retained. If you like to drink during a meal or right afterward, do so. (For more information on water, see Chapter 3.)

What's wrong with nightshade vegetables? I've heard they're dangerous.
Tomatoes, potatoes, peppers (red and green bell peppers, chili peppers, paprika), and eggplant belong to the nightshade family, a botanical group that also includes tobacco and some other very toxic plants like belladonna (deadly nightshade), henbane, mandrake, and jimsonweed. Some of these dangerous species have a long history of use in shamanism and witchcraft in Europe and the Americas. There has been much suspicion about the edible members of the family, especially when they have been introduced to cultures unfamiliar with them. For example, Europeans thought potatoes were poisonous when they first arrived from Peru, and in fact all parts of the plant except the tuber *are* poisonous. Even when Europeans began to accept tomatoes from the New World as food, they thought they had to be cooked to make them safe. As recently as the early 1800s most Americans and Europeans thought raw tomatoes could kill you.

Today superstitious fears about nightshade vegetables persist, now mostly rationalized in terms of medical dangers. Followers of macrobiotic diets shun tomatoes, potatoes, peppers, and eggplants as unhealthy, and some medical practitioners warn patients with arthritis away from them. Actually a small percentage of arthritis sufferers are nightshade-sensitive and will experience benefit if they eliminate all foods containing these vegetables. Unless you have a specific allergy or sensitivity to these foods, there is no reason to avoid them or consider them dangerous (except for the pesticides they may contain).

All my life I've struggled with weight. I've tried many diets with no permanent success. What is your advice to people who want to lose weight?

All of my advice can be summed up in two words: Eat Less. That is the whole secret of losing weight; there is no other. Despite the simplicity of that statement, I do not expect to see an end to all the books, plans, clinics, and products that promise some other way.

There is no miracle diet that will enable you to shed pounds while eating all the foods you like. There are no foods with "negative calories" that magically burn fat, no supplements that speed up your metabolism to the same end.

Losing weight is a national obsession in our overnourished society, and people who are overweight encounter a lot of disapproval. Not only are they told that their excess poundage endangers their health, they must deal with the powerful influences of the entertainment and fashion industries, which have made most of us think that beauty and sexual attractiveness equate only with anorexic leanness. These attitudes cause much anxiety and discomfort in those who do not meet the impossible standards for body contour, and since overeating is a common response to anxiety and insecurity, the fat get fatter.

At other times and in other cultures, the ideal body has looked different, with large, rounded forms idealized as beautiful. Some of our cultural prejudice against obesity has probably distorted medical thinking. Being somewhat overweight may not be unhealthy at all, and since fat is our reserve of energy, individuals who carry some may be in better shape to meet the demands of severe or chronic illness and stress. If you are more than somewhat overweight, say more than 20 percent above your ideal weight, you probably do have increased risks of developing cardiovascular disease (heart trouble, high blood pressure), diabetes, gallstones, some kinds of cancer, and osteoarthritis.

The physiology of eating is regulated by a control center in the brainstem that acts like a thermostat for hunger. The set point of this control center determines how often and how much we eat. In many of us it seems to be set wrong, causing us to take in far too many calories. This may have a genetic cause. Many of our ancestors survived because they had the capacity to eat and store up calories very efficiently whenever food was present. The set point of our hunger center is right for a world with food available only some of the time ("feast or famine") or available in insufficient quantity most of the time. In a world with too much food available in tempting variety all of the time, it is a problem.

I know of only two ways to change the set point of the brain's hunger center. The first is to take stimulant drugs: caffeine, cocaine, amphetamine, or nicotine, for example. These drugs all promote weight loss by diminishing hunger and interest in food and by increasing metabolism; these effects result from the drug's action on the brain. This may sound good, but there is a steep price to pay: the certainty of addiction with regular use and a host of psychological and medical problems in its wake. Many people go this route thinking it is the answer to their prayers for controlling overeating and weight. It is not. Eventually you will have to get off the drugs, and all the weight you lost will be speedily regained.

Recently, products containing the herb ephedra (sometimes identified by its Chinese name, ma huang) or its active component ephedrine have become enormously popular as natural aids to weight loss. The products are said to produce a thermogenic effect, meaning that they raise metabolism to help burn fat while curbing appetite. This they do, but ephedrine is just another stimulant, and whether in herbal or chemical form can be just as problematical as the other drugs in its class.

The second way to change the set point is to increase activity through regular aerobic exercise. Not only does this burn calories, it can, over time, change the brain's regulation of hunger. Since the effects of aerobic exercise are all positive if you do it sensibly (see Chapter 5), I very frequently recommend it to people who want to lose weight. But exercise alone will not help if you do not also follow the cardinal rule: Eat Less. Since fat is the densest source of calories (nine calories per gram compared to five calories per gram for both carbohydrate and protein), the easiest way to eat less is to eat less fat. If you begin to cut down on fat as you increase aerobic activity, you will begin to lose weight. As long as you stay on a low-fat diet and continue to exercise, you will not regain. There is no advantage to losing pounds quickly on this kind of program. In fact, the more gradually you lose, the better your chance of maintaining your desired weight once you reach it.

Please do not fall for fad diets, quick diets, all-protein-and-no-carbohydrate diets, magical pills and powders, or other weight-loss gimmicks. Even if you do lose weight with them, you will certainly gain it all back. Do read the section on food addiction in Chapter 7.

Can you give some examples of low-fat recipes and ways to modify recipes to make them healthier?

I've been waiting for you to ask. From time to time I teach workshops on food and nutrition, in which participants make meals together. Here are some sample recipes from one such workshop.

LENTIL SOUP

Pick over 1 pound of green (regular) lentils to remove any stones, dirt, and other foreign objects. Wash them well in cold water. Place in large pot with enough cold water to cover lentils by 6 inches and add 1/3 of a bay leaf. Bring to a boil, skim off foam, lower heat, and boil gently, partially covered, till lentils are just tooth-tender, about 45–60 minutes. Add 3 large carrots, peeled and sliced, 2 stalks celery, sliced, and 1 large onion, halved and thinly sliced. Cook partially covered till carrots are tender, about 20–30 minutes. Add 2 tbsp flavorful olive oil, salt and pepper to taste, and 2 cups crushed tomatoes or tomato purée. Simmer, partially covered, until lentils become very creamy and soft, at least 1 hour more. Stir occasionally and add boiling water if necessary to prevent sticking. Add more pepper if desired, along with some vinegar (red wine, cider, or balsamic). Remove bay leaf before serving.

MISO SOUP

Heat 2 tsp canola oil in large pot. Add 3 slices fresh gingerroot and 1 large onion, thinly sliced; sauté over medium heat for 5 minutes. Add 2 carrots, peeled and thinly sliced, 2 stalks celery, thinly sliced, and 4 cups coarsely chopped cabbage. Stir well. Add 5 cups water, bring rapidly to a boil, then lower heat and simmer, covered, till carrots are just tender, about 10 minutes. Remove from heat. Place 4 tbsp miso (dark or light, available at natural food stores) in a bowl, add a little of the broth, and stir well to a smooth paste. Add more broth to thin the mixture, then add it to the pot of soup. Let rest for a few minutes. Serve in bowls with chopped raw scallions. You may wish to remove the sliced ginger before serving, and you can add a few drops of roasted (dark) sesame oil to each bowl if desired.

BLACK BEAN SOUP

Pick over 1 pound black beans to remove any dirt, stones, or foreign objects. Wash well, then soak for 8 hours in ample cold water. Add $1/3$ of a bay leaf and bring beans to a boil. Skim off foam, lower heat, and boil, partially covered, till beans are just tender, about 1 hour. Add 1 large onion, sliced, and continue to cook until onion melts into liquid, about 1 more hour. Add salt to taste and a few cloves of chopped garlic. Continue to cook, adding a little boiling water if necessary, until beans are very soft and start to melt into liquid, about 1–2 hours more. Remove bay leaf and turn off heat. Ladle beans in batches into blender or food processor and purée. Add 2 tsp dry mustard powder and 2 cups dry sherry (not cooking sherry). Correct seasoning. Reheat and serve, adding any garnishes you want.

GREEN BEAN SALAD

Trim and slice 1 pound fresh green beans. Cook in rapidly boiling water about 5 minutes or until crunchy tender. Drain beans, chill in cold water, and drain well. Toss with 1 tbsp finely shredded gingerroot and the following dressing: mix 4 tsp dry mustard powder and 1 tbsp cold water to a smooth paste; add 2 tsp sugar, 2 tbsp low-sodium soy sauce, 3 tbsp cider vinegar, and 2 tsp roasted (dark) sesame oil.

POTATO SALAD

Boil organic red potatoes in their skins, covered, just until they can be easily pierced with a sharp knife. Meanwhile prepare dressing: in a 16-ounce jar combine ½ cup good mustard (Dijon or Düsseldorf), ½ cup dry white vermouth, ½ cup white wine vinegar, 4 tbsp flavorful, extra virgin olive oil, salt and pepper to taste. Shake well. Drain potatoes, let cool enough to handle, then peel and slice thickly into a large bowl. Pour dressing over them while they are warm, tossing well. Add chopped raw onion, sliced celery, capers, finely chopped fresh parsley, chopped fresh dill, and, if you like, other chopped vegetables (red bell pepper, radish). Correct seasoning. Chill. Tastes best after 24 hours in the refrigerator. Lightly cooked fresh green beans (about ½ pound) are a good last-minute addition.

LOW-FAT SALAD DRESSINGS

Vinaigrette: put into blender container ¼ cup apple juice, ¼ cup cider vinegar, 2 tbsp fresh lemon juice, 2 tbsp water, 2 tbsp chopped onion, 1–2 cloves garlic, mashed, pinches of rosemary and thyme, ½ tsp dried whole oregano, ½ tsp dry mustard powder, ½ tsp paprika, and ½ of a roasted red pepper or pimiento from a jar. Blend thoroughly, add salt to taste, and chill overnight.

Sesame: put into blender container ¼ cup toasted sesame seeds (buy raw hulled sesame seeds and toast them in a dry pan over medium-high heat, stirring constantly), ¼ cup sliced, steamed zucchini, 4–6 tbsp water, 2–3 tbsp fresh lemon juice, 2 tsp soy sauce, 2 tbsp fresh parsley, and 1 clove garlic, mashed. Blend till smooth.

Tomato: put into blender container 1 small (6 oz.) can tomato paste, 1 whole roasted red pepper or pimiento from a jar, 2 tbsp red wine vinegar, 2 tbsp water, mashed garlic if desired, 1 tsp dried basil. Blend well.

Creamy: put into blender container 6 ounces tofu, drained, 2 tbsp fresh lemon juice, 1 tbsp canola oil, ½ tsp salt, ¼ tsp pepper, 1 tbsp chopped fresh parsley, 1 clove garlic, mashed, 1½ tbsp cider vinegar. Blend well. May be used as a base for blue cheese dressing, pasta salad or cole slaw dressing, or dip. Play with additions and seasonings.

(Note: try these dressings on baked potatoes instead of the usual butter or sour cream.)

PASTA SALAD WITH SPINACH PESTO

Cook 1 pound dry pasta (ziti, rigatoni, twists, or shells) as directed. Drain, cool in cold water, drain, place in large bowl, and add lots of sliced celery, diced red and green bell pepper, grated carrot, chopped scallion, chopped radishes, chopped pickles or olives, or anything else that appeals. Toss with spinach pesto sauce.

Spinach pesto sauce: wash and stem 2 pounds fresh spinach. Place leaves in large stainless steel pot with no additional water and cook, covered, over medium-high heat until spinach starts to steam. Remove lid and toss spinach just until all leaves are wilted and bright green. Do not overcook. Drain off excess water, then place spinach in food processor with 1 cup fresh basil leaves (packed), 2 tbsp extra virgin olive oil, 5 or more cloves garlic, mashed, 2 tbsp pine nuts (optional), and salt to taste. Purée thoroughly. Add a little grated Parmesan cheese if desired.

PASTA AND GREENS

Soak ½ cup dried tomatoes in boiling water till soft (10 minutes), drain, cut into pieces, and reserve. Begin cooking 1 pound dried pasta (shells, twists, rigatoni, etc.). While pasta is cooking, prepare greens. Use collards, kale, beet greens, chard, or a mixture of these, about 1 pound total. Remove and discard coarse stems and midribs. Chop greens coarsely and reserve. Cut a large onion in half and then into thin slices. Have ready ½ tsp red pepper flakes (or more, to taste), 1 tbsp dried basil, 2 tbsp capers, 2–4 peeled and mashed garlic cloves. Heat 2 tbsp flavorful olive oil in a skillet, add onion and red pepper flakes. Sauté over medium-high heat, adding a little water if necessary to prevent sticking. When onions begin to color, add the tomatoes and chopped greens, tossing well. Mash in the garlic, add basil, and toss just until greens are completely wilted and bright green. Add the capers with a little of their liquid. Drain the pasta and mix with vegetables. Sprinkle with a little grated Parmesan if desired.

KASHA WITH VEGETABLES

Soak a handful of dried shiitake mushrooms in hot water till soft. Remove and discard stems. Drain, saving the soaking water, and slice mushrooms. If buckwheat groats (kasha) are untoasted, toast them lightly in a dry skillet over medium heat, stirring frequently. Add 1 cup toasted groats to 3 cups boiling water (include the mushroom-soaking liquid), lower heat, and add 1 large carrot, peeled and sliced, 1 medium onion, coarsely chopped, and the sliced mushrooms. Cover and simmer until water is absorbed. Add salt or soy sauce to taste.

CILANTRO SAUCE FOR PASTA

Wash, clean, and stem 4 bunches cilantro (fresh coriander). Chop well. Heat 1 tbsp canola oil in a small skillet. Add 1 tbsp finely chopped, peeled fresh gingerroot and sauté for 1 minute. Add cilantro and stir-fry just until it turns bright green. Lower heat. Add 2 tsp sugar, ¼ cup low-sodium soy sauce, and a little water. Stir well over heat for 1 minute, then remove and pour over cooked, drained pasta.

BAKED SPAGHETTI SQUASH CASSEROLE

Place 1 whole spaghetti squash in a large pot of water (squash should float). Bring to boil, lower heat, cover, and boil gently for 50 minutes. If you do not have a pot big enough to hold the squash, you can bake it. Cut the squash in half lengthwise and place the halves skin side down in a baking dish containing an inch of water. Cover the dish with foil and bake in a 350-degree oven for about 45 minutes, until meat is tender.

While squash is cooking, peel and slice 2 large carrots, 2 stalks celery, 1 large onion, 1 bell pepper (red, green, or some of both). Heat 2 tbsp olive oil in a skillet and add onion, carrot, and a little water to prevent sticking. Sauté over medium-high heat for 5 minutes. Add rest of vegetables with some red pepper flakes and a little salt if desired. Sauté, stirring frequently, till vegetables are barely tender, about 10 minutes. Add 1 large can (28 ounces) crushed tomatoes, basil and oregano to taste, and a sprinkle of ground allspice. Squeeze in 2–5 cloves of garlic. Simmer mixture uncovered for 15 minutes. Meanwhile grate ¾ pound part-skim mozzarella and have ready ½ cup grated Parmesan cheese.

Remove squash from pot or oven and allow to cool until you can handle it. If it is whole, cut it in half lengthwise, then remove seeds with a spoon and squeeze any excess water out of meat. Remove meat and break it up into strands with a potato masher or the back of a large spoon. Mix squash well with vegetables and put half in the bottom of a large baking dish. Top with half the cheeses, rest of squash, and rest of cheeses. Bake for 30 minutes or until cheese is bubbly and slightly browned. Let rest 5–10 minutes before serving.

CHILI BEANS

Pick over 1 pound Anasazi beans, removing any dirt, stones, or foreign objects. Wash well and soak in large amount of cold water for 8 hours. Discard water. Rinse beans, cover well with cold water, and bring to a boil. Skim off foam, lower heat, and boil gently, partially covered, till beans are tender, about 1 hour. Add 1 onion, sliced, and 1 tsp ground red chili pepper. Continue to cook until onion is soft. Meanwhile heat 2 tbsp olive oil in skillet. Add 2 onions, sliced, 2 carrots, sliced, and any other vegetables you like (½ pound mushrooms or 2 chopped peppers, for instance). Sauté over medium-high heat, adding a little water if necessary, till vegetables are barely tender. Add salt to taste, 1 heaping tsp ground cumin, 1 tsp whole oregano, 5 or more cloves mashed garlic, ground red chili to taste, and ½ tsp ground allspice. Continue cooking for 5 minutes, then add mixture to beans along with 1 large can (28 ounces) crushed tomatoes. Simmer for at least another hour till beans begin to melt into liquid. Correct seasoning, adding a little vinegar (cider or red wine) if you like, and Tabasco sauce if you like it spicy.

PINK LENTIL CURRY

Pick over 1 pound pink lentils to remove any dirt, stones, or foreign objects, wash in cold water, and place in pot with enough cold water to cover well. Bring to boil, lower heat, and cook, partially covered, till lentils become a thick mush (about 1 hour). Meanwhile heat 1 tbsp canola oil in a skillet and add 2–3 cups chopped vegetables (onions, carrots, celery, cabbage, and whatever else you'd like), along with a little water. Cover and steam-fry until vegetables are barely tender. Add curry powder (or your own mixture of Indian spices) to taste, along with 2–4 cloves garlic, mashed, 1 tbsp chopped gingerroot, and salt or soy sauce to taste. Simmer covered till vegetables are tender, then add to lentils. Correct seasonings and simmer for 10 minutes to blend flavors. Serve with rice.

CORN BREAD

Heat oven to 425 degrees. Sift together into large bowl 2 cups yellow cornmeal (organic, not degerminated), 2 cups unbleached white flour, ¹/₂ tsp salt, 4 tsp baking powder (nonaluminum), ¹/₃–¹/₂ cup fructose (available at health food stores). Add to this 2¹/₂ cups boiling water mixed with 2 tbsp canola oil. Stir to mix the ingredients but do not overbeat. Add additional hot water if necessary to make a light batter. Spoon batter into hot cast iron skillet. (Heat skillet in oven and oil lightly just before using.) Batter should sizzle when it contacts the skillet. Bake 30 minutes.

APPLE-OAT BRAN MUFFINS

Heat oven to 325 degrees. Lightly oil muffin tin. Peel and core 2 large green cooking apples and chop coarsely. Reserve. In separate bowl sift together 2 cups whole wheat pastry flour, 1 cup unbleached white flour, 1¹/₄ cups oat bran, 2¹/₂ tsp baking soda, 1 tsp cinnamon, and ¹/₂ tsp nutmeg. Add 1 can (12 ounces), thawed, frozen pure apple juice concentrate, the chopped apples, and enough water (about 1 cup) to make a light batter. Mix just enough to moisten all ingredients. Divide batter among 12 cups of muffin tin and bake till lightly browned, 25–30 minutes. Remove muffins from cups while hot.

COCOA-BANANA FROZEN DESSERT

Peel 4 *very* ripe bananas and place them in blender or food processor with 4 heaping tsp pure unsweetened cocoa powder. Add 1 tsp pure vanilla extract. If you like, add a few tbsp rum or maple syrup. Blend till very smooth. Pour into individual cups or small bowls and freeze until just frozen.

Please try these recipes, and feel free to play with them. I came up with them by experimenting in my kitchen, and I encourage you to use them as starting points for your own experiments.

Please give me some suggestions for other readings in the area of diet and health.

Eat More, Weigh Less by Dean Ornish, M.D. (New York: Harper-Collins, 1993) contains 250 very low fat recipes contributed by a number of eminent chefs.

Laurel's Kitchen: A Handbook for Vegetarian Cookery and Nutrition by Laurel Robertson, Carol Flinders, and Bronwen Godfrey (Berkeley, Calif.: Nilgiri Press, 1976) is a good collection of basic recipes with excellent nutritional tables and discussions of nutrients. The information on fats is not up to date, and the book calls for much too much polyunsaturated oil.

Jane Brody's Good Food Cookbook (New York: Bantam, 1987) is a good guide to low-protein, high-carbohydrate eating, with ample discussion of nutrients. The fat content of many dishes can be cut further without losing flavor.

Diet for a New America by John Robbins (Walpole, N.H.: Stillpoint, 1987) is a sweeping indictment of the way most people eat. It documents all that is wrong with our reliance on animal foods, including how these foods are raised, what they do to our health, and what they do to planetary ecology. Robbins's writing is overly emotional at times, but the facts speak for themselves.

The Food Pharmacy by Jean Carper (New York: Bantam, 1988) is an interesting collection of facts about the beneficial effects of specific foods on health. The information is accurate, and the book is well referenced.

Food — Your Miracle Medicine, also by Jean Carper (New York: HarperCollins, 1993), is a newer book, filled with even more detailed information. It makes a strong case for adding omega-3 fatty acids to the diet and eating more fish and more fruits and vegetables.

Your Defense Against Cancer by Henry Dreher (New York: Harper & Row, 1988) includes a 100-page section, "The Diet Factor," that contains much useful material.

Health & Fitness Excellence by Robert K. Cooper (Boston: Houghton Mifflin, 1989) has a good section called "Nutritional Wellness" as part of an overall action plan for improving health.

Transition to Vegetarianism by Rudolph Ballentine, M.D.

(Honesdale, Pa.: Himalayan International Institute, 1987) is based
on an Indian/yogic tradition and therefore is biased in favor of using dairy products, including butter. Otherwise it is a useful guide
for those who wish to move away from diets based on animal protein.

Much Depends on Dinner by Margaret Visser (Toronto: McClel-
land and Stewart, 1987) contains an excellent discussion of salt in
chapter 2: "Salt: The Edible Rock." This book is delightfully infor-
mative.

3

WHAT WILL YOU HAVE
TO DRINK?

ONE OF THE QUESTIONS I ask in taking a lifestyle history from a patient is "Do you drink water?" So many people answer "Not as much as I should" that I am the habit of abbreviating this response in my notes as "NAMAIS." At least these people know they ought to be drinking water.

I do not know a better drink than good-quality water. Also the pleasure of drinking cold, pure water when you are hot and thirsty equals any other. Maybe I have a special appreciation of that pleasure because I live in a desert, where it can be very hot and very dry. I have many vivid memories of coming back to my house after a summer hike and drinking glass after glass of delicious well water, feeling total satisfaction. I have also been known to immerse myself in a mountain stream on a hot day and let the icy water run over me and into me.

Do I need to tell you why drinking plenty of good-quality water is as essential to health as eating properly? In a nutshell: one of the main activities of the body's self-healing system is filtration of the blood, a job performed mostly by the kidneys with a little help from the mechanism of perspiration. Kidneys are such efficient, compact, and miraculous filters that they put to shame the dialysis machines used to maintain patients with renal failure. The heart, blood, and kidneys are a single functional unit that constantly cleanses and purifies itself, removing all the toxic wastes of metabolism and the breakdown products of harmful substances that get into our bodies one way or another. *This purification system can operate efficiently only if the volume of water flowing through it is sufficient to carry away the wastes.* Dehydration is the greatest threat to the process of blood purification and the commonest stress on the kidneys. Many people go around in a state of mild to moderate dehydration just because they forget to drink fluids or because they drink beverages that stress rather than help the filters.

People who risk immediate trouble from not drinking enough water are those with fever, infection, diarrhea, urinary problems (including bladder and prostate infections), or asthma; those who take drugs; and anyone doing hard physical work or exercise, especially in a hot environment. The rest of us may not suffer immediately, but by preventing our blood purifiers from working at optimal efficiency, we increase the risks of disease in the future.

How much water should you drink? The health spa where I used to work had signs everywhere reminding guests to drink eight glasses of water a day, that is, two quarts or almost two liters. For people who don't like to drink that seems like an impossible prescription. I don't think you should force yourself to put away that amount of water, but I would like you to try to drink six to eight glasses a day of fluids that are mostly water. Many of the beverages people drink most often do more harm than good. Alcohol is a diuretic and a urinary irritant; it promotes fluid loss by inhibiting a pituitary hormone that helps us retain water. Caffeinated beverages (coffee, tea, cola) are also diuretics and urinary irritants. Fruit juice is a concentrated sugar source, which you should not consume in quantity or frequently. Milk is a protein food that may stress the kidneys more than it helps them, especially if the diet is already heavy in protein.

If plain water is unappealing to you, try hot or iced caffeine-free teas or mineral water, either unflavored or flavored (but not sugared) or sparkling water with a *little* fruit juice in it. If a whole glass of liquid seems like too much or makes you feel bloated, drink smaller amounts more frequently. Think about keeping a container of drink with you as you go about your daily routine, so that you have ready access to liquid in your car and at your office. Whether you drink it with meals or between meals makes no difference. Rather than focusing on the number of glasses you can get down, just remember to drink frequently, increasing the amount when it is hot or when you are more active and perspiring a lot. Always drink more water when you are sick.

One way to tell if you are really increasing the amount of water you are drinking is to be aware of your urinary output. You should notice an increase in frequency of urination. Think of that as a sign that you are boosting the efficiency of your blood purifiers and filters, not as a nuisance. Also the color of urine should lighten as you drink more water. Passing small amounts of dark, concentrated urine means you are not drinking enough.

I wish I could end this chapter here, having simply reminded you to drink more water and to guard against stressing your kidneys by allowing yourself to get dehydrated. Unfortunately, there is a big catch. I have urged you to drink more water *of good quality,* and that is becoming a scarce and precious commodity.

In the past twenty years a great deal of evidence has come to light about the health dangers of much of the water we drink, whether it comes from taps connected to wells or public reservoirs, from streams and lakes, or from bottles. In the not-too-distant past, waterborne infectious diseases were very common, and they still are in many parts of the world. In our part of the world safeguards in water supplies have mostly eliminated the danger of disease-causing germs, but they have not protected us from contamination by toxic chemicals. The number of chemicals in our water is large and increasing. A few come from natural sources, but most find their way into our water from products of human industry and agriculture. Industrial wastes dumped into lakes and rivers often turn up in drinking water, as do run-offs from mines and seepage from septic tanks, oil wells, and refuse sites. Toxic wastes spread on the ground can leach down into groundwater and the large aquifers that supply many of our wells. Many of the chemicals, drugs, and poisons used on farms get into groundwater, either directly or indirectly through animal wastes. Acid rain, the product of industrial pollutants released into the atmosphere, contaminates surface water quickly and groundwater more slowly. Toxic metals can dissolve out of pipes into the water flowing through them.

Water purification plants continue to focus on disinfection as the major concern, ignoring most chemical contamination. Even the most common method of disinfection — chlorination — is antiquated and probably dangerous, since chlorine is a very poisonous gas that produces toxic by-products called trihalomethanes (THMs). THMs are known to cause cancer and birth defects. Chlorine is also suspect as a possible contributing agent to coronary heart disease. A superior technology exists for disinfecting drinking water that relies on ozone, an active form of oxygen, instead of chlorine. Ozone breaks down to oxygen, leaves no awful taste like chlorine, and is even cheaper to use. Nevertheless, because of the high costs of changing their systems, water suppliers resist using ozone. Similar resistance exists to the new technique of air stripping, also called packed-tower aeration, in which water flows down through columns of air blown up from the bottom of a tower. This system removes volatile organic compounds that account for much of the pollution-related toxicity of our drinking water.

Only very recently, as a result of political action from concerned citizens, have Congress and state legislatures passed laws attempting to safeguard the quality of drinking water. These laws are not tough enough, and they remain poorly enforced, largely because powerful pressure from industrial lobbies and water providers has frustrated efforts to apply them vigorously. The only long-range solution to this problem is for more people to get involved in political action to guarantee the safety of our drinking water.

In the meantime you must know some of the common dangers of drinking water and how to protect yourself from them. Let's start with chlorine and lead, two of the most worrisome. Chlorine is one of the few contaminants you can smell and taste. I cannot now understand how people put up with this taste, but since I grew up drinking tap water in Philadelphia, a city notorious for its bad-tasting, heavily chlorinated water, I suppose I should know: it is a matter of what you get used to. Once you get used to drinking pure water, you will be unable to tolerate chlorination in any degree.

You can reduce the amount of chlorine in your water in two simple ways. The first is to let water stand in an uncovered pitcher or wide-mouthed container for several hours; chlorine is volatile and will slowly dissipate into the air. The second is to whir the water in an uncovered blender or mixer for several minutes. This is a kitchen version of the air-stripping process. If your tap water is chlorinated, however, rather than trying to reduce the offending chemical, you would probably do better to drink something else or invest in a home purifier that will remove the gas and its by-products. (I will discuss home purifying systems in a moment.) The alternative is to buy bottled water, but this presents a whole other set of problems.

First of all, bottled water is outrageously expensive. It makes no sense to pay so much money — a home purifier will quickly pay for itself. Second, there is no assurance that bottled water is of good quality. "Mineral water" is exempt from federal regulation, and only bottled water marketed across state lines is subject to federal drinking water standards, which, as I have said, are not adequate. Be suspicious of "spring water": whose spring did it come from? and what assurance do you have that it was not contaminated? Since most of the surface water and groundwater in our country *are* now contaminated with dangerous organic molecules — and this is just as true in rural as in urban areas — spring water is no prize unless the bottler can provide you with an analysis that sets fears to rest.

Much bottled water is simply tap water that has been put through a purifying process. As I will explain shortly, different methods of purification do better and worse jobs of removing different kinds of contaminants. One source of contamination that is not obvious is the containers themselves. These may or may not have been handled in sanitary conditions. Soft plastic bottles, the kind sold in supermarkets in sizes from one-half to two gallons, can impart a plastic taste, meaning plastic molecules, to water. When I am driving long distances I buy gallons of water to keep in the car, usually steam-distilled water, which, I think, is the best bet from the supermarket. It is likely to be cleaner than spring water or the more common water that has been purified by the ion-exchange method described below. I wish it were available in glass jugs.

Bottled water should be free of chlorine and sodium and should taste good. *Consumer Reports* magazine (January 1987) has published the results of tests of fifty brands of bottled water, and you can look these up in the library if you are considering buying water on a regular basis. Do not buy water from any bottler who will not provide you with test results for chemical contamination, heavy metal content, sodium content, and chlorination by-products if chlorine was used as a disinfectant. Do not buy water from any bottler who will not tell you the source of the water and the method of purification used.

Lead is the heavy metal most frequently encountered in drinking water. The major source of this toxic substance is plumbing. Our word *plumbing* comes from the Latin *plumbum,* meaning "lead," which is why the chemical symbol for this element is Pb. For much of history, water has flowed from reservoirs to kitchen taps through lead pipes, and even when copper or galvanized piping was used, connections were made with lead solder. Lead is particularly toxic to fetuses and young children. It stunts growth, damages the nervous system, reduces intelligence, and can cause severe retardation and death. In adults it can cause hypertension and damage to various organs. It doesn't take much lead to cause trouble. If your drinking water contains more than 10 parts per billion of lead, it will put enough of this metal in your blood to do harm. Recent laws have banned the use of lead for plumbing and plumbing repairs, but these do nothing for all the households with existing lead plumbing. You should find out what your pipes are made of and get your water tested for lead content. Or just get a home purifying system that will remove lead, copper, and other metals.

How much metal dissolves out of pipes and connecters depends on how corrosive the water is that flows through them, how hot it is, and how long it stays in contact with the plumbing. The corrosivity of water depends on its chemistry — how acid or alkaline it is and how many dissolved minerals are in it. The fewer minerals are in the water, the more it can take up, hence the more corrosive it is. Ironically, some kinds of purified water are more corrosive to metal piping than impure water just because they can hold more dissolved metals. This is an argument against attaching a purifier at the point where water enters the house; it's better to put it at the end of the piping, near the tap.

I recommend *always* taking two precautions to reduce the chance of ingesting lead and other contaminants from plumbing in the water you use. First, let water run from the tap for three to five minutes in the morning and evening and after any period of nonuse before taking water for drinking or cooking. This will flush out water that has had extensive contact with plumbing. Second, never draw water from the hot water tap for drinking or cooking even if you are going to use it to make tea or boil pasta. Hot water leaches out impurities much more readily than cold and, in addition, it has sat for long periods in a heater tank, which is probably not very clean inside. Water from the hot tap is unfit for human consumption, no matter what your pipes are made of.

As public concern about the safety of drinking water has grown, the bottled water industry has boomed. Now the home water purifier business is thriving as well. I recommend water purifiers to many of my patients, and I use one myself, but I urge you not to invest in one without doing some homework, since they vary greatly in quality, efficiency, and price, and salesmen will make many questionable claims for them. You might want to have your water tested to see just what impurities it contains and whether you actually need a home purifying system. State and local health departments will often do free tests for bacterial contamination, but that is not what most of us need to worry about. To find out about toxic substances, you will have to go to a private testing lab. Testing for a range of common contaminants can easily cost over $100.

You certainly should know about the different kinds of purifying systems available and the cost and trouble of maintaining them. Be especially careful to find out how often you need to change cartridges or filters, how much the replacements cost, and whether you can install them yourself. Although a few models of home airstripping purifiers have been developed, this system is mostly for large-scale commercial use at the moment. It is excellent for removing volatile organic compounds, which are common chemical pollutants from industrial wastes. Many of these compounds are toxic and injurious to DNA. Air stripping may not remove heavy metals and germs very well, but it can be combined with other systems of filtration and disinfection and should be in much wider use to protect public water supplies.

For home use, five systems of water purification are now available. I will not say much about purifiers that rely on ultraviolet (UV) light. They are designed to kill microorganisms that may be in water but have no effect on chemical contaminants. The oldest and one of the surest methods of ridding water of unwanted substances is steam distillation, a simple process invented hundreds of years ago and much used in chemistry labs to produce pure water for experiments. In steam distillation water is heated to boiling, the steam is conducted through glass or metal piping to a condenser, where it is cooled, and the condensate is collected. A few impurities cannot be removed this way because they boil over with the water, but most are left behind in the boiler. Steam-distilled water is very pure; however, there are several disadvantages to this process for home use. It uses power; the pure water dispensed from the unit is very hot; and all dissolved gases, including oxygen, are removed, making the water taste flat. Also production of water may be slow. I packed up my home distiller for good after all the steam it gave off caused the paint to peel from my kitchen ceiling.

The most common system in use for the home is the activated carbon filter. Usually attached under the sink or on the tap, these units contain a column of specially prepared, granular, porous carbon. As water flows through the column, contaminant molecules stick to the large surface area of the carbon. This method is very good for removing chlorine and all toxic organic molecules, including THMs. It takes bad odors, tastes, and colors out of water, but it does not remove heavy metals or mineral contaminants like arsenic and salts. Activated carbon filters are fast and effective; however, they have two problems. First, they work well only until the carbon becomes saturated with contaminants. If you do not change the filter at or before that point, you will be drinking contaminated water. You should find out how often you have to change the carbon and how much trouble and expense will be involved. Second, as organic contaminants build up in the filter, they provide an ideal breeding ground for bacteria. When you turn the unit on after a period of nonuse, bacteria will be washed out into your drinking water. You can minimize but not eliminate this problem by running water through the filter for a while to flush it before taking any for use. You can also buy silver-carbon units instead of plain carbon ones. In these versions the carbon has been impregnated with metallic silver to inhibit bacterial growth. Silver-carbon filters are more expensive and may contaminate your drinking water with unhealthy amounts of silver.

You can buy portable carbon filters to take to restaurants and hotels and on trips. They treat a glass of water at a time and are a great solution to the problem of chlorine and other foul tastes in water you are served away from home. You can also buy huge carbon filters for the water line going into your house. These are safe because carbon-filtered water is not corrosive to pipes. There are units for your shower, too. Don't laugh; a shower volatilizes many organic contaminants, and you can breathe in large amounts of them, depending on the nature of your water and shower and how much time you spend in it. For people who have severe chemical and environmental sensitivities or mysterious chronic diseases, showering in filtered water may not be a bad idea.

The fourth system for purifying water is a newer one called reverse osmosis (RO). It is the one I use in my home now that the distiller is retired. In an RO unit, water pressure forces water through an osmotic membrane, often called a semipermeable membrane because the holes in it allow small water molecules to pass through but not the contaminant molecules. This is a "reverse" process because by normal osmosis purer water would flow through the membrane to dilute the impure water. In an RO filter, water pressure on the incoming side overcomes this tendency, pushing water through the membrane and leaving a higher concentration of contaminants behind. These are carried off in waste water. RO filters require adequate water pressure to work well, and they produce a volume of waste water.

Reverse osmosis purification effectively removes toxic metals and minerals in addition to organic molecules. Unlike distillation, it does not degas water. Bacteria cannot pass through the membrane, and because there is no build-up of food for them in the filter, they cannot grow there either. Here are the disadvantages: (1) filtration may be slow, depending on the nature of the membrane and the water pressure in your house; (2) a lot of water is wasted, which may be a problem, depending on your water source and cost; and (3) RO water is very corrosive to metal pipes, so that these systems should be used near the tap, never on the main line leading into the house.

People sometimes ask me if it is all right to drink water that is mineral free, such as distilled and reverse osmosis water. I think it is fine. Water is not the source of your minerals. You get them from food, especially by eating a variety of vegetables. There is no truth to the belief that distilled water leaches minerals out of the body. The body is not like a metal pipe; it has elaborate ways to absorb, transport, and hold on to the various minerals it needs. One possible concern is the lack of fluoride in mineral-free water. If you live in an area with fluoridated water and switch to mineral-free drinking water, your children will not be getting the fluoride they need to form strong teeth. Let your dentist know this so that he or she can prescribe supplemental fluoride.

The final system of water purification is called ion exchange. It is used in the water-softening units popular in areas of the country where water is "hard" because of dissolved minerals, especially calcium and magnesium compounds. Calcium and magnesium are not hazardous to health, but people often object to hard water because it leaves deposits, and soaps do not work well in it. Much bottled water is purified by ion exchange as well. The method is simple. Water passes through a filter that exchanges charged particles (ions) in the water for charged particles in the filter. Ordinary salt is the commonest material used in these units, with sodium and chloride ions exchanging for contaminant ions in the incoming water. This system is very good at removing toxic metals and minerals, but it replaces them with sodium, which can be a health hazard for a significant fraction of the population (see the section on salt, pp. 58–61, and the section on sodium, p. 220). Unless the sodium is then removed by another process, water purified in this way may be harmful. Also, water from an ion exchange system can be corrosive to household plumbing, resulting in higher levels of copper, iron, and lead in the drinking water. Finally, ion exchange filtration does not remove the worrisome organic molecules as efficiently as other methods do. In short, I do not recommend it for home use. I agree that it is pleasant to shower and wash clothes in soft water, but if you decide to install a water softener, make sure that you do not get your drinking water from it. If you buy bottled water that is purified by this method, make sure that it is sodium free and check the analysis to see if testing was done for organic contaminants.

If you go camping or backpacking, you probably know by now that much surface water can make you sick, even if appears clear and clean. The commonest problem is a protozoan parasite, *Giardia lamblia*. Giardia infection can cause upper abdominal pain and significant intestinal disturbance, along with weakness and malaise. It usually requires treatment with antiprotozoal drugs. The parasite is transmitted by animals, especially beavers. It is frustrating to be in a beautiful wilderness area and have to worry about the safety of water in brooks and streams, but having had giardia once during a stay in Ecuador, I am inclined to take precautions. Backpacking and camping stores sell hand-pump filters that are much preferable to using iodine tablets or boiling water. The pumps force water through a filter element that mechanically screens out bacteria and protozoans. They may remove some chemical and mineral contaminants as well.

And you thought you were going to get a simple answer to the question "What will you have to drink?"

SUGGESTED READING

Consumer Reports magazine, January 1990, reviews home water purifiers and gives ratings of specific brands.

4

AIR AND BREATH

As I WATCH the air in our cities get dirtier and dirtier, I wonder whether we will soon be buying bottled air along with our bottled water, and I think about investing in corporations that make air filters. The world has always known air pollution from natural sources — volcanoes, forest fires, dust storms — but, as with water, the major problem now is the toxic emissions of human industry, including the exhaust fumes of cars. The technology exists to reduce or eliminate these emissions, but industry will not apply it unless coerced, and clean-air legislation has been too limited and too late to save the situation. We have compounded the problem by destroying the world's forests: trees protect us and the atmosphere by absorbing some toxic gases and releasing pure oxygen.

Polluted air is not only ugly, it is a significant threat to health. It increases the risks of respiratory diseases of all sorts, weakens our immunity, and makes us more susceptible to cancer. If some of the more dire predictions of environmental scientists are right, pollution also threatens the health and welfare of the whole planet by damaging the earth's protective ozone layer and upsetting the delicate balance of forces that maintains the earth's climates.

One of our basic needs for good health is clean air to breathe. Unfortunately, the problem of dirty air is not so easily remedied as the problem of dirty water. The only answer to air pollution is tough environmental policy and laws, but public apathy on this issue is great, and government has tended to side with industry. Ronald Reagan, our recent popular president, actually said that acid rain was produced by trees more than by industry.

I do not think it is wise to live and work full-time in an urban area where air pollution is bad. Try to find a way to move to a cleaner area, or at least visit one often. Even in New York, London, and Tokyo, you can spend time in city parks, where the microenvironment created by trees is significantly healthier. You can also make some changes in your house to minimize pollution. There are some good air filters available that you can put in a room of your home in order to create one clean-air zone. The best are called "high efficiency particulate air" (HEPA) filters. They force air through screens containing microscopic pores, which remove almost all particles. HEPA filters work very well and are not too expensive. I recommend them if you have to live with a smoker; if you have bad allergies to pollen, dust, or other inhalants; or if you live in an area with bad smog.

If the air outside is bad, you ought to do whatever you can to keep the air inside your home as clean as possible. Some common sources of indoor pollution are gas appliances (stoves, water heaters), air fresheners, aerosol sprays, moth crystals, stored paints and solvents, gardening chemicals and pesticides, bottles of perfume and household cleaning products, incense, chlorine and other volatile contaminants of shower water, radon gas from the ground, and formaldehyde from pressed-wood products used as construction materials.

At the end of this chapter is a list of readings on this subject, which go into much more detail about indoor pollution and what you can do about it. Nontoxic alternatives exist for every imaginable household product of questionable safety, and these books tell you how to find them or make them. In Chapter 11, "How Not to Get Cancer," I give specific recommendations about household chemical products.

Let's assume that you have cleaned up the indoor pollution in your house and that a strong thunderstorm has just swept through your town, giving the air a good electrical and mechanical scrubbing. When you step outside, you can see the distant horizon with crystal clarity. The air smells fresh, clean, delicious. Now all you have to do is breathe it. Would you believe that most people do not know how to breathe? Or at least that they do not know how to breathe so as to take full advantage of the nourishing, health-giving properties of the act of breathing? It's true, and for that reason I am now going to stop talking about the air and tell you what I know about breathing, including how to do it better.

This is not information I got in medical school, I'm sorry to say. There I learned about diseases of the respiratory tract, but I learned nothing about breathing as the bridge between mind and body, the connection between consciousness and unconsciousness, the movement of spirit in matter. Breath is the master key to health and wellness, a function we can learn to regulate and develop in order to improve our physical, mental, and spiritual well-being. I'm not making this up. A great many teachings from such diverse traditions as yoga, martial arts, Native American religion, natural childbirth, and osteopathic medicine all point to breath as the most important function of life.

In many languages — not English, unfortunately — the words for *spirit* and *breath* are one and the same (Sanskrit *prana*, Hebrew *ruach*, Greek *pneuma*, Latin *spiritus*). Native Americans, among others, believe that life enters the body with the first breath, not at the moment of birth or of conception. In this view the fetus and newborn have a kind of vegetative life, uninvested with spirit until the breath cycle begins.

What I know about breathing comes from my own experience, from reading, from studies of yoga, from working with patients, and from spending time with practitioners who focus on breath. One of the most interesting of these is a retired osteopath, Dr. Robert Fulford, perhaps the most effective clinician and healer I have met. He was eighty when I first got to know him, and still in practice, although he had moved to Arizona from Ohio in order to retire. He was so good that people would not let him retire; the demand for his services was too great.

Unlike most osteopathic doctors today, Bob Fulford practiced in the tradition of that system's founder, Andrew Taylor Still (1828– 1917). (See *Health and Healing*, chapter 11). He relied on manipulation alone for treating a variety of diseases, gave no drugs, used no diagnostic tests. After his brief retirement Fulford worked mostly with infants and children, because he said his energies went further by producing change in this age group.

Dr. Fulford worked from the principle that breathing is the key function of the organism and that restrictions in breathing lead to dysfunction and disease. He paid attention not only to the movements of the chest and diaphragm but also to subtle movements in the central nervous system that are not recognized by most medical doctors or osteopaths. These pulsations of the brain and its associated structures are another kind of respiration, perhaps the most fundamental rhythm of life. A skilled practitioner can feel them through the cranial bones as well as in the sacrum at the other end of the spinal column. Bob Fulford was a leading practitioner of craniosacral osteopathy. He has finally retired but continues to teach the method.

When he was in practice, he had great success with problems that most doctors could not solve. For instance, he regularly cured young children of recurring ear infections (otitis media) by simply, in his words, "freeing up their breathing and getting their tailbone [sacrum] unstuck" so that it could get back into normal respiratory motion. To do this he performed gentle manipulation with his hands, along with application of a vibrating instrument known as a "percussion hammer." A single treatment would often end cycles of ear infections that had previously required massive doses of antibiotics and decongestant drugs. Fulford explained that the underlying cause of recurrent otitis media is fluid stagnation in the middle ear caused by restricted breathing, since the motions of respiration mechanically pump the lymphatic circulation. When this motion is restricted, fluid backs up in the ear, providing a perfect breeding ground for bacteria. You can wipe out the bacteria all you want, said Fulford, but if you do not correct the underlying problem of restricted breathing, they will always come back.

Once I sent him a patient with a difficult problem, a man in his mid-thirties with a three-year history of worsening intestinal dysfunction: constant diarrhea, often with blood and mucus, abdominal cramping, food intolerance, and weight loss. The patient, who worked in Mexico part of the year, had been treated off and on for intestinal parasites and infections, but finally, the tests for infection were negative, and he presented a clearer and clearer picture of chronic inflammation of the lower bowel: ulcerative colitis or something like it. I sent him first to a gastroenterologist who did an expensive and invasive workup, culminating in a biopsy of the colon. After all this the gastroenterologist concluded that the case was "fascinating and mystifying." He determined that severe chronic inflammation of the colon was present but could not definitely call it ulcerative colitis without doing yet more tests.

At this point I sent the patient to Fulford. The young man had a long history of athletic injuries and trauma. I noticed that he habitually breathed through his mouth. Fulford assessed him as a critical case, told him that his breathing was completely off as a result of past trauma and that it was not adequate to nourish his nervous system. One consequence was malfunction of the vagus nerve, which controls the digestive system. He made this diagnosis after a very few minutes of observing the patient, moving his limbs, feeling his cranium, and asking him several questions about his history of injuries. He then gave him a twenty-minute treatment of craniosacral manipulation designed to restore normal respiratory function and cranial motion.

Six hours after this treatment the patient's diarrhea stopped for the first time in six months. It never returned, and he subsequently regained all the weight he had lost. He no longer breathed through his mouth. I tried to arrange a meeting with the patient, Dr. Fulford, the gastroenterologist, and me to discuss the case, but the gastroenterologist, though he said on the phone that he was interested, did not show up.

Seeing results like this on a regular basis motivated me to pursue my interest in breathing and to begin teaching patients how to do it better. Breathing is special in several respects. It is the only function you can perform consciously as well as unconsciously. Breathing can be a completely voluntary act or a completely involuntary act, because it is controlled by two sets of nerves, one belonging to the voluntary nervous system, the other to the involuntary (autonomic) system. Breath is the bridge between these two systems.

Much illness comes from unbalanced functioning of the autonomic nervous system. When the tone of this system is not right, it can produce irregular heart rhythms, high blood pressure, disturbances of blood circulation, stomach and intestinal disorders, urinary and sexual problems, and more, since autonomic nerves regulate all of our vital functions. Our conscious minds have no direct access to this system. We experience its activities as involuntary, so we cannot ordinarily influence them by acts of will. Medical doctors treat autonomic malfunctions with strong drugs that may or may not help. There is reason to believe that by working with breath, you can change your autonomic tone and affect many of the "involuntary" functions. Much of the evidence for this comes from India, where adepts at physical yoga often master this kind of control. All of them learn it by first learning to regulate the breath. Even if you do not wish to be a yogi, you may want to lower your blood pressure, calm a racing heart, or help your digestive system without taking drugs. Practicing simple breathing techniques can give you these abilities. I will teach you some of them in a moment.

Besides affecting the autonomic nervous system, breathing has direct connections to emotional states and moods. Observe someone who is angry, afraid, or otherwise upset, and you will see a person breathing rapidly, shallowly, noisily, and irregularly. You cannot be upset if your breathing is slow, deep, quiet, and regular. You cannot always center yourself emotionally by an act of will, but you can use your voluntary nerves to make your breathing slow, deep, quiet, and regular, and the rest will follow.

Try closing your eyes for a few minutes and practice moving your breath in those directions. Keep your back straight. Begin with a deep, audible sigh, then quietly inhale and see how slow and deep and quiet and regular you can make your breathing and still have it feel perfectly comfortable, with no sense of not getting enough air. Do this for at least eight breaths, then open your eyes and breathe normally. This is a simple exercise but an effective one. Do it whenever you can. In Chapter 6 I will give you a different breathing exercise to practice, one that is a specific antidote for anxiety, stress, and emotional upset.

Next pay attention to your exhalation. If you watch people breathe, you will see that most of them use effort to inhale but none to exhale. Exhalation is usually passive and takes less time than inhalation. When you breathe this way, you do not move nearly as much air in and out of your lungs as you can. The more air you move, the healthier you will be, because the functioning of all systems of the body depends on delivery of oxygen and removal of carbon dioxide. To get more air into your lungs, concentrate on getting more air out of them by attending to exhalation.

At the end of a normal breath try squeezing more air out. You will be using your intercostal muscles to do this, and you will feel the effort as they compress the rib cage. Try to make your exhalation as long or even slightly longer than inhalation. Whenever you think of it, practice this technique of extending exhalation and developing your intercostal muscles.

If you have ever had the "wind knocked out of you" — that is, lost the rhythm of breath as a result of an injury, even for a few seconds, or if you have ever been unconscious as a result of injury, or if your birth was difficult and you did not breathe on your own immediately after delivery, you may have restrictions in breathing programmed into your nerves and muscles. These are the sorts of problems Dr. Fulford identified and treated. The best therapy I know for restricted breathing is manipulation by an osteopath trained in craniosacral technique (see Appendix A for information on how to find one), but other types of body work can also help. For instance, both Rolfing and Feldenkrais work, two very different systems of retraining the body, can change breathing patterns for the better (see Appendix A). So can yoga practice.

Aerobic exercise is a wonderful tonic for the respiratory system. One of the many reasons to do it regularly is to work that system and help condition the nerves and muscles that control it. If you give yourself aerobic workouts, remember to practice breathing more slowly, deeply, quietly, and regularly, and work to extend exhalation, you will be well on your way to better breathing. More elaborate breathing exercises, such as those taught by some yoga instructors, are not necessary. The yogic practice of breath control, *pranayama*, is meant to be done under expert supervision as one part of a general program of physical and mental development and purification. Taken out of context, these exercises can be dangerous, especially to mental and emotional health. I use some of the principles of pranayama in my medical work, and the relaxing breath I will teach you in Chapter 6 comes from yoga, but I assure you that the general work I have outlined is all you need to do to harness your breath in the service of health.

One of the interesting ideas of pranayama is that breath is the perceptible aspect of basic life energy. The more we expand our breathing, the more of this energy we can concentrate and the more vitality we have. Here again is the mystical conception of breath as spirit or life force. The words *mystic* and *mystery* come from a Greek word meaning "secret rites" or initiation into knowledge hidden from general view. A mystery can be experienced but not explained to others or to oneself. It is experienced but not understood.

Breath is mysterious in this sense. At the very center of our being is rhythmic movement, a cyclic expansion and contraction that is both in our body and outside it, that is both in our mind and in our body, that is both in our consciousness and not in it. Breath is the essence of being, and in all aspects of the universe we can see the same rhythmic pattern of expansion and contraction, whether in the alternating cycles of day and night, waking and sleeping, high and low tides, or seasonal growth and decay. Oscillation between two phases exists at every level of reality, even up to the scale of the observable universe itself, which is presently in expansion but will at some point contract back to the original, unimaginable point that is everything and nothing, completing one cosmic breath.

Breathing is a natural object of meditation. By putting attention on your breath, you will change your state of consciousness, begin to relax, and detach from ordinary awareness. Many systems of meditation use focus on breath as the main technique. In the Buddhist and yogic traditions are many examples of people who reached enlightenment by doing nothing other than paying attention to the rising and falling of their own breath. In this sort of meditation you can try to experience the dimensionless point between inbreath and outbreath and to glimpse enlightenment in that space. You can come to know reality itself as an eternal oscillation between being and nonbeing. All this is possible from experiencing breath, which is the mystery of being unfolding right in front of our noses, connecting us to the universal rhythm.

If today you can be aware of breathing for ten seconds more than you were yesterday, you will have taken a measurable step toward enlightenment, will have expanded your consciousness, furthered communication between mind and body, become a little more whole, and so improved your health. In writing about diet and exercise, I point out that those factors, while important, are not the sole determinants of health. I know people who eat excellent diets and exercise faithfully and are not very healthy, and I know some healthy people who eat bad diets and do not exercise. I do not know any healthy people who do not breathe well. For that reason I urge you to concentrate on the information in this chapter and put it into action in your daily life.

SUGGESTED READING

Books on breathing are very rare. The best is *Conscious Breathing* by Gay Hendricks, Ph.D. (New York: Bantam, 1995).

The single most useful book on indoor pollution is *House Dangerous: Indoor Pollution in Your Home and Office and What You Can Do about It* by Ellen J. Greenfield (New York: Vintage Books, 1989).

An excellent practical work is *Nontoxic and Natural: A Guide for Consumers: How to Avoid Dangerous Everyday Products and Buy or Make Safe Ones* by Debra Lynn Dadd (Los Angeles: Tarcher, 1984). It tells you where to get nontoxic alternatives to almost everything.

5

A GUIDE TO EXERCISE
FOR PEOPLE WHO HATE
THE WHOLE IDEA OF IT

"I HATE TO EXERCISE." How many times have I heard these words from patients and others? How many times have I said them myself? I hear them less frequently today, now that exercise has become stylish. City streets are filled with joggers and cyclists, people flock to spas and health clubs, and whole new classes of professionals have sprung up, such as exercise physiologists, sports medicine doctors, fitness advisers, and aerobics instructors. Nevertheless, I still meet many people who think that exercise is only for athletes, and many others who go about exercise in ways more likely to lead to harm than to better health. I also hear and read a great deal of confusing, contradictory, and unhelpful information on this subject.

Let me say at the outset that I am a great believer in the benefits of *sensible, moderate* exercise. I ask all people who come to me for medical consultations questions about their exercise habits, and I frequently urge them to make changes, usually in the direction of increasing the time they spend at physical activity. In this chapter I tell you why you should exercise and how to go about it. The advice I will give you comes from my own experience as someone who hated exercise for much of his life and now does not feel right if a day goes by without some form of it. I have also been on the staff of a health spa, have talked with many fitness experts, and have had to deal with many medical casualties of exercise — injuries in people who exercised incorrectly.

The idea of "taking exercise" would have seemed ridiculous to our ancestors. Throughout much of history mere survival demanded a level of physical activity that made rest an ultimate luxury. Rarely have people been able to be so sedentary that they needed to exercise apart from their routine of daily living. But in today's industrialized world most people do not have to hunt, fish, or work the fields to get food. They do not have to walk or run long distances to get from one place to another, or chop down trees to build shelters and make fires. Most of us sit while we work, sit while we travel, and sit during our leisure time. The exercise period is a distinctly modern invention.

The news media tell us constantly that physical fitness is not what it should be in our society, that standards of fitness are lax, that children today are not physically fit. The term *fitness* refers to adaptation. A fit individual is well adapted to his or her environment, able to respond to its changing demands. Many people today who are physically inactive are fit enough for the minimal demands of their comfortable, nonchallenging environments. If you have enough energy and muscle tone to walk up the occasional flight of stairs, mow the grass on weekends, walk the dog, and bend down to open the dishwasher, you may feel you have no reason or need to take up an exercise program. I hear this argument often.

The flaw in it is that our bodies evolved in very demanding environments and are meant to be used. If they are not used, they deteriorate faster than they should. Many of the illnesses that plague our society result from underuse of bodies. Clearly the prevalence of heart and artery disease correlates as much with lack of aerobic exercise as it does with unhealthy diets. Insufficient aerobic activity also predisposes us to musculoskeletal disorders, gastrointestinal problems, nervous and emotional illnesses, and a long list of other ailments.

The vast majority of people who start exercise programs do not stick with them. Health clubs make a lot of money selling yearlong memberships to men and women who make resolutions to get into shape. Most of them will stop using the club's facilities after a few months. Others buy expensive indoor equipment — stationary bicycles, rowing machines, weights, and the like — only to have them gather dust in the garage following an initial period of enthusiastic use.

These common patterns of behavior are like dieting to lose weight. You cannot get down to your ideal weight and stay there by making resolutions to diet, going on the latest fad diet, joining a diet center, or buying pills and drinks that promise magical results. You can do it only by changing your ways of eating permanently, by building up good, sensible food habits that you can stick with for the rest of your life. In the same way you will improve physical fitness by developing good, sensible habits of exercise that you can stick with for the rest of your life.

Exercise physiologists tend to make this subject unnecessarily complicated, probably because their field is new and rapidly changing. Some of them identify six or more kinds of exercise and say you must include detailed routines for each of them in your program. In fact, at the outset you need to pay attention to only two kinds of exercise, aerobic and nonaerobic. Aerobic exercise is any activity that increases your heart rate and respiratory rate, the kind that feels like work and makes you huff, puff, and sweat. Aerobic exercise does not just mean aerobics, the classes offered at most health clubs and spas. Aerobics classes are one kind of aerobic activity; there are many others, including running, some kinds of walking, cycling, swimming, cross-country skiing, jumping rope, dancing, and climbing stairs.

Aerobic exercise conditions our hearts and arteries and respiratory systems. It increases stamina and general fitness. It promotes cleansing of the blood by stimulating circulation and perspiration. It gives a sense of strength and well-being, in part by releasing endorphins, the opiatelike molecules in the brain that can make us high, happy, and more tolerant of discomfort. It increases the flow of oxygen to all organs, enabling them to work more efficiently. It burns calories, undoing some of the damage we do by eating too much. It strengthens the immune system. It reduces stress. It lowers serum cholesterol. It tones the nervous system. It is the type of exercise most people need to concentrate on first. With all those benefits, how could you not want to?

But in fact some part of us resists, even hates the whole idea of exercise. It is our lazy self, the principle of inertia in us, that tells us we do not need to exercise or do not have time for it. The only way to deal with this voice is to pay no attention to it. If you listen to it, you are certain to sabotage your best efforts. Here is a practical tip: if you want to unlearn old habits and develop new ones, spend time with people who have the habits you want. Your choice of friends and acquaintances is a powerful influence on your behavior. If you want to change your eating habits, spend more time with people who eat healthy food. If you want to be a habitual exerciser, keep company with people who exercise regularly and enjoy it.

Patients often ask me, "How much exercise do I need? How often should I do it?" The simplest answer is that you should do something aerobic every day, some activity that gets your heart beating faster and your breathing going, some sweat appearing on your skin. That does not mean attending an exercise class or putting in an hour on a stationary bike every day. It just means doing something vigorous or finding ways to make ordinary activities more vigorous. Gardening and yard work can be aerobic, housework can be aerobic, going out to get the mail can be aerobic. It all depends on how you do it.

For maximum benefit to your cardiovascular system, aerobic activity should be continuous and sustained for more than a few minutes. My recommendation is to work toward the goal of doing thirty minutes of some type of aerobic activity at least five days a week. Frequency is important; exercising for sixty minutes once or twice a week will not give you the same results. You don't have to begin at the recommended level, especially if you have not been exercising at all. Just keep in mind that you want to work toward that duration and frequency, then get there at your own pace. If thirty minutes seems like a lot of time, think about how much time you spend sitting and being inactive. Aerobic exercise is one of the key pieces of a program of preventive health maintenance. Thirty minutes of it five days a week is a sensible and moderate prescription.

I get bored doing any one aerobic activity and find that I am more likely to stick with my program if I make it as varied as I can. I like to run, hike, cycle, swim, dance, jump rope, and jump on a mini-trampoline, and I try to mix all of these up. Not only does variety help fight boredom, it develops your body in better ways. Just as a highly varied diet is important to get all the nutrients you need and to avoid getting too much of substances you don't need, a varied aerobic diet makes sure that your body is worked in all the ways it needs and reduces the chance of overworking or injuring any parts.

Many experts say you should calculate your "target heart rate" and take your pulse frequently during aerobic exercise to make sure you are getting an adequate cardiovascular workout. I do not find this to be necessary, and I feel it can make workouts less fun. If exercise is not fun or if you do not see benefits from it fairly quickly, your motivation to continue may erode. If a period of aerobic exercise does not leave you feeling that you have labored, with your heart beating faster and your breathing stimulated, you have not done it vigorously enough. If it leaves you collapsed on the ground painfully gasping for breath, you have overdone it. I think most people can figure out the right level of intensity without taking their pulse, consulting tables and charts, and worrying about whether they are in the target heart rate zone.

Making aerobic exercise more fun and less boring is your greatest challenge, because if you fail to do this, you are likely to let your program slide before it becomes established as a good habit. Let me tell you about some of the ways I've found to make workouts more fun. One is to exercise outdoors in interesting surroundings. If you run, walk, or cycle in a visually interesting environment, your concentration on the sights around you will take a lot of the drudgery out of that thirty minutes. Another is to exercise with a companion. Aerobic time spent with a friend goes much faster than the same time spent alone.

If you are exercising indoors, experiment with doing it to music. Having pleasant, stimulating sounds to attend to can be as helpful as beautiful sights, with the added advantage of rhythm to synchronize your movements. Of course, you can take a cassette player and headphones along when you go outside. I have listened to books on tape while exercising and have gotten so absorbed in the narrative that I have gone past thirty minutes without noticing. If you have an exercise machine at home, try reading while using it or put it in front of the television or turn on the stereo. I know some people who listen to foreign language lessons while pedaling their stationary bikes.

No matter how much you try to make it fun, and no matter what the experts tell you about how great you will feel, when you first start regular aerobic exercise, you will probably dislike it. Developing this habit takes time and effort. In the beginning it *will* be difficult, and time may move much more slowly than you'd like. You must force yourself to stick to your routine during this stage. A common pitfall is to forgo exercise on days when you feel tired and lethargic because you think you do not have enough energy for it. A secret, known to those who have become habitual exercisers, is that effort creates energy. Do not wait for energy to come when you are tired; create it by expending effort. You can easily prove to yourself that this principle works. Just try it.

The inner voice that says you don't have time for exercise is lying. You can make time for it once you realize its priority in an overall program of preventive health maintenance. In fact, regular exercise, by giving you more energy and a greater sense of well-being, will help you work more efficiently, so that you use your time better and have more to spare. I promise you that eventually you will move beyond the initial stage into a different relationship with aerobic activity. It will make you feel good both physically and mentally, at first after you finish exercising and later while you are doing it as well. Days without exercise will not feel quite right or complete. Then you will know that your good habit has begun to take solid form, and the chance of your abandoning the program will be much diminished.

Let me take you through the different forms of aerobic exercise, pointing out what I see as advantages or disadvantages of each.

Walking offers the great advantage of requiring no skill or practice. Everyone knows how to do it, and the only equipment you need is a good pair of shoes. You can walk outdoors or indoors (in shopping malls, for example). It is probably the safest option of all, with the least chance of injury.

The main problem with walking as a principal aerobic activity is that you can easily fail to do it strenuously enough to get the conditioning benefits of exercise. Aerobic walking cannot be casual or intermittent, and it takes a little more time than the other options. You should be able to walk about three miles in forty-five minutes. If, after building up to that, you still do not get a good workout, you will have to walk faster, do some uphill walking (long, gradual hills are best), or carry hand weights. (Never use ankle weights, which can stress joints and lead to injury.)

Good posture is important during walking exercise, and swinging the arms opposite to the movement of the legs makes for a better stride. Athletic supply stores can give you advice about good walking shoes. The right shoes are as essential for aerobic walking as for running. If you become accomplished at walking, you can join walking tours throughout the world or look into race walking, an advanced technique taught at some fitness clubs.

Running has become very popular in our society in recent years. I see people of all ages running along roadsides in the desert where I live, and I like to run myself. The great advantage of this form of exercise is its intensity. It promotes fitness quickly and efficiently and burns more calories than other activities, making it attractive to people who want to control their weight. Because of its intensity, running releases endorphins in many people, creating the runner's high that some describe as an "energy buzz." The runner's high — like aerobic highs in general — is a good antidepressant.

Running has some potentially serious disadvantages that you should consider before choosing to do it on a regular basis. The chance of injury is greater than for any of the other aerobic activities listed here. Running traumatizes the body, especially joints in the legs, knees, and back, as well as the kidneys. You can minimize this possibility by taking several precautions. Never run on concrete. If possible, run on cinder tracks or dirt paths. Asphalt is not as bad as concrete but not as good as dirt. Always wear well-made running shoes designed to minimize shock to the joints, and get a new pair whenever your present ones start to wear out. Women should wear athletic bras or other breast supports. Warm up before you start a run, not by stretching but by running in slow motion.

Above all, listen to your body. If you develop pain in any joints, stop running or cut down on it until you determine the reason for the pain. I have seen too many people who ignored warning signals of this sort and now are unable to run at all because of damage to vertebrae, hip joints, and knees. Of course, this caution applies to any form of physical activity, but because running subjects the body to so much trauma, it is of special importance here.

Running also seems more open to abuse than other forms of

exercise, probably because of its stressful nature and consequent effect on the endorphin system. Many people run addictively, that is, with a compulsive quality that takes over their lives. If circumstances prevent them from running, they may be impossible to live with. Others approach running as a form of self-punishment. In Tucson during the burning hot days of May and June, I often see middle-aged men running on city streets in the midday sun with looks of agony on their faces. They must believe they get more benefit from an aerobic workout if they make it as torturous as possible. I should not have to tell you that this idea is silly. The extreme stress of running in heat can damage the body, especially the cardiovascular and urinary systems. Be sure to replace fluids if you run in hot weather and sweat a lot. Also try not to run on streets with heavy traffic. You can take in a lot of exhaust fumes when your breathing is stimulated by aerobic exercise.

You can run indoors on an automatic treadmill. Fitness clubs usually have these machines, and you can buy one for the home. Many models allow you to vary the speed and the incline and give you continuous information about your work output on a video display screen. Treadmills greatly reduce the possibility of injury because the running surface has the proper springiness for safety. I find them quite boring, though, and really need to find ways to entertain myself while using them.

Swimming is another familiar activity. For most people it is less convenient than walking or running because it requires a pool and some skill. Exercise in water offers several advantages that other forms cannot. Water neutralizes the force of gravity, allowing free movement of joints and muscles. This makes swimming the activity of choice for anyone with musculoskeletal problems, such as arthritis or traumatic injury. Many people get into a desirable altered state of consciousness while swimming, brought about by the feelings of freedom and buoyancy water provides and by rhythmic breathing. Unlike walking and running, swimming uses the upper body as well as the lower, giving a more balanced muscular workout. It does not provide as intense a cardiovascular workout as running does.

To use swimming well as aerobic conditioning, you should develop good form, meaning good posture in the water, an efficient stroke, and breathing synchronized with movement. It may help you to work with a trainer for a while to improve your form if you intend to use this as a major exercise. The freestyle or crawl is the best stroke for aerobic swimming. Water aerobics, a combination of swimming, dance movements, and calisthenics, is taught in classes at many health clubs and can be much more interesting than swimming laps.

The disadvantages of swimming have to do mostly with pools. Unless you are lucky enough to live near a swimmable body of water in a favorable climate, a lot of your swimming will be done in pools. These environments are often not inspiring, and chlorinated water can be very bad for your eyes, skin, and hair, as well as for the membranes of your nose, mouth, and upper respiratory passages. Definitely wear good-fitting goggles or even a mask and snorkel, which can also help you achieve better posture in the water. I do not recommend ear plugs. If you get water in your ears, put a little rubbing alcohol in them when you dry off; it will remove the water. If you swim a lot, you will want to find a heated pool. This is especially important for people who have arthritis or injuries, because cold water can make those conditions worse. Another caution: try to get in the habit of turning your head both to the right and to the left to breathe, or swim with a mask and snorkel so that you do not have to turn your head at all. If you always turn to one side, you may develop neck and shoulder problems from unequal strain on muscles.

Cycling is also growing in popularity, and the promise of radical new cycle designs in the near future may mean that more and more people will come to use these leg-powered devices for transportation as well as for sport. As with walking, cycling must be done quite vigorously if it is to work as an aerobic conditioner. That means a speed of about fifteen miles an hour, never less than ten miles an hour, on a flat surface. Cycling can provide an exhilarating feeling of speed and freedom and give you access to beautiful surroundings that will make your exercise time more enjoyable. It is also the preferred activity for those with bad knees. By strengthening knee muscles without traumatizing the joint, cycling leads to greater stability and a lesser chance of injury in the future.

A major disadvantage of cycling is the need to buy an expensive piece of equipment. Before you invest in a cycle, you should try out different kinds. Many that are designed for racing sacrifice comfort for a degree of speed you will never need. I much prefer to sit upright rather than hunched over the handlebars, a position that stresses my neck and shoulders. A cycle must be designed and sized correctly for your body, or it will cause you problems. Cycle seats are a particular difficulty. Uncomfortable ones can irritate your skin, leave your bottom very sore, and even injure nerves by compression. Even with the right bike and seat, jarring motion to the spine can aggravate prostate trouble in men and back problems in anyone with a history of them.

Although the actual physical activity of cycling is much safer than running, cycling can be very hazardous, depending on where you do it. The main danger is from motor vehicles, which greatly detract from the pleasure of a ride if you always have to share the road with them. Not only do you have to keep most of your attention on the cars rather than on the scenery, you also have to breathe their fumes. Cycling is much more attractive as a regular exercise if you have access to bike paths or roads with little traffic.

Outdoor cycling may not be available to you throughout the year, but you can always use a stationary bike in a health club or at home. These come in many models, some of them very expensive and with a lot of computerized gadgetry. The stationary bike is a good aerobic option for the home if you shop for one carefully. Try putting it in front of the television, or read a book while pedaling.

Cross-country skiing is rated as the best aerobic exercise by many fitness experts because it works more muscles than other activities and is very efficient at conditioning the cardiovascular system. Risk of damage to the body is low, and mastery of this sport can give you a great deal of pleasure. The disadvantages are obvious. You can do it on a regular basis only if you live in a suitable area, and then only seasonally. Most people have to learn how to ski, probably from an instructor. You have to buy and maintain the necessary equipment.

Indoor cross-country ski machines are available at many health clubs and can be installed in the home. They are slightly harder to learn to use than stationary bikes but somewhat less boring and give a better workout.

Rowing has similar pluses and minuses. It's great if you have the time, place, and equipment, but few of us can rely on it as our main aerobic activity. Rowing machines are another indoor option. I am more cautious about them than about the other machines because of the possibility of overstressing the back. This is more likely with some models than others and with overuse of arm and back muscles instead of reliance on leg muscles. Have an instructor supervise you when you learn to use a rowing machine and pay attention to any signs of unhappiness from your back.

Dancing is one of the best aerobic activities of all, in my opinion, often slighted by exercise physiologists. It is perhaps the most fun, a tonic for the mind and spirit as well as the body. If you don't like rock music, try country swing, folk and ethnic dancing, or the old reliable, square dancing. In many areas you can find dancing classes, clubs, and societies that delight in teaching beginners. Dancing can give as thorough an aerobic workout as any of the activities mentioned so far, is never boring, and definitely promotes health. Some of the healthiest old people I see are those who dance regularly. Since dancing is usually a social activity, people are likely to forget that they can do it by themselves. Sometimes on bad-weather days I put on a favorite record or tape and get my aerobic workout by dancing around my living room, interspersing a few minutes of jumping rope, jumping on a mini-trampoline, and romping with my dogs. We all have a good time.

Aerobics classes are usually combinations of warmup stretches, aerobic movement, and muscle toning exercises done to music under the leadership of an instructor. If you are a member of a fitness club, you are familiar with these classes. Usually different levels are offered for beginner, intermediate, and advanced participants. Because aerobics classes are organized and structured, they are good for people who are not very motivated about exercise.

Regular aerobics classes usually include jumping and running of a sort that may traumatize joints. For this reason some clubs now offer the option of "low-impact aerobics," modified to avoid jarring. To my taste, aerobics classes are less fun than spontaneous, free-form dancing, but I recognize that they work well for many people. Be careful to start off at the level of difficulty you are comfortable with. If you have not been practicing this kind of activity, some of the more intense classes can leave you exhausted and with very sore muscles.

Rope jumping is another of my favorites. Although athletes have long used it as an efficient aerobic conditioning exercise, it is not nearly as popular as most of the activities I have listed here. It has several advantages, among them extreme portability. Jump ropes are inexpensive compared to other exercise equipment, and you can take them anywhere. I jump rope in hotel rooms and roadside rest areas when I am on the road, in my house and other people's houses as well as outside. The rhythm of this activity, when you become proficient at it, is hypnotic in a way that makes time pass quickly and smoothly, offsetting the monotony. Rope jumping gives an excellent cardiovascular workout and uses both arm and leg muscles.

It takes a bit of practice to master rope jumping. You want to be able to sustain a steady rhythm and use a smooth dance step (one foot at a time rather than both together) without lifting your feet very high. You will probably not want to jump rope continuously for thirty minutes, but you can intersperse it with other exercise routines.

Climbing stairs is surprisingly strenuous if you go up more than one flight at a time. If you are lucky enough to have stairs in your home, use them frequently. When possible, walk up stairs instead of taking elevators and escalators. One of the most demanding exercise machines is the stair climber. Look for it at fitness clubs and consider one for the home if you like it. Even using this machine at relatively slow speed, I am quickly drenched in sweat and obviously working hard during a thirty-minute climb. Skip this exercise if you are significantly overweight. It can be too much effort for your heart and can traumatize your joints.

Let me give some more general advice about aerobic exercise, including a few cautions.

• Any aerobic exercise is better than no aerobic exercise. I would be happy to see you doing even a few minutes of it on a regular basis, but if you want to experience all the benefits I mentioned at the beginning of this section, please try to do some continuous aerobic activity for thirty minutes a day, on average, five days a week.

- Remember to work up to this level gradually and at your own pace, especially if you have not been exercising.
- Remember also that I am recommending an *average* amount of activity over time. It is not the end of the world if you miss a day or two here and there. You can make it up later. Feeling bad about missing exercise probably does you more harm than missing it.
- In addition to these workouts, find other ways to increase your daily activity, such as using stairs more often, parking farther from your destinations to walk more, and doing more physical work yourself instead of delegating it to others.
- If you exercise with others, try not to do so competitively. Competitive thoughts negate some of the benefits of exercise, especially on your cardiovascular and immune systems and emotions. If you cannot avoid competitive thinking, exercise by yourself. (See Chapters 9 and 12 for information on how thoughts can affect the functions of your body.)
- Competitive sports like racquetball, handball, and tennis are not substitutes for the aerobic activities listed above. In these sports aerobic work is of a stop-and-go nature rather than continuous. It is regular, continuous effort that tones your cardiovascular system best.
- Always warm up before you get into the full swing of aerobic activity. The best warmup is a slowed-down version of the activity you are about to perform. For example, walk, run, or cycle in slow motion. You will see many people stretching as a warmup, but this does not prepare muscles for aerobic exercise as well as slow movement does.
- Give yourself a few minutes of cooldown at the end of the activity. Repeat the same movements in slow motion.
- If you have never exercised, get a medical checkup before you start an exercise program. If you have a history of heart trouble or high blood pressure or a strong family history of such problems, a cardiac stress test may be in order.
- Pay attention to your body! Discontinue exercise if you develop unusual aches or pains.
- Stop exercising immediately if you develop dizziness, lightheadedness, fainting, chest pains, or difficulty in breathing. Get a medical checkup promptly.

- Your heart rate and breathing should return to normal within five to ten minutes after the end of aerobic exercise. If they do not, get a medical checkup.
- Do not exercise if you are sick. Wait until you feel better, then resume gradually. Don't worry about losing fitness; it will come back quickly enough. Strenuous exercise at the onset of illness can cause you to be sicker longer.

Once you are on the way to establishing good habits of aerobic exercise, you can experiment with the many varieties of nonaerobic exercise. This category includes stretching, muscle toning, muscle building, and activities designed to improve balance, flexibility, agility, and coordination. I have saved all these for last, because I want you to work on your aerobic routines first. They require more effort, are often perceived as less fun, and demand real commitment at the outset until you are able to feel the benefits. It is often easier to use weight machines, do floor exercises for body trimming, or go to yoga classes than to put in thirty minutes of cardiovascular work. Therefore I urge you to concentrate first on aerobic exercises.

Stretching is a totally natural conditioning exercise that improves the tone and health of muscles; limbers up tendons, ligaments, and joints; changes the dynamics of the nervous system; and just feels good. You can learn a lot about our need to stretch by watching dogs and cats do it. All of us tend to stretch after being in one position for a long time, and students of the human body tell us we ought to make a habit of stretching in opposite ways from the positions we spend the most time in during the day. For instance, if you work leaning over a desk, when you get home you should spend a few minutes with your head, neck, and shoulders arched backward.

Muscles contain stretch receptors, special groups of cells that inform the central nervous system about their state of tension. This may be why stretching can change our level of arousal and mood. Stretching feels good, but it is a sensation that borders on both pleasure and pain. Although some kinds of formal stretching exercises, like yoga, may seem painful when you first try them out, your perception of the sensations will change fairly quickly if you practice.

Stretching is so natural that you can easily invent your own forms of it. If you feel the need to do it formally, you can find stretch classes at many fitness clubs (aerobics classes usually include some preliminary stretching, too), or you can learn from books. I strongly recommend that you stretch frequently, especially if you suffer from stiff muscles or spend a lot of time sitting or working in one position.

Yoga does much more for the body than just stretch muscles, but since most beginners will experience stretching as the main sensation, I will mention it here. In India this ancient science is a philosophical-religious system for attaining unity of consciousness. The physical aspect of it, known as hatha yoga, includes a number of *asanas* or poses. These are what most of us think of when we hear the word *yoga,* and these are what most yoga instructors in the West teach. In the larger context the yoga asanas are intended to facilitate concentration and meditation by quieting the body and nervous system. They are not meant to be an end in themselves, since it is possible to become very proficient at the postures without making any progress at the more important job of learning to still the mind.

You can learn yoga from books, but it is easier to learn it from a teacher. Yoga classes are widely available through health clubs, community centers, and universities. You can practice on your own once you learn the basics, and you do not need to spend any specified amount of time at it.

Looked at only as a very structured form of nonaerobic stretching exercise, yoga offers a number of advantages. It is an excellent muscle toner that balances all parts of the body. It increases flexibility and is a good practice for anyone with chronic back pain. In addition to promoting muscular health, yoga has definite beneficial effects on the nervous system. It leads to deep relaxation and is a powerful stress reducer. For this reason, I will mention it again in Chapter 6 as a relaxation technique. You can learn to do yoga at any age. Children who take it up can easily become as skillful as adults. For older people it is a great nonaerobic conditioner. For anyone yoga is a wonderful complement to the aerobic routines I have described above.

I have seen some cases of joint problems from the overenthusiastic practice of yoga. Certain postures can stress the neck, knees, and lower back if you do them too strenuously or hold them for too long, especially if you do not increase your flexibility slowly through gradual practice. One man who returned from a stay with a yoga master in India reported that his teacher forcibly bent him into difficult asanas, leaned on him with full weight to increase the strain, and even jumped on top of him while he was posing. These techniques gave him a great deal of pain at the time and left him with a great deal more pain for a long time after he left India. With yoga, as with any form of exercise, you must listen to your body. If you notice that one posture gives you persistent pain, stop doing it. Recently some unusual forms of yoga have appeared in the West that are much more dynamic and strenuous than hatha yoga. "Kundalini" and "ashtanga" yoga both emphasize vigorous movement as well as difficult poses. They are more stimulating than relaxing and are not for beginners.

Weight lifting and bodybuilding work muscles against resistance and have been the main activities at health and fitness clubs in the past. A great many people still do workouts that consist mostly of weight training, either with machines or with free weights, and most fitness experts still recommend this as part of an overall exercise program. At the risk of offending these people, I must tell you that I am not in favor of weight training as a way of promoting health. There may be other reasons for doing it, but I assure you that you can attain optimal health without ever pumping iron.

Weight lifting increases muscle bulk by a simple physiological principle: use any muscle more, and it will increase in size; stop using it, and it will decrease. This is an example of the body's quick responsiveness to the changing demands of the environment. In my experience most people who lift weights are attracted by the vision of having larger muscles and appearing more beautiful and more powerful. It is this focus on appearance that I find unwise. In fact, some of the most powerful, fittest people I have met have bodies very unlike those of bodybuilders, with none of the muscle bulk and definition that are so fashionable in health and fitness clubs. I do not believe there is any necessary correlation between this appearance and the realities of strength, fitness, and health.

To my eye, the bodies of many weight lifters look more interesting than beautiful. Often the upper portions are overdeveloped and disproportionately large, especially the shoulders, upper arms, and chest. At its worst, bodybuilding actually sacrifices health for super-ficial appearance by encouraging unsound dietary practices (con-sumption of high-protein foods and protein and amino acid supplements), the use of dangerous drugs (anabolic steroids), and neglect of the real work of preventive health maintenance. The bodybuilders I have known are not as a group any healthier than other people, and some of them are less healthy because of the ways they think about and treat their bodies.

Nonetheless, if I find myself in a health club, I usually do a circuit of the weight machines and some work with free weights, because this activity feels good to me. You might want to do the same. If you are drawn to this kind of exercise, I would ask you to examine your motives carefully. If you do decide to lift weights on a regular basis, beware of instructors who try to persuade you to eat more protein or take protein powders, amino acids, or expensive herbal supplements that are supposed to give the muscle-bulking effects of steroids in a natural way without any side effects.

One benefit of working muscles against resistance is that it will increase your bone density, providing an antidote to the hormonal and metabolic changes that can cause calcium loss and development of osteoporosis. Women become susceptible to this debilitating dis-ease earlier than men, but women who have good habits of weight-bearing exercise have more protection than those who do not. Weight lifting is one kind of weight-bearing exercise; some of the aerobic activities discussed above, like running, dancing, and using aerobic machines, also strengthen bones while they condition your heart and lungs.

Calisthenics, the familiar routines of physical education classes and military training, are muscle-conditioning exercises that can also be aerobic, depending on how fast and long you do them. Push-ups are probably the most popular variety, followed by pull-ups, jumping jacks, toe touches, and so on. A practical problem with calisthenics is that most of us have bad associations to them: some-one — a gym instructor, a camp counselor, an army sergeant — made us do them. When we take them up again on our own, we usually do so in fits of righteous determination to get into shape. These efforts are doomed to fail, much like crash diets. If you have a good relationship with some calisthenic exercises, by all means continue with them. Otherwise try to get the same benefits in more enjoyable ways: by dancing, hiking, or playing.

Muscle trimming, the "floor work" of aerobics classes, is intended to increase muscle tone and improve body contours. Beware of promises from books and instructors that this activity will firm up sagging bodies, make bulges disappear, and melt away "cellulite," the ugly fat deposits that no beautiful person can afford to be seen with. Would that all those leg lifts and abdominal crunches could accomplish such miracles, but the truth of the matter is otherwise. Fat disappears only by gradual weight loss through permanent changes in diet and general attention to all the principles of health stressed in this book. Even so, this sort of exercise can make you feel good and like your body more.

Abdominal exercises are a type of muscle trimming, but I put them in a special category because they may help prevent lower back trouble. For example, sit-ups can strengthen and balance the muscles that support the spine. Some male bodybuilders work at developing boardlike abdominal muscles. This is not healthy if the muscles cannot relax, because such extreme tone may interfere with the function of the digestive organs. The abdominal muscles should have good tone but also should be soft and yielding, a principle taught in most of the martial arts. I recommend moderate, sensible abdominal exercises for those who have had back trouble, abdominal surgery, or multiple pregnancies.

Martial arts, traditional disciplines of China, Korea, and Japan, have become very popular in the West. They emphasize agility, balance, and coordination in addition to fighting and defense. Some are much more aggressive than others (karate), and some regularly lead to injury (aikido). Of all of them, the only one that I recommend as part of a program of health maintenance is tai ch'i. Sometimes called "Chinese shadow boxing," it is a formal series of flowing, graceful, slow-motion movements designed to harmonize the circulation of energy (ch'i) around the body. In any city in China you can see thousands of people of all ages practicing tai ch'i while waiting at bus stops in the morning. Like yoga, tai ch'i is a good method of stress reduction and relaxation, and it also promotes flexibility, balance, and good body awareness. It is beautiful to watch and to do and is free of the problems of the other forms.

Martial arts schools like to represent themselves as teaching spiritual disciplines that raise consciousness and promote health and healing. Those who master the fighting arts, they say, are less likely than the rest of us to engage in violence. All of this sounds nice, but in actual practice martial arts training often contributes to unhealthy attitudes and emotions by making people more defensive, more likely to view others as potential assailants, and more committed to the wrong idea that violence is the solution to violence. If you are drawn to this activity, select your instructor and school carefully.

Just as you can develop varied aerobic routines and not be tied to any one activity, so you can be innovative about nonaerobic conditioning. For instance, one of the best ways to improve coordination, agility, and balance is to walk, run, or even dance over rough and uneven terrain. If you have never walked over rocks or up stream beds, try this cautiously at first and then be more daring. Playing in ocean surf is also effective, as are many ball games — if you do not get caught up in a competitive frenzy.

I cannot overemphasize the importance of play in relation to exercise, whether aerobic or nonaerobic. Ideally exercise should be fun, not drudgery, and you should be able to do it without being conscious of the passage of time. If you are always counting the minutes till you can stop, you are not having fun. Young children will wrestle playfully for hours, developing strength, coordination, and agility while getting a terrific aerobic workout and having the time of their lives. It is a pity that more grown-ups don't do the same. I try to give grown-ups permission to play in this way and have even taught workshops in noncompetitive (that is, fun) wrestling. It beats pedaling a stationary bike any day. Do not get locked into dull routines in classes and clubs with fancy equipment. Use these facilities if they help you develop good exercise habits, but also find ways to increase your activity that are creative and playful, using the resources of your own environment.

Before leaving this subject, I must point out a few pitfalls of exercise that are seldom discussed, especially in our fitness-obsessed age. Exercise is not the sole determinant of health any more than diet is. Some people who exercise vigorously drop dead of heart attacks. Others are unable to rest and relax. Aggressive, competitive people tend to approach exercise as they approach their work and life in general; they may have good-looking bodies, but they are sadly undeveloped emotionally and spiritually.

Many people who run or work out in gyms and spas become too dependent on exercise for their sense of well-being. An important aspect of real health is the awareness that you can feel complete and whole without any external aids, including an aerobics class or a dumbbell. When calamities befall exercise-dependent persons, they frequently respond by exercising even more (unless the calamity is a physical injury, in which case they are really in a pickle). I want you to get into the habit of exercising your body sensibly and moderately. I do not want the habit to become a compulsion. Exercise dependence and exercise abuse are not uncommon. They do not contribute to health and wellness.

SUGGESTED READING

Health and Fitness Excellence: The Scientific Action Plan by Robert K. Cooper, Ph.D. (Boston: Houghton Mifflin, 1989) contains a very detailed guide to all types of exercise.

Two good books on yoga, both by Richard Hittleman, are *Introduction to Yoga* (New York: Bantam, 1969) and *Yoga for Health* (New York: Ballantine, 1983).

6

RELAXATION, REST, AND SLEEP

A WOMAN in her early fifties consulted me for help with chronic constipation and poor circulation, problems I felt were probably related to her obvious anxiety. In the course of questioning her about her moods and feelings, I asked, "Do you have any unusual stress just now?" She hesitated for a moment, then looked at me and said, "You know, *life* is a stress."

I agree. We can no more eliminate stress from our lives than we can eliminate tension from our muscles. If muscle tension dropped to zero, we would fall to the ground in a shapeless heap. If all stress disappeared, we would not be alive. Stress is inherent in our interactions with the world around us and, unless it is overwhelming, it keeps us growing and developing.

One series of questions I ask in taking a medical history is "Do you consider yourself a nervous person? Are you tense? Do you worry? What do you do to relax? Have you ever had any kind of relaxation training?" Most people describe themselves as being under stress. Some say that they are outwardly calm but carry a lot of internal tension. Others say they think they are relaxed, but their spouses and friends say it's not so. Some look at me blankly when I ask "What do you do to relax?" Others give answers like "Drink wine" or "Watch television." There are better ways.

The word *stress* comes from the same Latin word that gives us *strict,* which originally meant "narrow" or "tight." Stress is the discomfort or distress caused by forces that limit our freedom and movement. The suggestion is that sources of discomfort are external. It is outside forces acting on us that keep us from ease: a demanding boss, an unhappy spouse, difficult children, the commute to work, mounting bills, the threat of crime, political unrest, pollution, the risk of cancer, and on and on.

In fact, stress has two aspects, one external and one internal. Life is full of challenges and disappointments that continually threaten to disrupt our ease, and we have to deal with them in order to survive, grow, and reach our full development. Just as muscles become stronger and bigger when they work against resistance, so our minds and spirits enlarge by meeting the difficulties life presents. Without difficulty, there is no growth.

The internal aspect of stress is our reaction to the obstacles and reverses of living. If we become anxious, fearful, angry, or depressed about them, those states can certainly do us harm. Internalized stress keeps the mind agitated, throws the nervous system out of balance, interferes with the functioning of the immune system, and produces the many stress-related disorders so common in our society. It is easy to think that external "stressors" are the cause of your tensions, but, in fact, you have a choice as to how they affect you, and you can learn to change your reactions to them.

By the way, it is not just our society that is plagued by stress-related illness. A former student of mine, now a doctor, spent part of a year in rural Kenya in an isolated hospital, the only medical facility serving a large region of tribal peoples who lived in traditional ways. She went there expecting to immerse herself in an exotic world of tropical medicine, where she would learn how to deal with sleeping sickness, parasites, snake bite, and jungle fever. Instead she found 90 percent of the patient population suffering from ulcers, hypertension, headaches, and other physical expressions of anxiety. The commonest drugs given out were Valium and Tagamet (for ulcers). The simple lives of our ancestors may not have been so simple.

For a number of years Valium, Tagamet, and drugs like them have been the most widely prescribed drugs in the world. That fact emphasizes the importance of learning how to neutralize stress or process it in ways that do not make you sick. As doctors and patients have become more aware of the role of stress in causing illness, stress reduction has become big business. We tend now to blame stress for any illness we do not understand or for which we cannot find a cause. This tendency can lead doctors to make mistakes in diagnosis.

A few years ago I saw a man in his early thirties whose only complaint was decreased sexual functioning. He said sex was not enjoyable; he did not get full erections and had diminished sensation in his penis. This problem had been with him a long time, almost eleven years. Before that all had been well. He was otherwise in excellent health, ate a good diet, was a fitness buff, liked his work, but had trouble with relationships because of his sexual difficulty. He told me he did not think it had a psychological basis. Over the years he had consulted a few doctors, but none of them had an answer. All told him he should see a psychiatrist. Once he had a possible urinary infection and went to a urologist who did rounds of tests, all of which came out normal. This doctor told him his problem was in his head, caused by stress, and recommended psychotherapy. Finally the patient did go to a psychologist, but after a few sessions he decided that it was a waste of time. Since then he had resigned himself to "living with it."

I asked him for more detail about his habits, how he ate, slept, relaxed, exercised. Exercise was a big part of his life, especially cycling on a ten-speed bike. He cycled long distances, twenty to thirty miles, almost every day. How long ago had he started this kind of cycling, I asked. He thought about it and replied, "Eleven years." This patient's problem was not all in his head. A good part of it, in fact the cause of it, was a compression injury of the perineal nerve, the nerve that carries sensation from the penis. Hard bicycle seats can press on this nerve enough to put it to sleep. I know because I once did this to myself after just a few days of riding a new ten-speed bike with an uncomfortable seat. By the time I realized what the pins-and-needles sensation meant, it was too late, and I was impotent for a week till the nerve recovered. If you keep compressing a nerve for eleven years, it will take a lot longer than a week to wake up, but recovery is possible. I told the patient to stop cycling and find another form of exercise or to get a split seat that would put no pressure on his perineum. Once the cause was removed, I recommended vitamin B-6 to speed healing of the nerve compression injury.

Of course, that was an odd case. Much more often doctors attempt to treat by physical methods problems that have nonphysical causes. My sense is that in many patients stress *is* a primary cause of disease, and in many more it is an aggravating factor.

It is always worth trying to change external situations that are destructive. I sometimes counsel patients to look for a new job, move to another part of the country, or get out of a bad personal relationship, but I know that simply making those kinds of changes does not give people tools for managing future problems any better. Therefore I also give all patients suggestions about how to relax and protect themselves from the harmful effects of stress. Nearly everyone can benefit from learning how to relax.

In order to approach these goals, you need to ask two broad questions: (1) what am I now doing that prevents me from relaxing? and (2) what am I not doing that could help me relax?

Let's start with the first question. Without realizing it, many people are influenced by factors that increase their anxiety and internal tension. These obstacles to relaxation should be removed. I will mention four of the most common ones.

Caffeine and other stimulant drugs activate the sympathetic nervous system, which prepares us for emergencies, for "flight or fight" responses. These drugs make us more jumpy, anxious, and fearful and thus often interfere with relaxation, rest, and sleep. Coffee, tea, cola, and chocolate are used so unconsciously in our culture that most users have no idea they are mind-altering drugs. I discuss them in detail in the following chapter, "Habits." Caffeine is an ingredient of many over-the-counter and prescription drugs. If you want to lower your level of internal stress and develop your ability to relax and let go of external annoyances, a good place to begin is to eliminate caffeine and its relatives from your life. Cocaine and amphetamines (speed) are illegal stimulants with similar effects. A legal stimulant to watch out for is phenylpropanolamine (PPA), the chief ingredient of over-the-counter diet pills and a common drug in over-the-counter cold remedies. Another is pseudoephedrine, usually sold as a decongestant (as in Sudafed). Some products sold in health food stores as tonics, energizers, and diet aids contain stimulant plants, especially guaraná (a caffeine source from South America), yerba maté (ditto), and ma huang or Chinese ephedra (source of ephedrine). Because of their action on the sympathetic nervous system, all stimulants, whether natural or synthetic, in the form of teas or pills, are obstacles to relaxation.

Sound has a profound influence on the nervous system. Some kinds of sound increase our level of arousal and make us tense and anxious. Consider the noise of sirens outside your window or the sounds of people arguing. How do they make you feel?

Music has special power to affect consciousness. It is often the soundtrack of a scary movie more than the images on the screen that gives you chills and goosebumps. Many cultures around the world recognize this power of music. Some forbid it (Islamic fundamentalists), others use it in rituals designed to alter consciousness (voodooists). The essential tool of the shaman is a drum. By using the right rhythms, he or she can leave the physical body and journey to the spirit realm. In Bali ensembles of gong players and drummers have roused warriors to frenzied violence. In African religions drumming is a highly developed art, capable of inducing spectacular changes in awareness, including sexual excitement, trance, spirit possession, and even complete loss of consciousness.

It is well documented that some of these African rhythms have found their way into our popular music through the development of jazz and rock 'n' roll. I have no objection to this music as entertainment, but I worry about its effect on the human nervous system when it is background noise, taken in unconsciously. For example, when I am stopped in city traffic I am often next to cars that have music with an exciting beat blaring from the tape deck. Drivers and passengers act as if nothing is amiss, just some music to make the drive more interesting. City driving is usually stressful enough without having the nervous system roused further by stimulating rhythms. When I flip through the bands of my car radio, a great deal of the music I receive is the sort that promotes internal tension and interferes with relaxation. I do not mean to imply that only rock music has this effect. Often I keep my radio tuned to a classical music station while I write in my home. Sometimes I switch it off in exasperation when I become conscious of the jangling effect on my mind of some dissonant composition. The danger here is that it is easy to listen unconsciously to sounds that directly and powerfully push the nervous system away from calmness and centeredness.

In a way, choosing which sounds to let into your consciousness and which to exclude is like making choices about foods. It is a question of nutrition in a broader sense, of mental nutrition, if you will. If you want to be excited, stimulated, sexually aroused, or prepared for physical violence, by all means listen to the readily available sounds that move you toward those states. If you want to relax and dissipate the tension resulting from external stress, do not make it harder for yourself by receiving those influences.

News can also affect our mental state profoundly. Most news reports increase anxiety, give us new possibilities for worry, and play on our desire for emotional stimulation. Many people are addicted to reading newspapers and news magazines and to listening to news on radio and television. Like caffeine addiction, news addiction is a major roadblock to learning to relax.

Is it really necessary to know about murders in a distant city or about the latest oil spill or the hideous acts of terrorists? My experience is that a great deal of the most upsetting news is of no relevance to our daily lives and that when an event is important enough to concern us, we find out about it soon enough. During the years of my studies of plants, drugs, and medicine in Latin America and Africa, I was often out of touch with news for weeks or months at a time. When I returned to it, the world was essentially the same. All I had missed was the chance to worry. Mark Twain once designed a universal front page for a newspaper to illustrate this point. Lead stories dealt with a revolution in Central America, rising crime in the city, and government assurances that the economy was in good shape. That was over one hundred years ago.

Be aware that news producers select and edit events for "journalistic value." Stories that excite and titillate, that cause anxiety and concern over developments to come have greater journalistic value than those that do not. Do not absorb this information unconsciously and habitually. Notice the effect it has on your mental equilibrium. Experiment with breaking the news habit, then use your power of choice to tune into news selectively and consciously.

Agitated minds of other people will agitate your mind. A kind of resonance takes place in the realm of consciousness. If you are in the presence of calm, centered persons, your internal tension diminishes, and you let go of some of your stress without making any effort to do so. If you are in the presence of people who are excited, angry, and anxious, you will naturally move toward those states. Pay attention to your internal responses to the people you associate with. As much as possible, avoid the company of agitated minds.

I assume that you are going to work to remove obstacles to relaxation. Now what you want to know are the positive actions you can take to reduce internal stress. You have many options here, and I will review a number of them for you.

Breathing, as I wrote earlier, strongly influences mind, body, and moods. By simply putting your attention on your breathing, without even doing anything to change it, you move in the direction of relaxation. There are many worse places to have your attention — on your thoughts, for one, since thoughts are the source of much of our anxiety, guilt, and unhappiness. Get in the habit of shifting your awareness to your breath whenever you find yourself dwelling on upsetting thoughts.

The single most effective relaxation technique I know is conscious regulation of breath. I will teach you a yogic breathing exercise I give to most of my patients. It is utterly simple, takes almost no time, requires no equipment, and can be done anywhere.

Although you can do the exercise in any position, to learn it I suggest you do it seated with your back straight. Place the tip of your tongue against the ridge of tissue just behind your upper front teeth, and *keep it there through the entire exercise.* You will be exhaling through your mouth around your tongue; try pursing your lips slightly if this seems awkward.

> First exhale completely through your mouth, making a *whoosh* sound.
>
> Next close your mouth and inhale quietly through your nose to a mental count of four.
>
> Next hold your breath for a count of seven.
>
> Then exhale completely through your mouth, making a *whoosh* sound to a count of eight.
>
> This is one breath. Now inhale again and repeat the cycle three more times for a total of four breaths.

Note that you always inhale quietly through your nose and exhale audibly through your mouth. The tip of your tongue stays in position the whole time. Exhalation takes twice as long as inhalation.

The absolute time you spend on each phase is not important; the ratio of 4:7:8 is important. If you have trouble holding your breath, speed the exercise up but keep to the ratio of 4:7:8 for the three phases. With practice you can slow it all down and get used to inhaling and exhaling more and more deeply.

This exercise is a natural tranquilizer for the nervous system. Unlike tranquilizing drugs, which are often effective when you first take them but lose their power over time, this exercise is subtle when you first try it but gains in power with repetition and practice. I would like you to do it at least twice a day. You cannot do it too frequently. Do not do more than four breaths at one time for the first month of practice. Later, if you wish, you can extend it to eight breaths. If you feel a little lightheaded when you first breathe this way, do not be concerned; it will pass.

You may also notice an immediate shift in consciousness after four of these breaths, a feeling of detachment or lightness or dreaminess, for example. That shift is desirable and will increase with repetition. It is a sign that you are affecting your involuntary nervous system and neutralizing stress. Once you develop this technique by practicing it every day, it will be a very useful tool that you will always have with you. Use it whenever anything upsetting happens, before you react. Use it whenever you are aware of internal tension. Use it to help you fall asleep. I cannot recommend this exercise too highly. Everyone can benefit from it.

People often ask me the reason for keeping the tongue in that position. Yoga philosophy describes two "nerve currents" in the human body, one positive, electric, and solar, the other negative, magnetic, and lunar. These begin and end at the tip of the tongue and the ridge behind the upper front teeth. Putting those structures in contact is supposed to complete a circuit, keeping the energy of the breath within instead of letting it dissipate. I don't know if there is any correlation between these ideas and Western concepts of physiology, but since yogis have been doing this exercise for thousands of years, it seems worth following their instructions exactly.

Progressive relaxation is a way of releasing tension in muscles. It is often taught in yoga and exercise classes, on self-help tapes, and by various instructors, from massage therapists to psychologists.

There are many variations of it. Most begin by having you lie on your back in a comfortable position. Take a series of deep slow breaths and then focus your awareness on different parts of the body in turn, becoming aware of any muscular tension and releasing it. One way to do this is to first tense a muscle deliberately and then relax it. You can start with the front of the body, tensing and relaxing the muscles of the upper face, then moving on to the jaw, neck, chest, front of the arms, abdomen, thighs, lower legs, feet, and toes. Then do the same down the back of the body. Finally, lie still with the eyes closed, concentrating on your breath and enjoying the feeling of peace and freedom from tension. You can easily learn to do this on your own, but it is pleasant to follow spoken instructions from someone with a soothing voice. You can incorporate progressive relaxation into your daily routine and find ways to make it more portable. For instance, you can modify it for a sitting position and do it at your place of work.

Exercise can be relaxing, and many people tell me it is their main method of reducing stress. One of the reasons I recommend regular aerobic exercise is for its moderating effects on emotions. This is a long-term benefit, but exercise, both aerobic and nonaerobic, can also work in acute situations. If you feel angry or upset at other people, yourself, or the world in general, a brisk walk or run or a half hour of lifting weights will often put you back in a good mood. In this case exercise is a symptomatic treatment. It burns up excess energy but does not teach you how to process stress differently. For that reason I do not recommend it as the sole method of relaxation. Whenever someone answers my question "What do you do to relax?" by saying "Exercise," I always urge the person to learn some other technique as well: breathing, visualization, or yoga, for instance.

Yoga, as mentioned earlier, is an excellent promoter of relaxation as well as a good form of nonaerobic body conditioning. It perfectly complements aerobic exercise. Yoga requires commitment to a formal practice and is best done with an instructor, at least at the start.

Massage and body work can be wonderfully relaxing. In order to gain full benefit, you need to be totally passive and surrender to the touch of a skilled therapist. There is a great deal of evidence that the state of the mind and nervous system is reflected in the state of

the musculature, also that body work is one route into the unconscious mind. Some kinds of massage are more relaxing than others.
One of the best for this purpose is Trager work, a system that uses
rocking and bouncing movements to lull the recipient into a very
dreamy altered state (see Appendix A).

Like exercise, massage is more a symptomatic treatment than a
lasting change. It is also limited in its application, since few of us
are able to go to a massage therapist on a daily basis, and most of
us need to practice relaxation skills every day.

Visualization and guided imagery have you concentrate on images
held in the mind's eye. We all look at our internal images from time
to time, especially when we daydream or have sexual fantasies, but
few of us have learned how to develop our imaging capacity and
take advantage of its ability to affect our minds and bodies. Visualization and guided imagery work with the connection between the
visual brain and the involuntary nervous system. When this portion
of the brain (the visual cortex at the back of the head) is not occupied with input from the eyes, it seems to be able to influence physical and emotional states. Moreover, a great many people in different
parts of the world believe that images held in the mind's eye shape
our experience of reality, and that learning to sharpen these images
puts us more in control of our destiny. Whether you find that to be
true or not, you can experiment with images to promote relaxation.

You can learn the technique from books, from self-help tapes, or
from an instructor, especially psychologists and hypnotherapists
who specialize in it (see Appendix A). You may have read of the use
of visualization as an adjunctive treatment for cancer and other
serious diseases. In some people with some kinds of diseases it can
trigger healing, possibly through effects on the nervous, endocrine,
and immune systems. For this purpose the images should be the
patient's own, and one of the functions of the therapist is to help
patients find the images that are right for them.

For relaxation and stress reduction it is all right to start with
images you get from books or tapes, as long as they feel right for
you. Or simply recall a scene from the past when you were su-
premely content, secure, and centered. Close your eyes, take a few
deep breaths, and picture yourself back there. Try to make the image
bright and clear and try to hear, feel, and smell the surroundings

too. How long you focus on it is less important than how regularly you do it. If you spend a few minutes every day practicing your visualization, you will reap greater benefits than if you spend an hour at it every so often.

The best times for practice are the transition states between sleeping and waking. Just before falling asleep and just after waking up, try to concentrate on your peaceful image. At these times it passes more easily into your unconscious mind, where it can relax your nervous system and body. Of course, try it during the day, too, especially if external stress gets you down and you become aware of internal tension.

Biofeedback uses technology to help you learn relaxation faster. The idea of biofeedback is clever and simple: if you can develop sensory awareness of an involuntary function, you can learn to change it. In a common biofeedback setup, temperature sensors are connected to your fingers, and skin temperature is converted to an audible signal, perhaps a beep tone: the faster the beeps, the higher the temperature. Your job is to make the beeps go faster by raising your skin temperature. The tone gives your ears and brain feedback from a body function that is ordinarily unconscious and beyond the reach of your will. Skin temperature is a measure of blood flow into the hands, and that is determined by the size of little arteries. The autonomic nervous system regulates this flow by causing arteries to constrict (sympathetic influence) or dilate (parasympathetic influence). In order to raise your skin temperature you have to relax your sympathetic nervous system.

If I were to tell you to relax your sympathetic nerves or let more blood flow into your hands, you would not have a clue where to begin, because your conscious mind has no way of perceiving these functions, but in the biofeedback arrangement just described, you will quickly discover that you can influence the rate of the beeps and make them go faster. You will not know exactly what you are doing. Instead you will learn what it feels like when you relax the right area, and the reinforcement of faster beeps will soon have you doing it better and better. Learning in this way is interesting and fun.

The rewards of mastering the relaxation response are much greater than warm fingers (although that might be reward enough for people with cold hands and disorders like Raynaud's disease, in which excess sympathetic tone causes severe spasm in the arteries when hands are exposed to cold). Changing the balance of the autonomic nervous system away from dominance by its sympathetic division has a large spillover effect throughout the body, leading often to lowered heart rate and blood pressure and better digestive function, for example.

You can use other modes of biofeedback to work on muscle tension (as in cases of tension headache or of bruxism — involuntary grinding of the teeth at night) or on brain waves. The applications of this method are many, limited mostly by the imagination of therapists and the willingness of trainees to practice. Once you get the feel of the state you want to create, your work has just begun. Now you have to go home and recreate it on your own without the machine. Unless you do this on a regular basis, you will have wasted your time and money, because the point is to incorporate what you learn into daily life. Ideally you should spend fifteen to twenty minutes a day at this practice, preferably after a few minutes of progressive relaxation, visualization, or meditation to set the stage.

Biofeedback works best for people whose tension is expressed in bodily complaints and who like machines with dials, lights, and beeps. I recommend it often to people with migraine, hypertension, cardiac arrhythmias, ulcers, chronic intestinal problems, Raynaud's disease, and bruxism. I also recommend it to people who feel they need outside help in learning to reduce anxiety and internal stress, who doubt they can do it on their own. Of course, when you do biofeedback you *are* doing it on your own, and much of the fun comes from realizing that fact. Brain-wave biofeedback, now becoming available to the public at specialized centers, can be a powerful technique to change your state of consciousness, advance a meditation practice, and overcome psychosomatic problems.

A typical biofeedback training program consists of ten hourlong sessions, often spaced a week apart. You can find biofeedback therapists in the yellow pages of the telephone directory or on the staffs of hospitals and spas (also see Appendix A). Shop around and do not get involved with anyone who does not seem interested in you. Some therapists do the training mechanically with little attention to individual needs. Medical insurance may pay for biofeedback, especially if a medical doctor prescribes it. I do not recommend using home biofeedback devices on your own without first training with a therapist.

Meditation is directed concentration. Meditators learn to focus their awareness and direct it onto an object: the breath, a phrase or word repeated silently, a memorized inspirational passage, an image in the mind's eye. Researchers have documented immediate benefits in terms of lowered blood pressure, decreased heart and respiratory rate, increased blood flow, and other measurable signs of the relaxation response.

Teachers of meditation usually recommend it for greater goals than mere relaxation. They promise that it can calm an agitated mind, creating optimal physical and mental health; that it can undo our sense of separateness, which is the common root of fear and misery; and that it can unify consciousness, putting us in touch with our higher self and connecting us to higher consciousness. They say meditation restructures the mind, allowing us to achieve our full potential as human beings. They admit that this is hard, long work. Buddhists say the untrained mind is like a drunken monkey stung by a bee — a wild, unruly force, the source of all our unhappiness.

I believe in these potentials of meditation and practice it myself, but I do not recommend it to everyone looking for a way to relax. In the first place many people are not ready to meditate. They must first work to improve their diets, develop good exercise habits, and learn how to breathe properly. Some people need simpler techniques for relaxation that give immediate results with less effort, like the breathing exercise I described earlier. Others harbor negative associations to meditation as an aspect of religion, especially of Eastern religion, with images of yogis on beds of nails and greedy gurus come to the West to fleece devotees.

In fact, there are as many varieties of meditation as there are of exercise. Some are religious practices, some are not. Some are complicated, some are not. If you want to give meditation a try, shop around for a form of it that seems comfortable, that suits you and does not conflict with your belief system. All forms of meditation require regular, daily practice over a long period of time before they deliver the big rewards.

You can learn to meditate in a number of ways. I know a few

good books and instructional tapes on meditation, which are listed at the end of this chapter. You can sign up for meditation classes at some schools and yoga centers or go on group meditation retreats. However you learn a method, you then have to practice it.

You can meditate in any position, but most systems recommend a seated posture with the spine straight. It is perfectly all right to sit in a chair if you cannot find a workable position on the floor. All sorts of meditation aids are available, too, from firm cushions to benches, stools, and pads. Try to meditate every day without fail, twenty to thirty minutes being a reasonable length of time. The best time for me is first thing in the morning. If I miss that opportunity and get caught up in the day's activities, I am unlikely to do it. Usually I am too sleepy at the end of the day to sit, but if I force myself to do even a little meditation before going to bed, that feels good too.

Many newcomers to meditation think the goal is to stop all thoughts. That is not possible. What you want to learn is to withdraw attention from the endless chains of associated thoughts that stream through the mind, putting attention instead on the object of meditation. Whenever you become aware that your attention has strayed — to images, sensations, thoughts of dinner, or whatever — gently bring it back to your chosen object. The tedious work of meditation is just this constant running after your attention and bringing it back.

If you want to get a feel for this challenging work, I suggest you try your hand at breath counting, a deceptively simple technique much used in Zen practice. Sit in a comfortable position with the spine straight and head inclined slightly forward. Gently close your eyes and take a few deep breaths. Then let the breath come naturally without trying to influence it. Ideally it will be quiet and slow, but depth and rhythm may vary. To begin the exercise, count "one" to yourself as you exhale. The next time you exhale, count "two," and so on up to "five." Then begin a new cycle, counting "one" on the next exhalation. Never count higher than "five," and count only when you exhale. You will know your attention has wandered when you find yourself up to "eight," "twelve," even "nineteen." Try to do ten minutes of this form of meditation.

It may not be a good idea for people who are mentally ill to meditate without supervision. Otherwise, meditation is for anyone willing to commit to a discipline that makes training the body look like child's play. By the way, Buddhist teachers would say that we are all mentally ill, and that meditation is the one and only cure for our dis-ease.

Mantram is the practice of repeating over and over in the mind certain syllables, words, or phrases that help unify consciousness and counteract negative mental states. *Mantram* is a Sanskrit word, and the technique is especially prominent in Hinduism, yoga, and Buddhism, although it occurs in many Western traditions as well. Repetition of a verbal formula is a way of focusing the thinking mind and counteracting the damage done to both mind and body by thoughts that produce anxiety, agitation, and unhappiness. You can get some of this benefit by repeating anything: "Peace, peace, peace, peace . . ." or "The sky is blue, the sky is blue . . ." or "Day by day in every way I am getting better and better." If you choose a holy name or spiritual formula from a religious tradition, you may get added benefit from the special power of those words and the field of consciousness created by millions of persons repeating them.

In India a guru will often give a disciple an individual mantram to be used by that person alone and not revealed to anyone else, but some very well-known mantrams are believed to have great transformative power on consciousness. Here are a few:

Rama, Rama, Rama, Rama (a Hindu name of God)
Om mani padme hum (the Buddhist formula, referring to the "jewel in the lotus of the heart," a symbol of enlightenment)
Lord Jesus Christ, son of God, have mercy on us . . . (the Jesus prayer from the Eastern Orthodox tradition)
Hail Mary, full of grace . . . (the Roman Catholic prayer)
Allah, Allah, Allah, Allah (the Muslim name of God)
Shema Yisroel, adonai elohenu, adonai ehod . . . (Jewish: Hear, O Israel, the Lord our God, the Lord is One!)

Repetition of a mantram provides a comforting focus for the mind. It is a totally portable technique, requires no training or equipment, and can be used in any circumstance, though you should be cautious about doing it while driving, operating machinery, or engaging in other hazardous activities that require undivided attention. Mantram is especially helpful for people with restless minds, whose turbulent thoughts keep them from relaxing, concentrating, and falling asleep. I recommend experimenting with it.

Hypnotherapy, the contemporary name for hypnosis, has fallen in and out of favor over the past few hundred years. Currently it is accepted as a useful method of relaxation, pain control, and management of habits like smoking and overeating. In fact, the use of trance and suggestion to affect the unconscious mind and through it the regulatory systems of the body has many more potential applications in the treatment of disease, but few hypnotherapists are willing to tackle interesting physical ailments. Most limit themselves to control of pain, stress, and habits.

Hypnotherapists do not put you into a trance. They just arrange circumstances to increase the likelihood of your shifting into a trance state, which is part of the normal repertory of human consciousness. About 20 percent of the population has a high capacity for trance; these people may go very deep under hypnosis and not remember the experience afterward. Another 20 percent has a very slight capacity for trance and may not respond to hypnotherapy at all. The rest of us fall somewhere in between these extremes.

I emphasize that the hypnotic state is one of your own potentials, because many people fear losing control to a hypnotist and being made to do things they would never do in a normal state. In a similar expression of this fear, yoga philosophy says that hypnosis is dangerous because it weakens the will. I often send patients to hypnotherapists, but I always sound them out first to make sure they do not have fears of loss of control that will get in the way of successful therapy. Also I urge people not to enter into this work unless they feel totally comfortable with the therapist. Finally I tell them, as with biofeedback, that it is up to them to implement the program by committing to regular practice on their own. That may mean taking fifteen or twenty minutes a day to reproduce the feeling and concentrate on the images you learn in sessions with the therapist. At its best hypnotherapy gives you a sense of what it feels like to be relaxed and open, along with the tools to re-create that state on your own.

Hypnotherapy is a good choice for people who think they have no idea what it feels like to relax and for those with stress-related health problems. A few sessions of hypnotherapy can also teach you how to use visualization for self-improvement and can help you begin a meditation practice.

Drugs are used by many to relax, but they are not as safe or effective as the methods I've already described. Alcohol is the most common drug taken for this purpose; think of how many people drink at the end of the workday to unwind. I discuss alcohol in the next chapter, explaining its toxicity and the many reasons not to use it regularly or immoderately. If you come to rely on it as a relaxant, you are likely to become addicted to it.

Medical doctors hand out millions of prescriptions for tranquilizing drugs. Like alcohol, most of them are depressants that interfere with mental function and carry strong risks of addiction. The most common are the benzodiazepines, a family that includes such well-known members as diazepam (Valium), chlordiazepoxide (Librium), alprazolam (Xanax), and lorazapam (Ativan). In my opinion these are all dangerous drugs. Most doctors who prescribe them and most patients who take them do not understand their effects or appreciate their dangers. Benzodiazepine addiction is one of the most difficult forms of drug dependence to treat.

I never prescribe these tranquilizers, but I do recommend a few natural substances. Spearmint and chamomile teas are both mildly relaxing. You can drink as much of them as you want. A stronger remedy is passionflower, made from a plant *(Passiflora incarnata)* native to southeastern United States. Tincture of passionflower is available at herb and health food stores. The dose is one dropperful in a little water up to four times a day as needed. You may be able to find capsules of the freeze-dried plant as well; take one or two of them one to four times a day as needed. Passionflower is not sedating.

Remember that relaxing substances are not substitutes for the techniques I've described in this chapter. You can use them as aids to relaxation, but you still have to work to learn how to neutralize the effects of external stress.

It should be obvious that adequate rest and sleep are also basic needs for optimal health. Many people do not rest even on vacations. They carry their concerns and agitation with them. Again, this points up the need for relaxation training by any of the methods recommended in this chapter. Yoga philosophy says that dreamless sleep is the highest state of consciousness, only we are not aware of it. It is not at all clear why we need to sleep, by the way. The idea that the body repairs and regenerates itself while we are sleeping is not a medical fact.

Many patients tell me they do not sleep well. Almost always the cause is internal tension. An agitated mind will not let you drift off into easy sleep and will wake you up long before you have slept enough. Doctors prescribe many drugs for the sleepless, and again these are all depressants, more or less closely related to alcohol, all of them addictive, and all dangerous if taken regularly. Triazolam (Halcion) is the benzodiazepine most commonly used as a sedative. I try to get people off it whenever I can. The only justifiable use of these drugs is for short periods, when sleep is disturbed as a result of external trauma, such as a death in the family or intercontinental travel. Regular use for more than a few nights running is not a good idea. In the section on insomnia in Part IV, I give a number of natural remedies to promote sleep. None of these will work by themselves if the root of underlying tension is not addressed by practicing stress-reduction techniques.

FURTHER READING

The Relaxation Response (New York: Avon, 1975) and *Beyond the Relaxation Response* (New York: Times Books, 1984) by Herbert Benson, M.D., are good overviews of the physiology of stress and relaxation, including results of research on effects of meditation.

Minding the Body, Mending the Mind by Joan Borysenko (Reading, Mass.: Addison-Wesley, 1987), discusses the mind/body connection and ways to influence it.

Getting Well Again by Carl Simonton, Stephanie Matthews-Simonton, and James Creighton (New York: Bantam, 1980) discusses visualization as a healing technique. *Healing Yourself: A Step-by-Step Program for Better Health Through Imagery* by Martin L. Rossman, M.D. (New York: Walker, 1987) offers specific instruction on visualization to promote health; a companion version on six audiocassettes is available from Insight Publishing, P.O. Box 2070, Mill Valley, Calif. 94942.

Meditation: An Eight-Point Program by Eknath Easwaran (Petaluma, Calif.: Nilgiri Press, 1978) is a straightforward introduction to the subject, free of religious dogma.

How to Meditate: A Guide to Self-Discovery by Lawrence LeShan (Boston: Little, Brown, 1974; available in Bantam paperback edition) reviews different systems of meditation and gives directions for practice. The same author has made an instructional tape, also called *How to Meditate,* available from Audio Renaissance Tapes, 5858 Wilshire Boulevard, Suite 205, Los Angeles, Calif. 90036.

Meditation: An Instructional Cassette by Daniel Goleman (Psychology Today Tapes, Box 059073, Brooklyn, N.Y. 10025) is another good audio tape for beginners.

The Mantram Handbook: Formulas for Transformation by Eknath Easwaran (Petaluma, Calif.: Nilgiri Press, 1977) is the only book I have seen on the use of mantram as a centering technique.

7

HABITS

"ADDICTION," "codependence," "addictive personality" — all are popular terms today. In every city twelve-step programs modeled on Alcoholics Anonymous offer help to people who compulsively use cocaine, narcotics, marijuana, or food or who compulsively gamble, shop, fall in love, or have sex. We would appear to be a nation of addicts. In fact we are a planet of addicts, because addiction is a basic human problem that all men and women experience in some form. I reject the concept of "addictive personality" unless it includes everyone. The only reason we do not see the universality of this problem is that some kinds of addictive behavior, such as making money, drinking coffee, falling in love, exercising, and working compulsively, are socially acceptable and do not attract attention.

Addiction is not a psychological or pharmacological problem and cannot be solved by the methods of psychology or pharmacology. It is at root a spiritual concern because it represents a misdirected attempt to achieve wholeness, to experience inner completeness and satisfaction.

Why do we think we need something to make us feel content: another slice of pizza, a piece of chocolate, a cigarette, a drink, a snort, a lover, another possession? How do we allow the objects of our addictive behavior to get such power over us that we lose all resistance and will power in their presence? Is there a way to feel complete and whole in ourselves without reaching for an external source of satisfaction? These are hard questions. I will try to answer them at the end of this chapter.

Since the roots of addiction penetrate deeply into the very essence of our humanness, changing addictive behavior is not easy. For some of us it may be the work of a lifetime. A basic strategy for wellness is to be free of harmful habits. If we cannot easily change our addictive nature, at least we can try to be aware of our addictions and work to move them in directions that are less harmful. For example, a cigarette addict who stops smoking and becomes an exercise addict is no less an addict but is a much healthier one.

Many of the most common and least noticed addictions interfere with health. Doctors often ignore these habits and fail to urge patients to change their ways, even though a great deal of illness could be prevented by doing so. I will discuss in this chapter three kinds of behavior that you must learn to control if you want to enjoy optimal health: compulsive eating, addictive use of legal drugs (alcohol, tobacco, and caffeine), and compulsive sex.

FOOD ADDICTION

Compulsive eating is much more difficult to change than drug addiction. You do not have to take drugs, but you do have to eat.

The study and treatment of eating disorders now constitute a hot field of clinical medicine. When I was in school bulimia (cyclic binging and purging) was a rare condition. Today it is so common that in some populations (women in college) it is almost accepted as normal behavior. In fact, what doctors call "eating disorders" are one end of a spectrum of difficulties people have with food. Many people I know and many who come to me as patients would not be diagnosed as having eating disorders, yet they have trouble limiting their food intake to what their bodies need. This problem takes an infinite variety of forms.

A single man in his mid-thirties came to me for a wellness consultation. He was in good health and just wanted my analysis of his lifestyle from a preventive point of view. I encourage this kind of visit and wish more people would call on me *before* they get sick. This man worked as a commodities trader in Chicago, a fast-lane life with lots of excitement and stress. He ate well, had good habits of exercise and relaxation and no major health risks. He said he liked himself and his life except for one odd behavior pattern that puzzled and worried him.

On days when he "took a hit" on the market — that is, ended up with a signficant net loss — or otherwise felt depressed and insecure, he would stop on his way home to buy a big steak, a bottle of vodka, tomato juice, and salted potato chips. Once in his apartment he would cut the steak into little pieces, settle into his favorite chair, and consume the entire plate of raw meat, interspersed with gulps of vodka and tomato juice and mouthfuls of potato chips. He said he realized this was "weird" but found it always made him feel powerful again. He worried that he might be doing himself harm.

I told him not to worry, at least not about physical harm. I do not recommend eating raw steak and drinking vodka, but this was an occasional binge, much in contrast with his normal habits. The real problem was that this man relied on food to comfort himself and experienced a compulsive need to eat in a way that he himself felt was strange. I urged him to practice other techniques of centering.

A woman lawyer in her mid-forties told me she used one particular brand of vanilla ice cream as her comfort food, in large amounts. She never ate less than a quart at one sitting, often a half gallon and sometimes a whole gallon. She did this in the dark in a closet of her home, and she was quite articulate in describing the state she got into. She said it was "regressive" and "infantile" and thought it took her back to the experience of nursing at the breast, the perfect antidote to anxiety and insecurity caused by the storms of the outside world. Frequent ice cream binges are probably worse for you than an occasional dinner of raw meat and vodka, since ice cream delivers a whopping load of saturated fat, sugar, and calories.

Some people cannot pass a bakery without buying pastry. Others cannot make it through an evening without eating quantities of peanuts, chips, and candy. Still others spend most of their time and energy preparing and consuming rich gourmet meals. Compulsive eaters are not feeding their bodies. They are attempting to feed their souls, to fill up an emptiness inside and feel complete, whole. Food cannot do that for us, unfortunately. It can only give us temporary satisfaction, pleasure, and sensory delight. If you bring full attention to bear on it, you can optimize the experience of eating, but in addictive eating the mind isn't even able to focus on the present moment. It is usually anticipating the next bite or thinking about the next item to eat, so that even the sensory pleasure of the experience recedes, and craving increases. It is very, very difficult to change these patterns, especially in a culture that glorifies food and that offers it up in endlessly tempting variety. Food addiction is stubborn and resistant to treatment. It can also be a significant threat to health, both because it is the principal cause of obesity and because it leads people toward foods that increase specific risks of heart disease and cancer.

More likely than not, some of your eating is addictive, not a response to bodily needs but an attempt to satisfy emotional and spiritual cravings. Here are some suggestions that will help protect your health:

• Read over the nutritional guidelines in Chapters 1 and 2. Try to adhere to them even if you are eating when not hungry, even if you are on a binge.

• In particular, learn the fat content of foods you eat and try to eat only low-fat foods (no more than 30 percent of calories as fat), especially when you are eating compulsively. A fruit ice binge is much healthier than an ice cream binge.

• Practice keeping your full attention on the sensory experience of eating. Focus on the taste, smell, and texture of the food you are consuming. Don't let your mind wander to anticipation of the next bite or the next item to eat.

• Maintain a good routine of aerobic exercise: thirty minutes a day at least five days a week to help burn up excess calories.

• If you cannot control your compulsive eating, seek help. Join Overeaters Anonymous. Consult an expert in food habit management. Try hypnotherapy. Spend more time with people who are in better relationships with food. Remember, you are not alone.

ADDICTION TO LEGAL DRUGS

Alcohol is the strongest and most toxic of the common psychoactive substances. It is a "hard" drug, harder than heroin, cocaine, LSD, and all the other illegal drugs. Our culture promotes and encourages the use of alcohol and gives the false impression that it is not as dangerous as the disapproved drugs.

Periodically some research group will report that moderate use of alcohol improves health. Often this research is biased, either consciously or unconsciously. For example, a Canadian study recently concluded that people who drink one to two beers a day have less illness than people who drink none. The study was financed by the Canadian brewing industry. Even when this kind of obvious self-interest is not present, the researchers themselves, like most people in our culture, are likely to be alcohol users. Users have an unconscious need to legitimize the drugs they choose to take.

Except for improved serum lipid profiles due to increases in HDL cholesterol, most of the alleged health benefits of alcohol are really benefits of relaxation, since most people drink to relieve anxiety and dissipate tension. The beneficial effects of relaxation can easily overshadow the direct effects of alcohol, which are toxic. Alcohol is poisonous to nerve and liver cells and irritating to the upper digestive tract and urinary system; in women it may be a significant risk factor for breast cancer. If moderate drinkers could learn to relax by other means, they would be in even better shape.

I am not a nondrinker. Very occasionally I have a beer, some Japanese sake, or a sip of something stronger, but mostly I use wine and liquor as flavorings in cooking, since I no longer like the effects of alcohol on my mind and body. When patients tell me they drink moderately and occasionally, I do not object, but a patient who reports drinking every day or drinking heavily or drinking as a main method of stress reduction is sure to get my lecture on the health hazards of alcohol. It is easy to become dependent on alcohol for your sense of well-being and easy to become physically addicted to it if you depend on it over time. This is most likely to happen if you drink to relieve depression or control anxiety, because alcohol will never teach you how to change those states, and you will have to take it frequently to keep them at bay. Alcohol addiction produces serious disease with irreversible damage to the liver and nervous system.

Most doctors can spot full-blown alcohol addiction and know where to point people for help in overcoming it, but few pay attention to the milder forms of alcohol dependence or appreciate the health consequences of ordinary social drinking. Here are my suggestions:

• *The best way to protect yourself from the hazards of alcohol is not to use it every day.* People who tell me they drink wine with dinner every night or have a beer every day or a mixed drink or two after work, all get the same advice from me: *give yourself two or three alcohol-free days a week.*

• Do not rely on alcohol as your main method of relaxation. Learn to relax using your own resources through breath control, yoga, meditation, or one of the other techniques discussed in Chapter 6.

• Do not use alcohol at all if you have liver disease, urinary problems, prostate trouble, ulcers or other problems of the upper digestive tract (esophagus, stomach, duodenum), or any nervous or mental disease.

• Never drink alcohol on an empty stomach. It is highly irritating to the lining of that organ.

• Alcohol burns up B-vitamins, especially vitamin B-1 (thiamine). If you drink, take a B-complex vitamin supplement plus extra thiamine (100 milligrams) on days you use alcohol. This will protect your nervous system, because the nerve damage seen in alcoholics is partly the result of thiamine deficiency.

• Alcoholic beverages, which are exempted from labeling requirements, may contain harmful additives. Wines frequently have sulfite preservatives and other allergens that can precipitate attacks of asthma, migraine, and various allergic reactions. The best beers are made only from barley malt, water, yeast, and hops, but many beers on the market have dozens of other ingredients. Liqueurs may be dyed with artificial colors. Try to buy quality brands of alcoholic beverages that advertise the purity of their composition.

• Alcohol has calories. They behave like carbohydrate calories, but the body cannot store their energy. It must burn them immediately. As a result, the calories of food you eat at the same time will more readily end up as fat, because the body will tend to store them. If you are trying to lose weight, cutting out alcohol will make the job much easier.

• If you find you cannot control your use of alcohol, get help from Alcoholics Anonymous or a professional counselor who specializes in substance abuse.

Tobacco in the form of cigarettes is the most addictive drug in the world, even more addictive than heroin. Two factors account for this: the pharmacological power of nicotine, one of the strongest stimulants known, and the efficiency of smoking as a drug delivery system. Smoking puts drugs into the brain more directly than intravenous injection. Almost everyone who uses cigarettes is addicted, and the addiction is difficult to break. Cigarette addiction is the greatest public health problem in our nation because it is the single most preventable cause of major illness. It is also far and away the most serious form of drug abuse in our society, alongside which the abuse of illegal drugs pales into insignificance. *The best defense against the harmful effects of tobacco is never to use it.* Its extreme addictiveness makes it too dangerous to experiment with.

Not every cigarette addict will get lung cancer or emphysema. Some people have strong respiratory constitutions to begin with, and individuals vary in their susceptibility to the harmful effects of any drug. Still, tobacco injures many systems of the body, and respiratory disease is only one of the possible results of addiction to it. It also causes bladder cancer and cancers of the head and neck, and raises risks of leukemia. It is very dangerous to use tobacco if you are diabetic or are taking birth control pills or if you have any heart or circulatory problems, respiratory disease, urinary or prostate trouble, digestive disorders, a family history of cancer or increased risk of cancer for any reason, high blood pressure, seizure disorder, or a family history of coronary heart disease.

Second-hand smoke endangers the health of nonsmokers. Smoke coming off the end of a cigarette contains more harmful compounds than inhaled smoke because it has not been filtered through a mat of tobacco. If you are forced to work or live with smokers, protect yourself with a good HEPA filter to remove this material from the air (see Chapter 4). Also join the political struggle to get smoking out of all public places, including airplanes, restaurants, and work areas; to ban all advertising of tobacco products; and to end government subsidies of the tobacco industry.

In the early part of this century cigarette smoking was accepted and encouraged as a healthy way to promote mental alertness, efficiency, and relaxation. In fact, one of the appeals of smoking is temporary, brief relief of internal tension. Unfortunately, twenty minutes after the last cigarette, the tension returns stronger than before, and the brain demands another fix. Aside from this minimal benefit, tobacco does nothing good. No one argues for the health benefits of moderate smoking.

Nicotine powerfully constricts blood vessels throughout the body, interfering with circulation in the brain and the extremities. It stimulates the heart, raises blood pressure, agitates the digestive system, and irritates the urinary system. Addiction to nicotine maintains the tobacco habit, but tobacco contains many substances besides nicotine, and many of them are also harmful. Tobacco smoke is one of the richest known sources of carcinogenic agents.

Low-tar, low-nicotine cigarettes offer no great advantages. People tend to smoke more of them or inhale more deeply to keep the brain supplied with the amount of nicotine it wants. Pipes and cigars, if not inhaled, do not cause lung cancer and emphysema but greatly increase the risk of oral cancers. So do the smokeless tobaccos (formerly called snuff) and chewing tobaccos that teenagers and baseball players like to put in their mouths.

I feel so strongly about the health risks of tobacco that I am unwilling to accept patients who are users unless they commit to attempting to quit. Many programs are available to help people quit, from acupuncture and hypnotherapy to support groups, but none of them work reliably for everyone. Most successful quitters do it on their own after one or more unsuccessful attempts, and most find that stopping completely ("cold turkey") is better than trying to cut down gradually. Do not be discouraged if you start again, because what counts is the attempt. You get credit for every attempt to quit you make. One day your reservoir of motivation will be full enough for the next attempt to be the one that works.

• Practice the breathing exercise on pages 119–120. It will help motivate you to quit smoking and help you deal with cravings for cigarettes.

• If you smoke or have been an addicted smoker any time in the past ten years, you should take antioxidant vitamins and minerals (see pp. 185–188). Antioxidants reverse to some extent the changes in respiratory tissue caused by smoking and so help protect against lung cancer. Also try to increase dietary sources of carotenes, such as carrots, sweet potatoes, yellow squash, and leafy green vegetables. These substances, related to vitamin A, may offer further protection.

• Never smoke and drink alcohol at the same time. Both substances increase the risk of developing cancers of the mouth, throat, esophagus, and stomach, but the carcinogenic potential of the combination is greater than the sum of the parts.

Coffee is another strong drug, one that is used unconsciously by millions of people. It is the strongest of all the caffeine sources, the one that is most irritating to the body, and the one most associated with addiction. I estimate that 80 percent of coffee users are addicted to it. The addiction is physical, with a prominent withdrawal reaction when use is suddenly discontinued. Here are the major characteristics of coffee addiction:

• The drug is used every day, typically in the morning. There are no days without coffee. The amount used is not a determining factor. I have seen true addiction in people drinking only one cup a day.

• Without morning coffee the user cannot function, experiences mental and physical slowness, and is irritable and unable to concentrate.

• The user is dependent on coffee to move the bowels.

• The user's energy cycle is controlled by coffee: typically he or she is energized early in the day but becomes lethargic and slow in the late afternoon.

• If no coffee is drunk for twenty-four to thirty-six hours, a withdrawal reaction begins: lethargy, irritability, and a distinctive throbbing (vascular) headache that can become severe. Nausea and vomiting may occur. These symptoms will last from thirty-six to seventy-two hours. They disappear rapidly if the user takes caffeine in any form.

Because our culture so strongly approves of coffee and encourages its use, most coffee addicts have no idea that they are taking a drug, let alone a strong one that can affect many systems of the body. Since many doctors are coffee addicts, they often fail to see this drug for what it is or stop to consider that it may be a cause of medical problems. I have in front of me a pamphlet from the American Heart Association titled "What Should I Put in My Coffee?" It describes a man named Larry who is concerned about his cholesterol. Larry drinks "4 to 5 cups of coffee a day, and in each cup he uses a spoonful of whatever creamer happens to be handy." The pamphlet goes on to describe the hazards of cream and recommends nondairy creamers made with polyunsaturated oils (and a host of additives). The American Heart Association appears to consider this sort of addiction quite normal and of no medical interest. In fact, coffee itself can contribute to elevated cholesterol and increased risk of heart disease.

My files are filled with dramatic cures of long-standing conditions, brought about simply by getting people off coffee. Here are some typical stories.

A thirty-three-year-old woman lawyer came to see me with a complaint of urinary dysfunction of twelve years' duration. She did not like doctors and let me know at the start of our meeting that it had taken a lot for her to come to another doctor for help. Her problem had started as urinary frequency and urgency, which got steadily worse. She began consulting physicians, but none of them could find anything wrong with her. Nevertheless, they put her on courses of antibiotics and urinary anesthetics because they had nothing else to offer. When she failed to get better, the doctors treated her as a difficult, complaining female whose problem was all in her head. She would leave in disgust and try to manage on her own until the urinary trouble got worse. Then she would take herself to a new doctor. She had seen twenty different physicians in twelve years and had had unsatisfactory experiences with all of them.

After several years she developed a new symptom, pain during sexual intercourse, that threatened to disrupt her marriage. Again no cause was found. After persistent complaining, she was pushed into having urethral reconstructive surgery. This operation was painful and expensive, and not only did it give her no relief, it gave her two new problems. As a direct result of the surgery, she had stress incontinence (loss of urine on coughing or sneezing) and dribbling at the end of urination. She was very angry at the medical profession by the time she reached my office door.

I began by asking her what had been happening in her life twelve years before when all this started. It turned out to have been a significant time. She had left home to go to college and had begun a high-pressure academic course leading to law school. All of her routines changed. Her eating patterns became irregular. She began staying up late to study. And she began drinking coffee. My ears perked up at this information, and I asked her in detail about her coffee habit. She drank "only" one to two cups of regular coffee a day, which in her mind was nothing. She had never gone a day without coffee since she started using it. She did not drink more than two cups a day because if she did, her hands shook and she got diarrhea. That told me she was very sensitive to the effects of the drug.

Shaking hands and diarrhea are symptoms of coffee's toxicity to the nervous and gastrointestinal systems. This woman did not know that the urinary system, especially in females, is another common target. I told her she would have to stop all coffee, that she would probably experience withdrawal and so should wait till she had a three-day weekend to attempt it. I told her to expect a headache and to use aspirin or another analgesic for it, as long as it did not contain caffeine. I also gave her an herbal remedy that helps promote healing of the urinary tract, and I suggested a visualization exercise.

When I next talked to this patient, she was a different woman. She said the withdrawal had lasted three full days and had surprised her with its intensity. All of her urinary symptoms disappeared after this and had not returned. She also reported that her anxiety level had dropped by 90 percent and told me, "I didn't even know I'd been anxious." Then she asked, "How could twenty doctors in twelve years not have told me coffee was the cause of my problems?"

Here is another case. A forty-year-old man who worked as a metallurgist for a mining company came to see me because he was experiencing "bad headaches." He had had them for twenty years and was now getting them every day. The pain was throbbing and could be relieved only by Excedrin. He took two Excedrins per headache and had one to two headaches a day. He also drank one to two cups of coffee a day. Doctors had been unable to help him with his headaches and had recently told him he needed a full-scale neurological workup to determine their cause.

The throbbing pain of vascular headache results from dilation of small arteries in the head. Caffeine constricts arteries. (It can actually be used as an immediate treatment for vascular headache, but only in nonaddicted persons.) In caffeine addiction the arteries are subjected to a constant constrictive force; in response they constantly try to dilate (which is why vascular headache is the main symptom of caffeine withdrawal). Any vascular headache that is relieved by Excedrin but not by aspirin must be a *caffeine-caused* headache, since Excedrin contains caffeine. I told this man he had to eliminate caffeine from his life and gave him the usual pep talk about how to handle withdrawal (rest, distraction, patience, plain aspirin for headache).

He went at it the next weekend and called me right afterward to tell me the results. "It was spectacular," he said. "I think I finally had the headache I've been trying to have for twenty years." That was a very accurate way of putting it. He has not had headaches since.

One more. A fifty-year-old woman consulted me at Canyon Ranch spa with the complaint of "diarrhea for the past six months." The diarrhea was painless and seemed unrelated to diet. She had no history of foreign travel, said she was not having any new or unusual stress, and had no other symptoms except for increasing anxiety about her health. She had been in excellent health, ate well, exercised regularly, and had good habits, except for drinking four cups of coffee a day.

After having constant diarrhea for two weeks, she went to her family doctor, who prescribed a drug that did not control it and caused uncomfortable side effects. She stopped taking the medicine and went to see a naturopathic physician. He told her to stop drinking milk and eating sugar and gave her a homeopathic remedy. The diarrhea persisted. She returned to her family doctor, who did a number of tests; although the results were all normal, he told her she still might have a parasite and put her on a course of Flagyl, a drug that kills amoebas. No change in the diarrhea occurred. She then went "with great reluctance" to a gastroenterologist, who did a lot more tests, including an upper and lower gastrointestinal (GI) series of X rays and sigmoidoscopy. His conclusion was that there was "no organic reason" for the diarrhea.

As the woman recounted her story, she became more and more upset. Finally she started crying as she said, "And now I think my whole digestive tract must really be messed up, because since I got out here four days ago, I've been *constipated*." My ears perked up again. The spa does not routinely serve caffeinated beverages. "Are you drinking coffee here?" I asked. No, she had not had any since her arrival. Had she had headaches? Yes, as a matter of fact, she had had an awful headache for two days but thought it was due to all the exercise. I explained that her diarrhea was a symptom of coffee toxicity; there was nothing else wrong. Without the drug it would take a while for her colon to regain its natural tone. I recommended that she drink a lot of water and take powdered psyllium seed husks as a source of bulk.

I assure you I could fill this chapter with similar accounts of chronic conditions that made patients miserable and baffled doctors. All went away when the addictive use of coffee stopped.

Here are my cautions about this substance:

• Coffee is a strong drug. If you like it and can use it occasionally as a useful stimulant without experiencing adverse effects, do so. If you use it every day, you are likelier than not to become addicted to it.

• Do not drink coffee at all if you have any of the following conditions: migraine, tremor, anxiety, insomnia, cardiac arrhythmia (palpitations), coronary heart disease or a strong family history of it, elevated serum cholesterol, hypertension, any gastrointestinal disorder, any urinary disorder, prostate trouble, fibrocystic breast disease, premenstrual syndrome (PMS), tension headache, or seizure disorder. If you are pregnant or planning to become pregnant, be aware that coffee may increase the risk of miscarriage.

• If you have reason to avoid coffee, stay away from decaffeinated coffee as well. It is not inert. In addition to small amounts of caffeine, it contains other active substances that are present in coffee beans and that can be irritating to the nervous, gastrointestinal, cardiovascular, and urinary systems. This is true of water-processed decaf as well as the less safe solvent-extracted brands, which may contain residues of toxic chemicals.

• Coffee addiction is easy to break compared to alcohol and tobacco addiction. Do not attempt it unless you have three days with no responsibilities and no demands on your time and energy. Arrange for ways to keep yourself distracted and comfortable. Prepare to be without energy and to have a headache for forty-eight to seventy-two hours. Take nothing with caffeine.

• Many coffee substitutes are available in both regular grocery stores and health food stores. They are made from roasted grains, roots, acorns, and other benign ingredients. Some (Cafix, Roma, Dacopa) are much better than others. Experiment with them or use a caffeine-free herbal tea in place of your habitual beverage.

Other caffeine beverages include tea, cola and other sodas, and two exotic drinks from South America, yerba maté and guaraná.

Tea addiction is rare in our culture but common in some parts of the world (Ireland, the United Kingdom, and parts of Asia). Tea contains much less caffeine than coffee but much more of a related drug called theophylline, which is used in pure form to treat asthma. Its side effects are the usual ones of stimulants: jitters, insomnia, anxiety, increased heart rate, and so on.

Tea contains tannins, which give a bitter, astringent flavor, especially after long brewing. Tannins irritate the lining of the upper digestive tract and account for the increased incidence of cancers of the oral cavity, esophagus, and stomach in some tea-drinking populations. Milk neutralizes tannins and protects from this risk. If you drink more than two cups of tea a day, add a little milk to it. Decaffeinated tea is largely inert and makes a good substitute for regular tea. Beware, however, of commercial "herb teas" that are actually herb-flavored regular teas with caffeine. Read labels to determine if you are getting a caffeine-free product.

Recent publicity on health benefits of Japanese green tea reports that it contains a group of compounds called catechins that are largely destroyed by the fermentation process used to make ordinary black tea. Catechins have significant anticancer effects and may also lower serum cholesterol. If you want to use a caffeinated tea, green tea looks like your healthiest choice.

Addiction to caffeine-containing soft drinks is common, to both the sugared and diet versions, and some people drink enough of them to experience all of the adverse effects of the drug. Cola nuts, native to Africa, are a stimulant and caffeine source. Very little cola nut goes into cola beverages, but they contain added caffeine from other sources. Children are especially susceptible to these drinks because of their sugar content and pleasant flavors. If you consume cola beverages, use caffeine-free ones when possible, unless you want an occasional stimulant effect. Remember that caffeinated sodas are drugs, not just "soft drinks."

Yerba maté and guaraná are caffeine-containing plants, often sold in health food stores, herb shops, and fancy groceries. Yerba maté comes in tea bags or as a loose tea. Guaraná is an ingredient in some tea mixtures and is also sold as a powder, either loose or packed into capsules. Both are sometimes deceptively labeled as caffeine free or nonstimulating.

Chocolate is a special case, since it is a food as well as a drug. It contains only a small amount of caffeine but has a lot of theobromine, a close relative with similar effects. Chocolate is usually thought of as a flavoring for desserts or a treat by itself, but it is also a mood-altering substance that can have strong effects on body and mind and can certainly be addictive. By itself, theobromine cannot account for all aspects of chocolate addiction, because chocolate addiction appears different from other forms of stimulant dependence. Most "chocoholics" are women, and many of them crave chocolate most intensely just before the onset of menstruation. Women who develop an addictive relationship with chocolate usually eat it in cyclic binges rather than continually and often say it acts as an instant antidepressant for them. There is no reason to think that theobromine affects men and women differently.

I have been collecting cases of chocolate addiction for some time. Here are two interesting stories:

A twenty-eight-year-old Swiss woman, working in the United States as an assistant to a college president, wanted to discuss her eating habits with me. She ate one to two pounds per day of dark Swiss chocolate. Sometimes that was all she ate. She considered it a "health food" and thought she would get sick without it. She was athletic, a skier and backpacker, and not obese. The main problem her addiction caused was anxiety about her supply. She would not consider eating American chocolate and said that only a few brands of Swiss chocolate were good enough to make her feel right. She was so concerned about feeling right that when she came to America to work, she brought only the clothes she wore, filling her luggage with chocolate.

A fifty-three-year-old woman, who had gone through menopause three years before, told me she had never been interested in chocolate until recently, when her gynecologist had started her on hormone replacement. She was taking estrogen for three weeks of each month followed by ten days of progesterone. In her words, "Sometimes during the days that I'm on progesterone I get insane cravings for chocolate, to the point that I have to get up in the middle of the night and drive to a convenience store to satisfy them. Nothing like this has ever happened to me before. I finally went to the gynecologist and asked him if it could be related to the hormone. He laughed at me, told me that was ridiculous, and made me feel silly for having asked." I assured her she was not silly, since I have heard the same story from other women.

Very little research has been done on chocolate. Recently German scientists showed that chocolate-seeking behavior in rats and mice could be blocked by giving drugs that counteract the effects of narcotics. This finding suggests that the endorphin system is involved. My guess is that chocolate contains a number of substances affecting mood and that addiction to it is complex. Since chocolate contains a lot of fat and sugar, it would lend itself to compulsive eating even if it were not also a stimulant.

My recommendations about chocolate are:

• Do not eat it if you have migraine, fibrocystic breast disease, or PMS or are subject to mood swings.

• Chocolate can be very stimulating to some people. Pay attention to its effects on your moods, energy cycles, and sleep patterns.

• Chocolate is high in calories and fat. Consider its effect on your overall dietary program.

• Although cocoa butter may not be as bad for the heart and blood vessels as other saturated fats, it is often replaced in cheaper brands of chocolate by unhealthy fats like palm and coconut oil. Read labels to avoid these products.

• Pure cocoa powder is low in fat but high in chocolate flavor. Use it to make low-fat chocolate desserts to satisfy a craving.

• Some women who could not control their chocolate binges have reported that magnesium supplements helped them. Try taking 300 milligrams of magnesium twice a day.

• If chocolate puts you in a good mood, try using it as a way of rewarding yourself for good behavior. Eating good-quality chocolate consciously and occasionally is a healthy way to deal with cravings for it.

In general, be aware of the total amount of caffeine you ingest in the course of a day. Remember that caffeine is an ingredient of many prescribed and over-the-counter medications. If you take such products and also use coffee, tea, cola, and chocolate, you may be consuming much more of this drug than you think.

SEXUAL ADDICTIONS

Compulsive sex is an invisible problem in our society because we have been led to believe that it is healthy and desirable to have sex and orgasm as often as possible. Many people feel they do not get enough sex and envy those who have it a lot. In some of our subcultures men who adhere to the ethic of *machismo* acquire social status by their numerous sexual conquests and ability to have frequent orgasms. With these cultural values the concept of sexual addiction is not popular, to say the least, and those few experts who have tried to draw attention to it have not met with much success.

Like drugs and food, sex produces powerful alterations of awareness. Orgasm can give us a glimpse of a higher reality, a sense of connection beyond the finite self. On a more mundane level it can provide temporary relief from stress and internal tension. Not surprisingly, people can develop compulsive relationships with sex, again trying to fill an inner void, again finding that satisfaction recedes as they pursue it with greater desperation.

Sex is an overwhelmingly powerful drive for human beings and one of our great fascinations. We think about it a great deal, yet live in appalling ignorance of its nature and best uses. Of course, sex will always remain partly hidden from understanding no matter how we attempt to come to grips with it intellectually, but even on the most practical level there is little information to assist us. The lack of good writing about sex is remarkable. Most of us struggle to come to terms with this drive without help. Parents, teachers, and religious instructors often add to our confusion. Trustworthy guides are seldom found.

If sex is so great, what's wrong with doing it all the time? In the first place, addiction of any sort, even a relatively harmless one, limits our freedom. It ties up a great deal of our mental and physical energy in useless ways, keeping us from the full experience of life. Besides, in this age of AIDS, sex with multiple partners is increasingly dangerous. We used to think of sexually transmitted diseases as nuisances rather than serious threats, but that is no longer the case. Even when a disease is minor, like venereal warts, it may have long-range consequences: increased risk of genital cancers and compromised immunity.

What about compulsive "safe sex"? Or compulsive masturbation? You won't contract diseases, but you will still be limiting your freedom. Sex, potentially, is a doorway beyond the limited world of the ego. It can be a way of establishing meaningful connections with other people and with the higher self. In sexual addiction that potential is never realized. Instead of intimate partners you have sexual objects. Instead of transcending ego, you reinforce your sense of an isolated, insulated self. In the next chapter I will argue that you cannot attain optimal health unless you establish meaningful connections beyond the ego. Compulsive sex is a major obstacle to that process and therefore an impediment to health.

Changing a sexual addiction is no easier than changing a food addiction. These behaviors are intrinsically hard to alter, and the values of our society make it all the more difficult.

You will find some specific advice about safe sex in Chapter 11. Here are some general guidelines for sexual behavior:
• Moderately frequent sexual activity may be more rewarding than very frequent sexual activity.
• Pay attention to the results of your sexual activity. Does it make you feel more or less isolated? more or less connected to other people and to your higher self?
• Try to associate with people who seem healthy in their sexuality.
• Most cities have twelve-step programs for sexual addictions.

I will close this chapter with some general thoughts on addiction. We all come into the world with wounds; they come with human birth, no matter what kind of family we grow up in, no matter what kind of society we live in. Much of our human seeking is a search for healing. We long for a sense of completeness and wholeness and for an end to craving. Most often we look for satisfaction outside of ourselves. That is the root of addiction. Ironically, whatever satisfaction we gain from food, drugs, sex, money, and other "sources" of pleasure really comes from inside us. We project our power onto external substances and activities, allowing them to make us feel better temporarily. This is a strange sort of magic. We give our power away in order to achieve a transient sense of wholeness, then suffer because the objects of our craving seem to have power over us. Addiction can be cured only when we consciously experience this process, reclaim our power, and realize that wounds must be healed from within. Suffering and craving goad us into action, forcing us to discover who we are, to identify with our true selves.

SUGGESTED READING

The Natural Mind: A New Way of Looking at Drugs and the Higher Consciousness by Andrew Weil (Boston: Houghton Mifflin, revised edition, 1986) goes into more detail about the relationship between drugs and states of consciousness.

From Chocolate to Morphine: Everything You Need to Know About Mind-Altering Drugs by Andrew Weil and Winifred Rosen (Boston: Houghton Mifflin, 1993) looks at all mood-altering substances, legal and illegal.

When Society Becomes an Addict by Anne Wilson Schaef (New York: Harper & Row, 1987) is a good general book on addiction that synthesizes theories of feminism, chemical dependency, and mental health.

Codependent No More: How to Stop Controlling Others and Start Caring for Yourself by Melody Beattie (New York: Harper & Row, 1988) deals with the problem of being in relationship with addicted persons. It is full of helpful advice.

Twelve Steps for Overeaters: An Interpretation of the Twelve Steps of Overeaters Anonymous by Elizabeth L. (New York: Harper & Row, 1988) presents the OA philosophy in a clear, straightforward manner.

A Substance Called Food: How to Understand, Control, and Recover from Addictive Eating by Gloria Arenson (Blue Ridge Summit, Pa.: Tab, 1989) is a useful book for compulsive eaters.

8

CONNECTIONS

YOU CANNOT ENJOY full health as an isolated, separate being. Health is wholeness, and wholeness implies connectedness — to family, friends, tribe, nation, humanity, the earth, and whatever higher power you conceive of as the creator of the universe.

A great deal of human misery and disease derives from self-centeredness, from inability to transcend the confining limits of the ego world. For example, many of us find change stressful, and many of us get sick when we go through such major changes as the loss of a spouse, a forced move, or the breakup of an intimate relationship. Why is change so stressful and frightening? My sense is that fear of change grows out of fear of death, because death is the great change. To the ego it is the ultimate threat, and it is ego consciousness that creates fear of change.

Depression, anger, loneliness, and other emotions that suppress immunity and unbalance the nervous system are also rooted in the sense of self as an isolated, separate entity. There is ample medical evidence that people who fail to establish meaningful connections have more illness, even that susceptibility to heart attack correlates with how often people use the words *I, me,* and *mine* in casual speech.

All religions and spiritual traditions stress the importance of overcoming the illusion of separateness and experiencing unity. This brief passage from the Hindu "Song of God," the Bhagavad Gita, says it all:

> Free forever is he who breaks out of the ego cage
> Of "I" and "me" and "mine" to be united with the Lord of Love.
> This is the supreme state;
> Attain thou this, and pass from death to Immortality.

What we have to do is clear. How to do it may not be clear, since we have so much practice at viewing the world from our "ego cage" and so little practice at transcending it. Before I end this discussion of basic needs for general health, I want to tell you about some of the ways I have found to reduce self-centeredness.

1. Connecting with Nature and the Earth

If you think of nature as a hostile force, separate from yourself, you will go through life unnecessarily afraid and cut off from one of the great sources of spiritual nourishment. Whether you connect with nature on wilderness trips or lunch breaks in a city park, you can always slow down and observe the infinite variety of her ways. My particular connection is with plants. I delight in gardening, collecting plants from the wild, growing cactuses and flowering bulbs, having unusual and useful plants in and around my home. They enrich my daily life, bring me comfort and joy, and remind me that however else I think of myself, I am also part of the natural world.

2. Connecting with Animals

Research shows that people who have pets have less illness than people who do not. They also recover faster from serious illness. Ex-prisoners who form relationships with pets have lower recidivism rates than those who do not. Pets are a responsibility. They demand a certain level of attention and care. The rewards they give in return are often too great to be measured.

I have two female dogs, Rhodesian ridgebacks, mother and daughter. They are part of my life, and I cannot imagine being away from them for long. They often make me laugh, sometimes make me furious, and always take me out of myself. My connection to them is a special bond, difficult to express in words. On occasion, when I am feeling blue or overwhelmed by problems, I have a session of dog psychotherapy, which I recommend highly. I ask my older dog to sit down facing me while I talk out my feelings and troubles. She listens intently and is only slightly less interactive than the Freudian psychoanalyst I went to many years ago. She costs much less (one biscuit per session) and gives me unconditional love even when I reveal the most awful thoughts and deeds. This is true friendship and support. After just fifteen minutes of dog psychotherapy, even the worst problems seem not as bad. Loving and caring for a pet animal is a good practice.

3. Connecting with Family

An anthropologist friend of mine was once teaching a section of a course on Native American society at Harvard. In the class was a Native American, a young man. In talking about social organization, my friend kept referring to the "extended families" of Indians. Finally the Indian in the class interrupted him, saying, "Excuse me, but we don't have extended families. We have families. You have contracted families."

The nuclear family of our modern society is, indeed, contracted. Human beings want and need the intimate support of a real family. It is hard not to look at the "extended families" of other cultures with wistful longing, if not outright envy. Where I live in southern Arizona, the Hispanic population seems way ahead of the rest of us in providing for this need. For example, there are no Hispanics in the nursing homes here. Nursing homes are where we put our old relatives when we no longer want to care for them. In Hispanic families the old people, even when infirm, continue to be valued members and live at home.

A nurse at the University of Arizona medical center who attended one of my courses told me that she worked for a number of years in the pediatric intensive care unit. During her time there she saw twelve children recover miraculously from apparently fatal head injuries. They had been in bicycle or motorbike accidents, were in deepest coma, had flat EEGs (brain-wave patterns), and were given up for dead by the attending physicians. The organ-transplant teams hovered around, waiting to take kidneys and hearts. She saw twelve children in that extreme state come back to full consciousness and life, to the amazement of their doctors and the annoyance of the organ transplanters. What caught her attention most was that all of them were Hispanic. In her words, "I've never seen an Anglo kid recover from such an injury. And do you know what the difference is? When a Hispanic kid is in coma like that, the whole family is around the bed day and night, talking to him, praying for him, *loving* him. The Anglo kids are there all by themselves, unconscious children in beds in intensive care, all alone."

We are not meant to be all alone. We are meant to be parts of bigger families, bands, tribes. Don't settle for nuclear family contraction. Extend!

4. Connecting with Community

Community is the sense of living and working together for common goals. We are naturally communal beings and derive great satisfaction from the experience of belonging to a group with a common purpose. Our society often fails to provide for this need, so unless we work to create community, it does not happen. You can define community any way you want. It may be your neighborhood, your sports team, your environmental action group, your church, your social club. What makes it work is what you bring to it and the role you let it play in your life. The strength and comfort of community come from the principle that the whole is greater than the sum of its parts. This kind of connectedness gives us power to improve our lives and make the world a better place.

5. Serving

Many religious traditions extol the ideal of selfless service as one of the great aids to dismantling the ego cage and restructuring personality. Selfless service means giving of yourself to help others with no thought of return. You do not have to go off to a leper colony in Africa to do this kind of work, but you have to do something more than write out a check to your favorite charity. There are countless opportunities each day to practice putting others' interests ahead of your own, to give of your time, energy, and presence to reduce the suffering or increase the happiness of others. The goal is not to acquire spiritual merit, increase your chances of going to heaven, or earn the admiration of the community. You do service as a way of acknowledging that we are all one and that the happiness of each is connected to the happiness of all. The more you can experience the interconnectedness of all beings, the healthier you will be.

6. Loving

To love is to experience connection in its highest, purest form, but oh, how we abuse the word *love,* how we confuse loving with other feelings that take us back into the world of separateness and fragmentation.

Recently I read an unusual newspaper article on sexual addiction. It talked about the pitfall of confusing sex with love and came to what I thought was an insightful conclusion: "Sex is not romance, romance is not love, and love is not sex."

Popular songs today seem to be mostly about love, not about loving as connection, but about the joys and pains of romantic love, which is something altogether different. Romance is the exciting adventure of becoming involved with another person and the terrific high that comes with the early phase of that involvement. Falling in love or being in love is as much a drug as any that people swallow, snort, smoke, or shoot. Just as with drugs, the high of falling in love does not last. It *always* ends, and the grief of ending is as intense as the joy of beginning. Weil's Law of Romantic Love states that

$$J + P = 0,$$

where J is the joy of romantic involvement and P is the pain of its ending. In other words, however high you get from the joyful phase of romance, the grief that follows will always bring you down to where you started.

Our culture glorifies the J state and has little to say about the inevitability or meaning of P. Many people go from one falling-in-love state to another in an addictive pattern, never learning the lesson of their experience.

I cannot recommend too highly a short book on this subject written by a Jungian analyst. Robert Johnson's *We: Understanding the Psychology of Romantic Love* (New York: Harper & Row, 1983) uses the myth of Tristan and Isolde to analyze the in-love state and contrast it to loving. One of his main points is that falling in love is based on projection. We project onto the other person some part of ourself, an idealized image of the perfect love object that we carry around in our psyche. Being in love is a trick done with mirrors, since the real source of our joy is internal, not external. When the projective magic breaks down, as it must sooner or later, we all know the shock and pain of discovering that the person we thought so lovely is really just an ordinary person with all the usual faults and blemishes. Then comes grief over the loss of what we thought was the source of all our bliss. This is the same kind of trick we use to fool ourselves into thinking that highs come from drugs and satisfaction from food.

Loving is not a trick, and it does not end. To love means to contact the source of love within yourself and let it shine outward, unconditionally, with no thought of return. To love another person is to experience connection, to accept that person as he or she is, to give the blessing of your warmth and light without any expectations. That kind of love is ultimately nourishing and transformative to the giver as well as the receiver. (In the words of Saint Francis, "Lord, grant that I may not so much seek . . . to be loved as to love.") Many of us have never experienced this kind of love. We have mostly received conditional love: I will love you IF . . . (if you love me, if you behave, if you keep your distance, if you don't make trouble, if you make me feel important, etc., etc.). That is not the way of true love.

Learning to love takes practice and time, especially in a culture that is focused so intensely on romantic love. We have all been conditioned to believe that if we meet Mr. Right or Ms. Perfect, bells will ring, our hearts will skip beats, the world will change in a flash, and we will live happily ever after, even though we never see living examples of such happiness.

In intimate relationships that work, the in-love state is replaced by mutual loving. That can happen only if both partners are mature and committed to a life together. Many people today have no idea what to do when they fall out of love with their partners; they think it means there is no possibility of continuing in relationship, which is why divorce rates are now so high.

Realizing that you have within you a limitless source of love that can benefit everyone and everything will help you form the best and strongest connections of your life.

7. Touching

Human beings need to touch and be touched. A great deal of animal and human research shows that individuals deprived of physical contact are insecure, poorly adjusted, and more prone to illness. Some cross-cultural research suggests that sexually repressed and touch-deprived societies are much more given to violence. Our own society, unfortunately, is in that category.

Of course, sex is only one kind of touching. An aspect of our sexual repression is great confusion about the connotations of touching. Many of us think that touch implies sexual interest or expectation, which leads us to avoid it or to find ourselves in sexual encounters when what we really want is to be held, rubbed, and stroked. Loving touch is a wonderful, comforting, healing form of connection. To take advantage of it, you must learn to decondition its associations with sex.

It is hard to see how deprived we are in this culture until you step away from it and spend time with people who have healthier attitudes about touching each other. For a number of years I traveled in remote areas of Latin America, collecting information about medicinal plants and traditional methods of healing. Whenever I arrived in an Indian village in the Colombian Amazon, people would stare in amazement at my bald head and beard and without any self-consciousness begin rubbing my head and twining their fingers in my beard. I remember being uncomfortable in Cambodia thirty years ago when men I had just met would put their arms around my waist while we walked and talked. I would not be uncomfortable with that now. I do not hug all my patients yet, but I hug a lot of them, and I certainly hug all my friends as often as possible.

Touching is an easy connection to make because it feels so good. Please do more of it.

8. Connecting to a Higher Power

One reason the twelve-step programs work as treatments for addiction is that they encourage connection to a power greater than yourself. I do not think it matters much how you conceive of that higher power; what matters is the sense of connection to it. It can be the father-god of the Old Testament, Jesus Christ, the Compassionate Buddha, the Great Spirit, the Goddess, pure, undifferentiated Consciousness, or simply the Mystery. You are free to choose the way you conceive of the universe and your place in it. People who experience themselves as part of and supported by something larger than themselves are less fearful and more healthy than people who view the world through the bars of an ego cage, seeing the world as separate from them, disconnected.

SUGGESTED READING

Chop Wood, Carry Water by Rick Fields, with Peggy Taylor, Rex Weyler, and Rick Ingrasci (New York: St. Martin's Press, 1984) is an excellent resource book for those interested in personal growth and development and in learning to extend connections.

A Book for Couples by Hugh and Gayle Prather (New York: Doubleday, 1988) deals with the rewards and problems of intimate relationships.

Grist for the Mill by Ram Dass and Stephen Levine (Berkeley, Calif.: Celestial Arts, 1987) is a wonderful book about spirituality and our place in the universe.

Healing into Life and Death by Stephen Levine (New York: Anchor Books, 1987) is about love, life, dying, and the essence of human experience.

PART II

SPECIFIC PREVENTION:
OUTWITTING THE
KILLERS

9

HOW NOT TO GET
A HEART ATTACK

CORONARY HEART DISEASE is under strong genetic control, especially in men. If you are a man and have male blood relatives (father, grandfather, uncles, brothers) who have had heart attacks before the age of sixty, you have bad cardiac heredity. You can't do anything about that, but you can work to prevent the genetic potential from expressing itself. Heredity is only one risk factor for a heart attack. There are a number of other factors, all having to do with lifestyle. If your lifestyle includes these risks, I urge you to make changes whether or not you have a history of heart disease in your family.

If you are a woman, your female hormones protect you from coronary heart disease up to menopause. Thereafter, your risk increases sharply. It can be reduced by taking synthetic estrogen and progesterone, but there are arguments against using these powerful substances at all (see pp. 172–173 and 313–315). Whether you are male or female, it is worth starting at a young age to build good habits of eating, exercise, and relaxation that strengthen the coronary arteries and protect them from harm.

Another inherited factor that can contribute to coronary heart disease is diabetes. In diabetics atherosclerosis often develops more quickly along with the problems that follow from it, including early heart attacks. If you are diabetic, it is even more important that you follow the prescriptions in this book regarding diet, exercise, and stress reduction.

1. Keep Your Serum Cholesterol Low

The most important predictor of a heart attack is high serum cholesterol, because it leads to the deposition of cholesterol in the walls of
the coronary arteries, a condition known as atherosclerosis. As the
arteries become narrowed and roughened by this process, blood
supply to the heart is reduced, and it becomes more likely that an
artery will be completely blocked by a blood clot. Such blockages
cause the death of a portion of heart muscle, and that is a heart
attack.

Most people can lower their serum cholesterol dramatically by
following the suggestions given in Chapter 1 (especially the section
on fats, beginning on p. 14) and Chapter 2 (pp. 43–46). Cholesterol-
lowering drugs can be toxic and, in my opinion, should not be taken
unless other measures fail or you have a rare inherited disorder that
keeps your cholesterol level high independent of diet. Even moderate
and advanced atherosclerosis can be halted and reversed without
drug treatment if you make the dietary changes I recommend and
follow the other guidelines in this chapter.

2. Do Not Smoke

Tobacco addiction impacts the heart and arteries in many different
ways. Nicotine constricts arteries throughout the body, interfering
with blood circulation and raising blood pressure. Smoking reduces
the blood's capacity to carry oxygen and may increase its clotting
tendency. Nicotine directly stimulates the heart through its action
on the nervous system, adding to the heart's workload. It stimulates
the sympathetic nervous system, increasing the likelihood of arrhythmias (irregular heartbeats) and coronary artery spasms, which
can also precipitate heart attacks. Tobacco smoking definitely increases the risk of coronary heart disease and heart attack. So does
living and working with smokers, because you breathe the smoke
second hand. Remember that smoke from the end of a burning
cigarette contains more toxins than smoke inhaled through a cylin-
der of tobacco.

3. Do Not Use Caffeine Addictively

Caffeine addiction is unhealthy for the heart and arteries. It adds to the workload of the heart and increases sympathetic tone and adrenal activity, making arrhythmias more likely. It is an obstacle to relaxation and may contribute to elevated serum cholesterol. If you want to take caffeine, especially coffee, as a stimulant, do so consciously, purposefully, and occasionally rather than unconsciously and habitually.

4. Exercise Aerobically

Follow the guidelines for aerobic exercise in Chapter 5. An average of thirty minutes of aerobic activity five days a week will improve the efficiency of the heart as a pump, tone the entire arterial system, reduce serum cholesterol, reduce the chance of abnormal blood clotting, and help balance the activity of the autonomic nervous system (decreasing the risks of arrhythmia and coronary artery spasm). This kind of conditioning can also increase collateral circulation in the heart muscle so that if a blockage does occur in a coronary artery, blood can find alternate routes around it. Less heart muscle will be lost than in a heart unconditioned by exercise. People in good aerobic condition are more likely than others to survive heart attacks and to recover fully from them.

5. Practice Relaxation Techniques

Internalized stress can precipitate heart attacks through various mechanisms. It can increase serum cholesterol and blood clotting. It can step up the activity of the adrenal glands and sympathetic nervous system, thereby causing the heart to work harder and increasing the risk of arrhythmias and coronary artery spasm.

This last point needs more explanation. When a person dies of a heart attack, which can happen within seconds or minutes, the mechanism of death is usually ventricular fibrillation, a chaotic, disorganized beat that fails to deliver oxygenated blood to the brain. What determines whether or not the death of a portion of heart muscle from a blocked coronary artery sends the whole heart into this fatal arrhythmia? Apparently the state of the autonomic nervous system at the time of the blockage is a critical factor. In particular, if the sympathetic division of this system is dominant, it sensitizes heart muscle in a way that makes ventricular fibrillation more likely. The sympathetic influence is opposed by the parasympathetic division, whose relaxing influence extends to the heart. If parasympathetic nervous activity is dominant, the heart is protected from fibrillation, even if the blockage is major and a large portion of muscle dies.

Furthermore, in some deaths resulting from heart attacks, autopsies fail to demonstrate complete blockage of a coronary artery. The assumption is that an artery has gone into spasm, causing a functional blockage. This kind of disaster can also be brought on by overactivity of sympathetic nerves and excessive adrenal stimulation. Learning to reduce the dominance of the sympathetic division and the activity of the adrenal glands by any of the methods described in Chapter 6 can protect the heart from the damaging effects of stress. Relaxation reduces the risk of heart attack and reduces the risk of sudden death should a heart attack occur.

6. Maintain Normal Weight

Obesity increases the heart's workload and discourages people from doing aerobic exercise. It also predisposes adults to the development of diabetes, which can accelerate the progression of atherosclerosis. Keep your weight within 20 percent of the normal figure for your height, sex, and build.

7. Maintain Normal Blood Pressure

High blood pressure (hypertension) stresses the arterial system, increases the workload on the heart, may accelerate the development of atherosclerosis, and is often associated with increased activity of the sympathetic nervous system and adrenal glands. Most cases of mild to moderate hypertension can be managed without drugs by making changes in lifestyle as suggested in this chapter. I discuss the treatment of hypertension in Part IV (pp. 301–302).

8. "Thin" Your Blood

Formation of blood clots on arterial walls that are narrowed and roughened by atherosclerosis is the immediate cause of most heart attacks. The first step in this process is the clumping together of blood platelets. Blood "thinners" are substances, usually drugs, that reduce the clotting tendency, often by making platelets less likely to clump.

The best-known substance of this class is aspirin, and you have no doubt heard reports of the value of aspirin in preventing heart attacks. In fact, the medical profession is so enthusiastic about this new use of an old drug that most doctors are urging middle-aged men to take one baby aspirin a day or one every other day. But this therapy involves some risk. If you are willing to modify your patterns of eating, exercising, relaxing, and relating to the world, you may not need aspirin. I would urge aspirin on people who are unwilling to make the changes in lifestyle described here.

One of the risks of thinning the blood, logically, is increased possibility of hemorrhage, especially of a stroke due to hemorrhage in the brain. Many men who take aspirin to prevent heart attacks report that when they cut themselves shaving, they have trouble stopping the bleeding. So any sort of leak from a blood vessel inside the body will also take longer to stop. A friend and colleague of mine, an internist in his early fifties, suffered a serious intracranial bleed while in excellent health. He was an avid jogger and health enthusiast who ate carefully, meditated, and had no risk factors for hemorrhage except that he was taking an aspirin once a day to prevent heart attack. Intracranial bleeding is a medical disaster that can cause permanent neurological damage.

Aspirin is also a harsh irritant of the lining of the stomach. Be sure to use only enteric-coated aspirin if you have ulcers, gastritis, or other disorder of the upper GI tract. Aspirin's actions on the rest of the body are many and varied. If you decide to use it to reduce the risk of heart attack, I recommend taking a low dose daily, less than the 300 milligrams of a standard tablet. Enteric-coated, low-dose tablets are available at drugstores.

You should know that natural methods of thinning the blood also exist. One is to include in the diet omega-3 fatty acids from oily fish (see p. 46) or from linseed oil (p. 24). The principal benefit to the heart of the omega-3's may be their effect on blood clotting rather than on serum cholesterol. Research on this point is not clear, but it is clear that populations eating the fish sources of these unusual oils have lower than expected rates of heart attacks.

Raw garlic and raw onions, eaten regularly, decrease the clotting tendency and increase the body's ability to dissolve clots. The mechanism of these actions is not yet known.

Another possible preventive measure is vitamin E. In addition to its antioxidant properties (see p. 186), it is a natural blood thinner. I recommend a daily dose of 400 IU (international units) for adults under the age of forty and 800 IU for those above that age. If you take your vitamin E capsule with a meal that has some fat content, it will be absorbed better from the GI tract, because it is one of the fat-soluble vitamins. I have not seen any toxicity from vitamin E.

Yet another blood thinner is a Chinese mushroom, the tree ear, wood ear, *mo-er*, or ear fungus, all names for *Auricularia polytricha*, a rubbery, dark-brown species that is cultivated on logs. A common ingredient of Chinese soups and stir-fries, it has a distinctive crunchy texture and almost no taste. Chinese herbalists have long regarded it as a medicinal food, but its anticoagulant effect was discovered only recently by a researcher at the University of Minnesota and then by accident. He found that his own blood platelets were less likely to clump after he ate a particular Chinese dish and he was able to trace the change to this one ingredient. You can buy dried tree ears at any Chinese grocery store. To use them, pour boiling water over a small amount, let them expand (they will do so enormously) and become soft, then drain them, pick off any hard bits, and cut them in strips or pieces to add to your favorite soup or stir-fry. A tablespoon of the soaked mushroom eaten three or four times a week may give you the benefits of aspirin without risk of hemorrhage and certainly with much less irritation to your digestive system.

9. Open Your Heart

People throughout the world associate the heart with emotions. We talk about heartthrobs, heartaches, broken hearts. This is not a chance association. The physical heart responds strongly to emotional storms, because it is so intimately connected to the autonomic nervous system. Many researchers have tried to identify personality types that are most at risk for heart attacks. The pictures that emerge from these efforts are of people who are driven, unable to relax, unable to control anger, given to fits of rage when frustrated, unable to give and receive love in a nurturing way.

In yoga physiology the heart region is one of the seven great centers *(chakras)* that organize the flow of energy around the body. The fourth, or heart, chakra participates in emotional connections to other people and the world beyond the self. Since the three lower chakras have to do with survival, sex, and power, the heart chakra is the first of the centers concerned with "higher" matters, with altruism, for example, and with love. If energy is blocked at this level through failure to open the heart, it cannot reach and activate the fifth, sixth, and seventh chakras, which control higher spiritual development. In this sense, blocked hearts and heart attacks mirror our emotional life and our ability to manage our feelings.

I do not want to belabor this point, but I do urge you to look at emotional blockage as another risk factor for heart attack, one that, like diet, can be modified. If you are given to uncontrollable anger and fits of rage, you can certainly learn control. I recommend meditation practice and breath work as two techniques to help you. If you are unaware of your feelings altogether or unable to express them, you might try psychotherapy. Read the advice in Chapter 8, "Connections," about ways to overcome the kinds of emotional blockages that may favor development of physical blockages in the coronary arteries.

SUGGESTED READING

Dr. Dean Ornish's Program for Reversing Heart Disease by Dean Ornish, M.D. (New York: Random House, 1990) is an excellent discussion of the prevention and treatment of atherosclerosis by lifestyle modification. The author is the first doctor to demonstrate conclusively that atherosclerosis can be reversed.

10

HOW NOT TO GET
A STROKE

THE TECHNICAL TERM for stroke is "cerebrovascular accident" or "CVA," meaning an accident in a blood vessel in the brain. The two general types are hemorrhages and occlusions (blockages), both of which interrupt blood supply to a portion of the brain, causing the death of nerve cells.

This will be a short chapter because you already know most of what I'm going to say. You avoid strokes in much the same way that you avoid heart attacks: by eating a heart-healthy diet, exercising, practicing relaxation, avoiding high blood pressure, and not smoking. I'll add a few details to that information, but in general, if you follow the preventive advice given in this book so far, you will greatly reduce your risk of having a cerebrovascular accident.

Hemorrhagic strokes are relatively rare in the Western world. The factors that promote them include congenital malformations of arteries in the brain, high blood pressure, and impairment of the clotting mechanisms of the blood. You cannot do anything about congenital arterial malformations, but they are not common. High blood pressure is common, and you can do a lot about it (see the entry on hypertension in Part IV, pp. 301–302). Problems of blood clotting are due mostly to medical drugs (anticoagulants or blood thinners), including aspirin. If you take any type of blood-thinning medication, it is important to have your clotting time checked periodically to make sure it is not dangerously long.

Occlusive strokes are of two types, depending on whether the obstruction is caused by a blood clot that has formed at the site (a thrombus) or one that has formed somewhere else and traveled to the site (an embolus). Thrombotic strokes are the commonest kind, and the usual cause is the same atherosclerosis that damages coronary arteries. When cholesterol deposits narrow major arteries in the head and neck, and calcification and scarring roughen the artery walls, blood clots are more likely to form. If a clot occludes an artery completely, it may cause the death of brain tissue. Risk factors for thrombotic strokes include diabetes, high serum cholesterol, lack of exercise, smoking, and high blood pressure. That list should sound familiar. Anything that increases the clotting tendency of the blood also increases risk. Cigarettes and birth control pills both do that, and they do it even more when both are used. Women who smoke should not use birth control pills because of the danger of blood clots.

An embolic stroke usually results from a blood clot that forms on the wall of a chamber of the heart, then breaks off and travels up to the head, where it occludes an artery supplying blood to the brain. The two commonest causes of these dangerous clots are chronic atrial fibrillation and heart attack. In atrial fibrillation the upper chambers of the heart beat irregularly. This does not interfere much with the pumping dynamics of the heart, and were it not for the danger of embolism, you could live with this condition without concern. Usually doctors prescribe blood thinners to people with atrial fibrillation to prevent that possibility. The two commonest causes of atrial fibrillation are rheumatic heart disease and coronary heart disease. You already know how to prevent coronary heart disease. Rheumatic fever is an autoimmune disorder triggered by strep throat in genetically susceptible people; it damages heart valves and can be prevented by the use of penicillin

The other major cause of embolic stroke is heart attacks that damage the inner walls of the heart chambers. Clots can form on the damaged surfaces of those walls, then break off and embolize to the head. The previous chapter tells you how to prevent heart attacks.

I said that this would be a short chapter, and I meant it. Before I close, I would like to emphasize once again that diseases of the heart and blood vessels, principally coronary heart disease and stroke, have been major killers in our society. Although we all have to die of something, we do not have to die prematurely because our arteries are clogged, scarred, and inelastic. Except in the very old, most cardiovascular problems are diseases of lifestyle, not inevitable fate, and you can greatly lower your risk of getting them by modifying your lifestyle in the directions suggested in these pages.

11

HOW NOT TO GET
CANCER

CANCER OFTEN RUNS in families, but what is inherited is a predisposition to the disease, not cancer itself. For the predisposition to express itself, other risk factors have to be present. For example, cancer of the colon, one of the major killers in our society, sometimes runs in families, but it also correlates with diet, particularly with high consumption of fat, animal protein, and refined starch and low consumption of vegetables and fiber. Most cancers of the colon arise in polyps — benign, mushroomlike growths that push out from the intestinal wall. Some people develop polyps repeatedly, while others never do. Recent research suggests that polyp formation is genetically controlled. If you have not inherited the gene for polyp formation, your chance of ever getting colon cancer may be zero. If you do have this gene, your risk may depend on what you eat. Cells of the tissue covering polyps are unstable and tend to turn malignant, but the bacterial and chemical environment of the colon may promote or retard that tendency. The colon chemistry of people on high-fat, high-protein, low-fiber diets is very different from the colon chemistry of those on low-fat, low-protein, high-fiber diets.

Similarly, breast cancer shows a familial pattern. If you are a woman whose mother and mother's sisters have had breast cancer, your risks of the disease are increased. What is inherited here is not known, but again, environmental factors must interact with it.

Whether you are male or female, if there is cancer in your family, you are at increased risk. If there is cancer on both sides of your family, your risk is even greater. That does not mean you will get cancer. It does mean you should pay attention to the information in this chapter and put it into action in your life.

1. If You Are a Woman . . .

You should be aware that high levels of female sex hormones — estrogens — in your blood favor the development of cancers of the breast and reproductive system, because estrogens stimulate cells of these tissues to divide and proliferate. You can lower your estrogen level and reduce your risk by having a baby before the age of thirty-five, by maintaining normal weight, by doing regular aerobic exercise, by following a low-fat, mostly vegetarian diet, and by minimizing or avoiding consumption of alcohol. A diet that includes a lot of meat, poultry, and dairy products may be dangerous because these foods often carry residues of estrogenic hormones used to promote growth in animals raised for the table.

Recent research implicates a large number of chemical toxins, including common pesticides and industrial pollutants, as "xenoestrogens" (the prefix *xeno-* means "foreign") that increase estrogenic pressure on women. It argues for even greater caution in minimizing intake of toxins (see pp. 179–183). Some protection may be offered by eating foods derived from soybeans, which contain phytoestrogens ("plant estrogens") that may prevent xenoestrogens from occupying hormone receptors on breast tissue. The low incidence of breast cancer among Asian women could be due to their high intake of soy foods.

More obvious sources of estrogens are birth control pills and the hormone replacements given at menopause. Birth control pills on the market today are safer than those used a decade ago. Still, I never prescribe them and often take women off them because of toxic effects. In addition to their immediate toxicity is the real possibility that they increase the risks of cancer. I recommend against using oral contraceptive pills if you are in any of these groups:

Have a family history of breast cancer
Have a history of fibrocystic (benign) breast disease
Did not have a first child until after the age of thirty-five

Are over forty-five and still menstruating
Are at increased risk of cervical cancer because of a history of
multiple sexual partners

Estrogen replacement therapy at menopause is safer today than it was in the recent past. The doses are lower now, and they are combined with progesterone, another female hormone that offsets the stimulating effect of estrogen. Women today are under great pressure from doctors and pharmaceutical companies to take this hormonal combination at the onset of menopause and to stay on it. I give other suggestions for managing menopausal symptoms in the entry on menopause in Part IV. Here I will simply state my strong opinion that *you should avoid estrogen replacement altogether if you are at increased risk of cancer for any reason,* including a family history of cancer of the breast or reproductive system. If you do decide to take replacement therapy, use low doses of estrogen (1.25 milligrams a day maximum) and never take it without progesterone for at least part of the monthly cycle.

2. Stay in Good General Health

Of course, you want to stay in good general health or you wouldn't be reading this book, but there is a particular reason for doing so if you are at increased risk for cancer. We know of many factors that promote cancer — types of radiation, chemicals, viruses, physical irritants, genes, and so forth — but we do not yet know exactly how they act. The final common pathway seems to be mutation, some permanent, heritable change in DNA giving rise to a colony of cells that ignore their relationship to the rest of the body, do not die on schedule at the end of their normal cycle of activity, and escape the usual controls on growth. Research suggests that mutations can activate tumor genes that lie dormant in our DNA, can knock out regulatory genes that protect against tumors, or cause trouble in a number of other ways.

The important point is that mutations in DNA, even if they give rise to malignant cells, do not mean you get cancer. Malignant transformation of cells probably occurs all the time, given the number of cells in our bodies (300 trillion), the number that die and are replaced every second of every day (10 million!), and the many mutagenic agents known to exist in our bodies and in the environment. The body recognizes and eliminates these abnormal cells most of the time; that is one of the functions of the immune system. For such a cell to persist and give rise to a detectable tumor, a failure of immunity must occur, a failure of the body's defense system. The best way to keep your defenses in good working order is to stay in good general health.

3. Avoid Exposure to Harmful Radiation

Ionizing radiation, the kind that is energetic enough to knock electrons out of their orbits, can damage DNA, causing mutations that can lead to cancer. X rays and nuclear radiation are of this sort, and they are very dangerous. Doctors and government officials have been slow to recognize the dangers of radiation. They often try to assure us that we have nothing to worry about, when in fact we have plenty to worry about.

Radioactivity was discovered less than a century ago, and at first its dangers were not recognized. In fact, people tried to exploit it as a health enhancer. I once came across (in a museum of medical curiosities) a device from about 1910: a belt to be worn about the waist with two pouches that fit over the area of the kidneys. These were filled with radium ore and were designed to deliver "healthful radiation" to the kidneys to improve their function.

If that seems unbelievable, consider that when I was growing up in Philadelphia in the 1940s and 1950s, shoe stores had fluoroscopes to check the fit of new shoes. My friends and I used to spend as much time as we could with our feet in the fluoroscope, delighted to watch images of our bones on the glowing green screen. We would stay there as the salesman looked, too, then we'd have our parents look. That was not so long ago. Many people today are as unconcerned about medical X rays and radioactive materials as we were about fluoroscopes in shoe stores.

Ionizing radiation selectively damages dividing cells. Tissues with the highest rates of cell division are the skin and the epithelium that forms the outer surfaces of internal organs as well as the linings of all hollow organs (like the colon) and glandular ducts. Since surfaces and linings bear the brunt of environmental stress, they must constantly renew themselves. When cells divide, their DNA uncoils so that its genetic information can be copied. In its expanded state, DNA is most susceptible to injury, not only from radiation but also from mutagenic chemicals and from random accidents in the cell division process. It is not surprising that most cancers arise from epithelial cells. The other parts of the body with very high rates of cell division are the tissues of the blood-forming and immune systems, especially the bone marrow. These, too, are very susceptible to cancerous growth.

Radiation is a double threat, then. Not only does it lead to cancer by causing malignant transformation of cells, it also damages the immune system, weakening our defenses against malignancy. Yet both of these effects may take a long time to show up, which is one reason why people have been slow to notice that radiation causes cancer and have been complacent about its hazards. Radiation hazards may be hard to avoid. Besides the obvious threat from nuclear weapons and nuclear waste, radiation sources occur in many manufactured products, from smoke alarms to electronic instruments. Often consumers have no idea they are receiving radiation from these products, since manufacturers do not warn them and sometimes even withhold the information. How many people know that the porcelain jackets used by dentists to repair damaged teeth often contain radioactive minerals added only to improve the resemblance to natural enamel? These minerals can bombard the epithelial tissue of the mouth with radiation capable of inducing malignant transformation. In most instances, unless some public outcry forces government action, the regulatory agencies set up to protect public health will do nothing about these problems and will contine to safeguard the manufacturers' rights to sell their wares. In addition to taking political action, you can protect yourself by following these recommendations:

• *There is no such thing as a safe dose of radiation.* Your risk of genetic and immune system damage correlates with the total amount of radiation you have received over your lifetime, and any amount, however small, adds to that cumulative total and risk. *Never believe anyone who tells you that the amount of radiation coming at you from any source is too small to matter.*

• *Do not let doctors and dentists X-ray you without good reason.* Medical and dental X-ray and fluoroscopic examinations are invaluable diagnostic tools. They are also greatly overused. Radiologists often minimize the hazards and fail to inform patients of them. Radiologists also have a shorter life expectancy than other doctors and a higher incidence of cancers known to be induced by radiation. If X-ray equipment is faulty or inadequately shielded, the risk to the patient and to other people in the vicinity is increased.

Do not agree to X rays unless the doctor can make you understand why they are necessary. Never agree to repeat X rays just for legal or insurance purposes. Do not let dentists X-ray your teeth just because they want to. Dental X rays are helpful in looking for causes of specific symptoms. In the absence of past problems and present symptoms, with good preventive care of the teeth, there is no need for them except at infrequent intervals such as every two years. Chiropractors are often reckless in their use of X rays, taking unnecessarily large and frequent films of the spine. Not long ago, dermatologists liked to treat acne with X rays. Do not submit to radiation therapy without good reason.

Mammograms for early detection of breast cancer are a special case. The benefits probably outweigh the dangers in women at risk for this disease, especially for women of fifty and older, assuming the equipment delivers low-dose radiation (in the range of one rad, or 1,000 millirads). Do not submit to mammography unless your doctor or technician can assure you that new, low-dose techniques are being used and can tell you how many millirads of radiation you will receive to the center of your breast.

• *Do not live near a source of natural or man-made radiation.* Some places on the earth have high background radiation from natural sources, such as uranium deposits near the surface. Groundwater in these places may carry dissolved radioactive minerals. This is one reason to get a water filter for your home, not an activated carbon type but one that removes heavy metals and minerals (see Chapter 3.) The higher the altitude you live at, the greater your exposure to cosmic radiation, since there is less atmosphere to absorb it.

Most of us are in greater danger from man-made sources of radiation than from natural ones. Do not live near a nuclear power plant or nuclear waste disposal site or tailings from a uranium mine. Do not stay in the area if radioactive material is accidentally spilled near your place of residence.

Finally, beware of spokesmen for industry and government who try to ease your fears of the dangers of these sources of radiation. In the 1950s tailings from uranium mining and milling were used in the foundations of homes and schools in Grand Junction, Colorado, and other towns in the Rockies. The public was kept in quiet ignorance until twenty years after the fact and is still being told there is no cause for concern.

• *Do not suffer occupational exposure to radiation.* If you are a uranium miner, a worker in a nuclear power plant, a radiologist, radiology technician, or handler of radioactive materials, or if you do any other work that exposes you to ionizing radiation, your chances of getting cancer are increased. If you are also at high risk for other reasons (such as a family history of cancer) you should find a safer job.

If you cannot find safer work, or until you do so, put more effort into following the other recommendations in this chapter. Also do whatever you can to minimize your on-the-job exposure by modifying your routines and being conscientious about the use of protective clothing, shielding, and decontamination techniques. Do not put too much faith in the badges issued to you that are supposed to monitor your exposure to radiation; often they are inaccurate.

• *Inform yourself about radiation hazards of manufactured products and take appropriate precautions.* Radioactive materials are used in many familiar products, including luminous dials of instruments and watches, antistatic devices for cleaning records and photographic equipment, smoke detectors, some eyeglasses, some false teeth and dental porcelains, and some chinaware. Some of the books listed at the end of this chapter have information on this subject. If you feel you are at low risk for cancer, you may not care to worry about these sources of radiation. If you are at high risk, you should think about eliminating them from your life or minimizing your contact with them.

• *If you live in an area where radon gas is a problem, make sure your home does not have dangerous levels of it.* Radon is an invisible, odorless, radioactive gas, a natural element that seeps out of the earth and can enter basements of homes through cracks and pipes.

It is the second leading cause of lung cancer after smoking and may account for as many as 20,000 deaths each year in the United States alone. Health officials and government have been slow to acknowledge this danger, partly because there is no obvious remedy for it.

At this writing, the areas of the country where radon is worst are the eastern seaboard of the middle Atlantic states and specific regions of the Northwest, Rocky Mountains, and Southwest. You can find out whether radon is a problem in your area by calling your local health department and the regional office of the Environmental Protection Agency. If you are in a problem area, you should have your house tested for radon. The EPA can recommend contractors to do the testing or distributors of home testing equipment. You can also purchase inexpensive home testing devices, but their accuracy may be questionable. (See *Consumer Reports*, July 1987, for a review of radon-testing devices, or get this information from the EPA.)

If you find that radon is accumulating in your house, you can install ventilation systems to remove it, at least in part. The EPA can tell you about both simple and complicated systems to deal with the problem. If they seem too complicated or expensive to install or if they fail to lower the radon level sufficiently, you ought to consider moving.

4. Protect Your Skin from Ultraviolet (Tanning) Radiation

Ultraviolet light (UV) is not ionizing radiation, but it will damage DNA in cells of the skin. Unless you are black or otherwise darkly pigmented, radiation from the sun and from sun lamps can give you skin cancer. (It can also accelerate aging of the skin.) Tanning is the skin's protective reaction to minimize this possibility, not a sign of health. In tanning, certain cells in the skin become more active, producing a dark pigment (melanin) that absorbs UV radiation. People wrongly consider suntans a sign of well-being, because they associate them with healthful outdoor activity. It is exercise, fresh air, relaxation, and fun that promote health, not UV radiation.

Of course it feels good to be out in the sun on a fine day. I do not agree with some vocal doctors who try to make us feel that *any* sun exposure is bad. I do urge you to be aware that at some times of day, at some times of year, and at some places on the earth, sunlight is very dangerous. When the sun is at a high angle in the sky (around the middle of the day, nearer to the summer solstice, closer to the equator), and at higher altitudes, its rays follow shorter paths through the earth's atmosphere, and fewer of the harmful wavelengths are filtered out. Furthermore, it is possible that UV light reaching the earth is becoming more intense as a result of damage to the atmosphere's protective ozone layer by pollutants. If you are fair-skinned, you must remember to protect yourself in those circumstances. Red-haired, fair-skinned people have the least protective pigment and so are at greatest risk.

The best protection is clothing, including a wide-brimmed hat. Highly effective sunscreens are also available everywhere. If you cannot cover up, use a sunscreen on exposed areas of the body, especially on the head and face. Use a sunscreen with the highest SPF rating you can find, and read the label to make sure it blocks both UVA and UVB.

Don't forget your ears, bald spots on the head, and the skin over the cheekbones and nose; skin cancers occur there with greatest frequency.

If you tan easily and must spend time in the sun, acquire your tan gradually and still use protection. Be especially careful on beaches, in or on the water, and near other reflective surfaces, as well as at high altitudes, where cold air temperatures may deceive you about the burning strength of the sun.

• *Avoid tanning parlors.* The popularity of tanning parlors is an indication of widespread ignorance about this matter. The ultraviolet radiation used in them is not safe, no matter what their advertisements say. Most skin cancer is related to UV radiation. Don't expose yourself unnecessarily in tanning parlors or anywhere else.

5. Avoid Exposure to Harmful Chemicals

We have heard so much about cancer-causing chemicals in recent years that many people have stopped listening. They are tired of hearing about saccharin, sassafras, red dye no. 2, tobacco, dioxin, PCBs, and all the other items on the list of suspects. Some people shrug it off by saying, "Everything gives laboratory mice cancer," or "Why worry about what you do or don't get exposed to? It all causes cancer."

In fact, it does not all cause cancer. Only a small percentage of known substances are carcinogenic, and many of them fall into distinct chemical families. In general, any chemical capable of causing mutations is likely to increase the risk of cancer. Since DNA is the same in all forms of life, scientists screen chemicals for mutagenic activity by testing them on bacteria. The reproductive cycles of bacteria are so much faster than those of animals that mutations can be spotted without waiting for years. Unfortunately, a number of industrial chemicals now in widespread use give positive results in the tests.

Chemical carcinogens are probably responsible for more cancer than radiation is. They are also identifiable and often avoidable. As with radiation, no level of exposure to these substances can be considered safe. Any exposure might initiate the process of malignant transformation or promote one that has already begun. Also, *every* exposure adds to the burden on the body's systems of defense against malignancy. Breakdown of those defenses is the crucial event in the development of cancer.

We do not yet know all the details of chemical carcinogenesis. Some compounds interact with DNA directly, causing mutations and starting cells on the road to malignant transformation. Coal tar and tobacco smoke contain many of these compounds. Others, called cocarcinogens or promoters, do not initiate malignant transformation themselves but potentiate the activity of substances that do; asbestos is an example.

One of the difficulties in specifying the exact harmfulness of any of these substances is the long interval between exposure and first appearance of cancer. Five to thirty years may elapse between those events, obscuring the connection between them. Apparently chemical carcinogenesis takes place in two steps. The first, called initiation, is rapid alteration of DNA. The second, called promotion, allows the genetic change (mutation) to express itself as malignant transformation. Promotion requires repeated exposure over time to the same initiating carcinogen or to any of the cocarcinogens that enhance its activity. Without promotion, one-time exposure to a carcinogenic chemical will not result in cancer even if DNA is altered.

Here are some guidelines about hazardous chemicals:

• *Be wary of all the chemicals in your life.* Even when chemicals do not directly cause cancer, they may do so indirectly by adding to the cumulative stress on our immune systems. The liver bears most of the burden of metabolizing and detoxifying unwanted substances that enter the body. Although the liver is not part of the immune system, it is closely allied with and protective of it. When the liver fails, as in alcoholism, the organs of the immune system become more susceptible to damage and their function declines.

In the twentieth century our livers are sorely taxed. Not only do they have to deal with all the naturally occurring toxins, they now have to face a staggering array of man-made compounds: medical and recreational drugs, food additives, pollutants and contaminants of air and water, and the dangerous chemicals people are exposed to on the job and in the home. The sum of all this chemical stress may, over the years, contribute to decreasing immune system defenses against cancer.

Harmful chemicals are discussed in detail in the books listed in the Suggested Reading at the end of this chapter. Reduce or eliminate exposure to all the chemicals in your life you can do without. Take precautions with those you must use. When you work with them, wear appropriate clothing and protection for the face, breathe clean air and bathe after a period of contact, drink plenty of pure water and try to sweat more to help your body eliminate residues (see pp. 204–205), and maintain good habits of rest and nutrition.

• *Minimize exposure to pesticides, herbicides, and other poisons.* This is a highly dangerous group of chemicals. The only safe insecticide is pyrethrum, obtained from a flower in the daisy family. A few other botanical pesticides (neem, rotenone, ryania) are of low toxicity to mammals. Do not use any commercial pesticides containing arsenic, heptachlor, chlordane, or alachlor. Do not use any herbicides (like 2,4,5-T) that are likely to contain dioxin as a contaminant. In general I would like you not to use any chemical pesticides or herbicides and not to keep these products around the home. Do not let an exterminator or anyone else use them in your home either.

If you must use these products, do not use them in aerosol form, which is more likely to contain carcinogens. Use products that spray from a pumped container instead. Be careful not to breathe the fumes or contact liquids. Use a face mask and protective clothing and wash your skin well when you are finished.

• *Inform yourself of the dangers of household products and take appropriate precautions.* Carcinogenic chemicals are present in paints and solvents as well as in other products for home use, including arts and crafts supplies. Check labels on all cleaning products to make sure they do not contain benzene, carbon tetrachloride, or perchloroethylene. If they do, get rid of them. Check labels on paints, paint strippers, and lubricants to make sure they do not contain methylene chloride. If they do, get rid of them.

Books that give more detail on the dangers of household products are listed in the Suggested Reading at the end of this chapter. As much as possible, keep chemicals out of the home.

• *Beware of products containing dyes and colorings.* Dyes are also among the chemicals most suspected as cancer causers. I have already mentioned their dangers as food additives (see p. 48). Few people stop to think that blue, pink, yellow, and green medications do not get that way by themselves. Colored pills, capsules, and liquids are dyed with the same suspect chemicals, and if you consume a lot of them, you are adding to your risk of cancer. Dyes are also used in cosmetic products like shampoos, lotions, and makeup. They are less risky when applied topically but still may be absorbed through the skin. I recommend minimizing your use of all artificially colored products intended for use in or on the body.

• *Do not live near areas of heavy industrial pollution.* Chemical dust poured into the air by industrial polluters is often carcinogenic, and the incidence of lung and other cancers is higher in more polluted areas. If you smoke cigarettes, your risk of getting lung cancer is even higher if you live in an area of the country with high smog levels.

If you are at risk of developing cancer for other reasons, do not live near oil refineries, mining smelters, chemical factories, paper mills, coal-burning power plants, toxic waste dumps, or other sources of industrial pollution.

The drinking water in industrially polluted areas is likely to contain carcinogenic chemicals. If you cannot move away from contaminated air and water, protect yourself by installing a good air filter in your home, by purifying your drinking water, and by applying the other recommendations in this chapter.

• *Do not work in a chemically hazardous environment.* If you work at manufacturing leather, rubber, dyes, plastics, textiles, poisons, paints, metal, paper, or other products involving the use of industrial chemicals, your risk of getting cancer may by high. Miners are likely to inhale carcinogenic dusts, as are those who work with wood. Dry cleaners breathe the fumes of dangerous solvents. Agricultural workers are exposed to pesticides and herbicides. And so on.

Be informed about the dangers of products you use in your work. (See the Suggested Reading at the end of this chapter or contact your union or the Occupational Safety and Health Administration in Washington, D.C.) If your risk of getting cancer is increased for other reasons, change your job. If you cannot, take all possible precautions to minimize your exposure to the chemicals you work with and follow the other recommendations in this chapter.

6. Do Not Smoke!

Tobacco smoke is the single most important cause of cancer in the environment today. It is full of carcinogens and cocarcinogens, as well as radioactive particles. Cigarette smoking is *the* principal cause of lung cancer, an especially bad tumor because there are no symptoms in its early stages. By the time the tumor is discovered, it almost always has spread, killing most of its victims within a few years whether they are treated or not. The incidence of lung cancer has increased drastically in this century, paralleling the rise in cigarette smoking. It is now a major killer of both men and women. Probably one fifth of all cancer deaths in the United States are due to lung tumors directly caused by cigarette smoke.

Of course, lung cancer is only one of the medical consequences of the cigarette habit. It also causes bladder cancer and arterial disease. If you are a nonsmoker, be aware that living or working with smokers exposes you to significant risk, the equivalent of smoking four to twenty cigarettes a day by some estimates. You should also know that habitual smoking of any plant, including marijuana, increases the risk of lung cancer. Tobacco is far and away the greatest cause for concern because it is so addictive, gives off so many carcinogens, and is in such widespread use as a legally supported and commercially promoted drug.

7. Do Not Drink Alcohol Heavily

Heavy drinkers are at greater risk of developing cancers of the mouth, throat, esophagus, and stomach, probably because alcohol irritates those tissues directly. Heavy drinkers are also more likely to get liver cancer. The danger is compounded if you also smoke tobacco. Drink moderately or minimally or not at all. (I give specific recommendations about alcohol in Chapter 7.)

8. Do Not Eat Carcinogenic Foods

You are more likely to get cancer, especially of the gastrointestinal tract, if you eat a lot of salted, pickled, or smoked foods, particularly of animal origin. This does not mean you should not eat pickles or enjoy an occasional meal of smoked fish. Just be aware of these dietary carcinogens and don't eat them immoderately.

The same goes for the natural carcinogens in some vegetables. I recommend against eating a lot of cultivated white mushrooms, celery, peanuts, or peanut products. Also avoid any food that has become moldy, especially nuts, grains, and seeds. The molds that grow on these foods frequently make carcinogens as metabolic by-products.

Cured meats that look red because they have been treated with nitrite preservatives (ham, bacon, corned beef, etc.) may form carcinogenic compounds in the stomach. Vitamin C can block their formation and may generally protect against cancer-inducing substances in the diet (see below, pp. 186–187). Remember that meats and other proteins become carcinogenic when they are seared black over open flames or on a charcoal grill. Do not eat charred flesh or, if you do, cut away the charred outer layers. Never breathe the smoke of burning meat or burning fat. Please review the section on fats in Chapter 1. It contains a lot of information about the dangers of polyunsaturated vegetable oils, rancidity, and fried foods which you must know for your protection. Review also the section in Chapter 2 on pesticide residues on and in foods (pp. 51–52).

9. Eat a Healthy Diet

The nutritional guidelines in Chapters 1 and 2 offer significant protection against cancer. By cutting down on fat of all kinds, minimizing your use of polyunsaturated vegetable oils, and eating much less animal protein, more soy foods, more fiber, and more fruits and vegetables you will be eating an anticarcinogenic diet.

10. Take Antioxidant Supplements

In discussing the dangers of polyunsaturated fats in Chapter 1, I wrote about their tendency to oxidize and form dangerous chemical compounds. These compounds are called "free radicals." They are highly reactive and have the potential to damage DNA, causing mutations that can initiate malignant transformation of cells. Free radicals can easily cause harm to the immune system, whose cells divide often, and they may be responsible for some of the changes of aging. They can be generated in many ways, not just from the degeneration of fats, but the process always involves oxidation reactions.

The theory that free radicals are involved in cancer causation — and I emphasize that it is a theory, not a fact — has led researchers to look for ways to neutralize them. Actually the body has its own biochemical mechanisms that scavenge free radicals, finding them soon after their creation and destroying them before they cause harm. We can help the body in its task by supplying it with natural substances that act as antioxidants. These substances block the chemical reactions that generate free radicals in the first place and can help destroy already formed ones. Some of the safest and most effective antioxidants are familiar vitamins and minerals required in human nutrition. I discuss vitamins and supplements in detail in Chapter 14, but here I will suggest a specific antioxidant formula that I take myself and recommend to you as part of your cancer-prevention effort.

Beta-carotene, the water-soluble precursor of vitamin A, is one member of a large family of carotenes, yellow and orange pigments that may help prevent many kinds of cancer. The best dietary sources of carotenes are yellow and orange fruits and vegetables (mangoes, corn, sweet potatoes, carrots, squash), tomatoes, and dark, leafy greens (kale, collards, bok choy). If your diet is not rich in these foods, you should take supplemental beta-carotene, 25,000 IU a day, which is the same as 15 milligrams or the amount you would get by eating several large carrots. Supplements containing mixed carotenes from natural sources may soon be available, and I would recommend them over isolated beta-carotene. Until mixed carotenes come on the market, your best bet is natural beta-carotene obtained from marine algae. In doses above 50,000 IU a day, this antioxidant vitamin may produce an orangy pigmentation of the skin, noticeable first on the palms of the hands. Some people like this color change, thinking it looks like a nice suntan. To me it looks orange. But the color is harmless and will go away if the dose is reduced. You can take beta-carotene at any time of day.

Vitamin E is the second element of the antioxidant formula. I recommend taking 400 IU a day if you are under the age of forty, and 400 IU twice a day if you are over that age. Most vitamin E is synthetic dl-alpha-tocopherol. I do not recommend it. Look instead for natural d-alpha-tocopherol combined with other tocopherols (or mixed natural tocopherols), providing 400 IU of the d-alpha molecule plus some of the d-beta, d-gamma, and d-delta forms as well. To ensure absorption, vitamin E should be taken with your largest meal, because it requires some fat to be absorbed. It should also be taken together with selenium (see pp. 187–188).

Vitamin C is the third antioxidant, a powerful one, often used as a food preservative because of this property. The doses I recommend are large compared to those recommended by conventional nutritionists but not nearly so large as those taken by followers of Linus Pauling, the chemist and Nobel laureate who has tried to promote the use of megadoses of Vitamin C.

Vitamin C must be taken in divided doses through the day in order to keep blood levels of it up. The minimum dose I recommend is 1,000 milligrams (1 gram) twice a day. Taking 1,000 milligrams three times a day is even better, and if you eat an unhealthy diet, such as a lot of foods containing nitrites, or have increased cancer risk for other reasons, you would do better to make it 2,000 milligrams three times a day.

Vitamin C is not toxic, even in very large doses, but as you increase your intake of it, you will eventually reach a dose level that will give you unacceptable flatulence and then diarrhea. This is the limit of bowel tolerance of the vitamin. Stay under that limit. If the doses I recommend cause these problems, take smaller amounts more frequently and make sure you have food in your stomach when you do.

Ordinary vitamin C is ascorbic acid. It tastes very sour, can upset the stomach, and can damage the enamel of your teeth. I prefer nonacidic forms. Do not use sodium ascorbate; you do not want extra sodium in your diet. Calcium ascorbate is much better. It tastes somewhat bitter and costs more than ascorbic acid, but it will not bother your teeth or stomach; it also provides some calcium, which most of us can use. Large pills and tablets of vitamin C may not dissolve inside you. It is better and cheaper to buy soluble powder in bulk. One quarter teaspoon of calcium ascorbate powder equals 1,000 milligrams of vitamin C. You can dissolve the amount you want in a little juice. Or check out the various effervescent forms of vitamin C. As long as they are not too sour, do not contain sodium or sugar, and are reasonably priced, they are satisfactory. (See Appendix B for a source.)

Selenium, a trace mineral, is an antioxidant with significant anticancer effects. In areas of the world with high levels of selenium in the soil, the crops contain selenium, and those who live there have low cancer rates. However, selenium is toxic in not very large doses. The amounts I recommend, 100–300 micrograms a day (1,000 micrograms equals 1 milligram), are much smaller than those of the three vitamins. Take 100 micrograms if your cancer risks are low, 300 micrograms if they are increased for any reason.

Most brands of selenium are labeled as "organic, yeast-bound" or "yeast-derived." These may be preferable to inorganic sodium selenite. (The amount of yeast in one little tablet should not bother even those people who think they are very intolerant of it.) One other caution about selenium: it does not mix with vitamin C; in fact, they interfere with each other's absorption. Therefore do not take selenium within thirty minutes of taking vitamin C. Instead, take it with vitamin E at your largest meal.

That is my antioxidant formula. One way to follow it is to take beta-carotene and one dose of vitamin C at breakfast, followed by vitamin E and selenium with lunch or dinner, and a second dose of vitamin C before going to bed. I would like you to start this regimen and just stay on it. It cannot do you any harm, and it may safeguard your immune system and retard aging while giving you protection from cancer. When you take these supplements, try to keep the thought in mind that you are doing something concrete to reduce cancer risks. This is a good antidote to worrying about cancer. Instead of trying to stop the negative thoughts, put your energy into positive ones, in this case by reminding yourself that you are taking defensive action.

11. Exercise!

Not again, you say. Yes, it's true; exercise has anticancer effects, and, again, it is regular aerobic activity that does it. How it does this, we do not know. Aerobic exercise may protect women from breast, uterine, and cervical cancer by lowering levels of circulating estrogen. It definitely increases the efficiency of the immune system, and it counteracts negative moods that depress immunity. Here is yet another reason to be sure that regular aerobic exercise is part of your lifestyle.

12. Practice Safe Sex

As sexually transmitted diseases increase in our society, we have begun to see links between them and cancer. Sex is an easy way to transmit viruses between partners, and viruses play a role in cancer, either directly by altering DNA or indirectly by interfering with the immune system. For example, the sexually transmitted human papillomavirus (HPV), which causes genital warts, is probably the cause of cervical cancer. The virus that causes genital herpes, once suspected as the agent of cervical cancer, may act as a cofactor here, so if infection with both viruses is present, cancer may be more likely than with HPV alone.

It is the epidemic of acquired immune deficiency syndrome (AIDS) that has generated the concept of safe sex and made us aware of ways that unsafe sex weakens our defenses against disease, including cancer. The basic guidelines are very simple:

• *Limit the number of your sexual partners* in order to minimize your chances of contracting sexually transmitted diseases.

• *Know the sexual histories of your partners* and be especially careful with those who have had many partners, have used drugs intravenously, have had sexually transmitted diseases, or have practiced high-risk sex (that is, sex that is traumatic or involves exchange of bodily fluids).

• *Avoid exchanges of bodily fluids,* especially blood and semen, which are common carriers of viruses. *Use condoms whenever there is doubt about safety.* Condoms are not the final solution to the problem of sexual safety, but they can prevent the transmission of AIDS and other sexual infections, including viruses that increase risks of cancer.

13. Work with Your Emotions

Health professionals who see a lot of cancer patients often describe them as "nice" — that is, pleasant, inoffensive, unwilling to make trouble, apologetic for being sick. This frequent observation has given rise to the notion of a "cancer personality." In many ways it is just the opposite of the heart-attack personality with its tendency to rage. It is said that cancer-prone people bottle up their emotions, never expressing anger and often not even being aware of their anger. They are said to carry around a lot of deep, unexpressed sadness and grief, emotions that depress immunity and allow malignant cells to develop into deadly cancers.

The problem with these ideas is that they are based on retrospective reasoning. You see certain personality traits in a cancer patient, then try to reach into the past to make a causal connection between personality and disease. No one has come up with good prospective data to allow us to identify personality traits in advance and *predict* who will get cancer and who will not. Until that happens, the idea of a cancer personality is an interesting idea, nothing more. (Research linking hostility and rage with heart attacks is more solid.)

Still, given the growing body of research demonstrating links between the mind and the immune system, it is reasonable to assume that living with a lot of unexpressed or unfelt grief and anger doesn't do you or your immunity any good. Therefore I suggest that you work with your emotions, trying to become more aware of feelings and better able to express them. Whether or not this will specifically reduce your chances of getting cancer, it is a good prescription for general health and wellness.

14. Protect Your Immune System

Since your immune system is your main defense against all the natural and unnatural forces pushing in the direction of malignancy, you ought to know how to keep it in the best condition. I find that many people do not know what harms the immune system and what helps it. I present that information in the next chapter.

SUGGESTED READING

Your Defense Against Cancer by Henry Dreher (New York: Harper & Row, 1989) is the best general work on cancer prevention. It includes extensive discussion of dietary, lifestyle, and psychological factors relevant to cancer, including good information on hazardous chemicals.

Well Body, Well Earth: The Sierra Club Environmental Health Sourcebook by Mike Samuels, M.D., and Hal Zina Bennett (San Francisco: Sierra Club Books, 1983) is a detailed, practical handbook on environmental hazards, including chemicals to be most concerned about in the home and at work.

Radiation and Human Health by John W. Gofman (New York: Pantheon, 1981) is the best book on the health hazards of radiation.

12

HOW TO PROTECT
YOUR IMMUNE SYSTEM

YOUR IMMUNE SYSTEM is your interface with the environment. If it is healthy and doing its job right, you can interact with germs and not get infections, with allergens and not have allergic reactions, and with carcinogens and not get cancer. A healthy immune system is the cornerstone of good general health. Its problems are of two general sorts: underactivity, which predisposes to infections and cancer, and overactivity, which predisposes to allergies and autoimmunity. Although the advent of AIDS has made us very conscious of immunity and its failures, most people I meet do not have a clear picture of what the immune system is. I often hear references to the "autoimmune system." There is no such thing; autoimmunity is a disease process in which the immune system attacks the body's own tissues. (See pp. 259–260 for more information on autoimmunity.)

The immune system is hard to understand for several reasons. First of all, it was not recognized as a functional unit of the body until recent years. It is a sobering fact of modern medical history that doctors labeled many of the organs of the immune system "functionless" throughout most of this century, giving surgeons license to remove them with abandon. The medical profession has removed or destroyed countless tonsils, adenoids, appendixes, thymus glands, and spleens in the belief that these structures were useless, not worth the space they occupied. Second, the components of the immune system do not hang together in any neat arrangement that makes it easy to picture the whole, as we can picture the digestive system or the vascular system. Finally, the operations of the immune system are immensely intricate.

Let me try to cut through the complexity and tell you what I think you need to know to protect your body's defenses. The immune system comprises the tonsils and adenoids, the thymus gland, the lymph nodes throughout the body, the bone marrow, the circulating white blood cells and other cells that leave blood vessels and migrate through tissues and the lymphatic circulation, the spleen, the appendix, and patches of lymphoid tissue in the intestinal tract. The essential job of this system is to distinguish self from not-self, to recognize and take appropriate action against any materials that ought not to be in the body, including abnormal and damaged components. For example, it can seek out and destroy disease germs and cells infected by germs, as well as recognize and destroy tumor cells.

In deciding what belongs in the body and what does not, the immune system pays particular attention to details of protein chemistry, because of all the molecules that make up living organisms, proteins are the most distinctive and the most specialized.

Like the nervous system, the immune system is capable of learning. It analyzes its experiences, remembers them, and passes them on to future generations of cells. Because its tissues are very active and very involved in processing information, its cells divide very rapidly and so, as you learned in the last chapter, are unusually susceptible to injury by types of energy and matter that can alter (mutate) DNA. *All of the recommendations I gave you for decreasing your risks of cancer also hold for protecting your immune system.* Please follow them.

Here are some further guidelines:

1. Do Not Allow Infections to Persist

One of the greatest strains on the immune system is an infection it cannot eliminate. Never ignore such symptoms as unexplained fevers, night sweats, or tender, swollen lymph nodes ("glands"); they can indicate a hidden infection.

One area of the body where infection often goes unnoticed is the mouth. Pockets of germs in the gums and teeth may cause few symptoms yet use up a lot of the body's immune resources. It is important to maintain good oral hygiene and to have the teeth and gums examined regularly to detect any areas of infection.

Sexually transmitted infections may also go unnoticed while they drain the vitality of the immune system. Observe good sexual hygiene and good hygiene of body orifices. Limit the number of sexual partners and make a habit of practicing safe sex.

2. Do Not Use Antibiotics Indiscriminately

Whenever the immune system deals successfully with an infection, it emerges from the experience stronger and better able to confront similar threats in the future. Our immune competence develops in combat. If, at the first sign of infection, you always jump in with antibiotics, you do not give the system a chance to test itself and grow stronger. There are less drastic methods to try first with ordinary infections (see Chapter 13); you don't have to bring out the heavy artillery until simpler measures fail.

Antibiotics are powerful medicines that should be reserved for situations that demand them, for instance, when the immune system cannot contain a bacterial infection or when a bacterial infection establishes itself in a vital organ like the heart, lungs, or brain. Another strong reason to be cautious about overuse of antibiotics is the possibility of selectively breeding new strains of antibiotic-resistant, more virulent bacteria. Even people who are aware of that danger seldom realize that frequent use of antibiotics can lead in the long run to weakened immunity.

3. Avoid Immunosuppressive Drugs

Examples of immunosuppressives are the drugs used in cancer chemotherapy and those used to suppress rejection in patients receiving organ transplants. Another class of drugs with similar effects is cause for greater concern because it is much more commonly used. It is the corticosteroids, or steroids, derivatives and relatives of cortisone in widespread use for the treatment of allergies, autoimmune diseases, and inflammatory conditions. I consider them dangerous drugs, much misunderstood, abused, and overprescribed.

Cortisone is a hormone produced by the outer layer (cortex) of the adrenal gland. It has a distinctive molecular structure, called the steroid nucleus, that is shared by a few other natural hormones and many synthetic drugs with powerful effects on metabolism. Collectively these substances are known as steroids. Synthetic steroids, like prednisone, are widely used in allopathic medicine today. Doctors prescribe them in many forms: as pills, injections, inhaled aerosols, and topical creams.

Steroids cause allergies and inflammation to disappear as if by magic. In fact, the magic is nothing other than direct suppression of immune function. I have no objection to giving these strong drugs for very severe or life-threatening problems, but even then I think they should be limited to short-term use: no more than two to three weeks. I deplore prescription of steroids for illnesses of mild or moderate severity or for months and years at a time. I have known them to be given to patients with mild cases of poison ivy, infants with diaper rash, and adults with back pain and undiagnosable fatigue. Steroids are terribly toxic, cause dependence, suppress rather than cure disease, and reduce the chance of healing by natural methods of treatment. Moreover, they weaken immunity.

Even topical steroids are dangerous in my opinion. The medical profession is so unconscious of the hazards of these drugs that it allows steroidal ointments and creams to be sold over the counter. Many people apply them every day to skin rashes and irritations that could be much better dealt with by simple remedies. All of these products are absorbed through the skin to one degree or another, and all of them can suppress activity of the thymus, the lymph nodes, and the white blood cells.

In summary: *Do not use steroids in any form until you have exhausted all other possible treatments. If you must take a steroid for a severe problem, limit its use to a few weeks at most.*

4. Avoid Blood Transfusions

Blood transfusions and injections of blood products may transmit viral diseases — hepatitis, especially — that cannot be treated. They also stress the immune system by flooding it with foreign proteins. Obviously, in an emergency it may not be possible to do without blood, although synthetic blood replacers that are safer may soon become available. If you know in advance that you are going to have surgery, have some of your own blood drawn and stored for any replacement you might need.

5. Avoid Exposure to Radiation

Please read again the cautions on radiation in the previous chapter. In addition, be aware of a special danger to the immune system from any radiation treatments (usually for cancer), as opposed to diagnostic X rays, directed to the head, neck, or chest. The thymus gland, behind the breastbone, is very vulnerable. Insist that a lead shield be placed over it if you ever have to undergo radiation therapy. If the therapist will not comply, refuse treatment. Many doctors continue to believe that the thymus has no function in adulthood. It does; it is an integral part of your immune system.

6. Avoid Exposure to Harmful Chemicals

All of the chemicals that cause cancer may also damage the immune system. Please follow the recommendations about harmful chemicals in the previous chapter.

7. Eat a Healthy Diet

Follow all of the dietary guidelines I have given you so far. In particular:

• *Avoid polyunsaturated vegetable oils* and products made from them. Their tendency to form free radicals makes them dangerous to cells of the immune system.

• *Eat less protein.* Residues of protein metabolism can irritate the immune system, especially in people prone to allergy and autoimmunity. A low-protein, high-carbohydrate diet with plenty of fruits, vegetables, and fiber is good for immunity as well as general health.

• *Do not eat many foods of animal origin.* Meat, poultry, and dairy products often carry residues of antibiotics and steroid hormones that can weaken immunity.

• *Minimize consumption of milk and milk products,* especially if you are prone to allergy or autoimmunity. Milk protein is a common irritant of the immune system.

8. Take Antioxidant Supplements

The vitamin and mineral formula given in Chapter 11 (pp. 185–188) protects immune function as it reduces cancer risks. Use it.

9. Learn about Foods and Herbs That Enhance Immunity

Medical doctors know a lot of ways to hurt the immune system but few ways to help it. With AIDS and other manifestations of weakened immunity much on people's minds, a great many products have appeared in health food stores that claim to boost resistance. Usually, solid research to back these claims is nonexistent, but in some cases the evidence is there. The idea of immunopotentiators is appealing, especially if we can find ones that are natural, nontoxic, and effective.

Because of a long-standing interest in mushrooms, I came to learn of several mushrooms from China and Japan that may have the desired effects. Traditional doctors in those countries esteem many mushrooms as both foods and medicines. Some of the most prized remedies in the Chinese herbal repertory are mushrooms that act as tonics and that are believed to increase resistance to all kinds of stress as well as extend longevity. Traditional Chinese medicine did not know the immune system as a set of interacting organs and cells, but it understood the concept of a defensive function of the body and taught that a useful way to treat disease was to support that function. Tonic mushrooms are supposed to do just that. One of the most promising ones is *Polyporus umbellatus,* the source of a traditional Chinese remedy called *zhu ling.* This fungus grows wild on tree stumps in this country (although it is not common) and can be cultivated. Above ground it produces large clusters of fleshy mushrooms that are edible and delicious. Below ground it produces hard, tuberlike masses of fungal tissue that are the source of the remedy. Suppliers of Chinese herbal medicines sell dried slices of *zhu ling* to be boiled in water and drunk as a tea (see Appendix B for a source). Recently medical scientists in Beijing showed that extracts of *zhu ling* were effective against lung cancer in both animals and humans. The treatment also potentiated the effect of chemotherapy and had no toxicity of its own. Most interestingly, it worked only in living animals with intact immune systems. The extracts showed no activity against cancer cells growing in test tubes. The scientists concluded that *zhu ling* worked by stimulating an immune response against the tumor.

The National Cancer Institute included *Polyporus umbellatus* in a series of screening tests of natural products for anticancer activity, but the tests were done in test tubes and gave negative results. In the West we have focused on the development of cytotoxic drugs as weapons against cancer — poisons we hope will kill more tumor cells than normal cells. The complementary approach would be to look for nontoxic therapies that work by strengthening the host's defenses, and *zhu ling* might be one of these; more studies of it are needed.

A close relative of *zhu ling* is *Grifola frondosus,* known to mushroom hunters as hen-of-the-woods, a delicious edible species. Japanese know it as *maitake* ("dancing mushroom"), and Japanese scientists have figured out how to cultivate it on a commercial scale. You can buy fresh maitake in any Japanese market, but until now only the rare wild form has been available here. Recent research indicates that maitake has outstanding immunopotentiating effect. The dried form of the mushroom is now sold in some health food stores here, along with extracts in tablet form; these are imported from Japan and tend to be expensive. Mushroom cultivators on this side of the Pacific are busily working to introduce maitake to the American market, so it should become more widely available soon. Other mushrooms that may be effective, based on Japanese research, are the shiitake and the enokidake *(Flammulina velutipes),* both of which are good to eat and increasingly easy to find.

Another Chinese herbal remedy with similar properties comes from the root of a plant in the pea family, *Astragalus membranaceus.* This plant is a relative of our locoweed, which is toxic to livestock. The Chinese species is nontoxic, the source of a very popular medicine called *huang qi* that you can buy in any drugstore in China for use against colds, flus, and other respiratory infections. Recent studies in the West confirm its antiviral and immune-boosting effects, and *Astragalus* preparations are now available in most health food stores here.

American Indian medicine gave us a useful native plant that is another immune-system booster: purple coneflower, *Echinacea purpurea* and related species. The root of this ornamental plant is held in high esteem by herbalists, naturopathic doctors, and many laypeople because of its antibiotic and immune-enhancing properties. You can buy echinacea products in any health food store: tinctures, capsules, tablets, and extracts of fresh or dried roots. Although few medical doctors in America are familiar with echinacea, much research on it has been done in Germany, and the plant is in widespread use as a home remedy in Europe and America. (See pp. 238–239 for more information.)

Zhu ling, maitake, shiitake, enokidake, *Astragalus,* and echinacea share some common chemistry. All contain polysaccharides, long chain molecules composed of sugar units, which seem to be responsible for their action as immunopotentiators. Polysaccharides have never excited much interest among scientists who search for new drugs. They are structural components of many organisms and are not the kinds of molecules that usually have biological effects. Yet researchers are finding them in a whole range of plants and mushrooms that seem able to enhance our immunity. One possibility is that they resemble components of the cell walls of bacteria and stimulate immune responses for that reason.

However they work, it is good to know that safe natural products exist and are readily available to help us during periods of low resistance. I do not think you need to use them if you are in good health, but if you are having frequent colds or other infections, if you seem to "get everything that's going around," if your healing responses seem sluggish and your resistance low, you might consider taking one or more of these immune enhancers for a time.

10. Work at Improving Your Mental and Emotional Health

For many years immunologists maintained that the immune system was the only autonomous system of the body, the only one that operated free of external controls. This is a silly idea. No system of the body is autonomous. All are interconnected, especially with the nervous system. In addition, the clinical experience of doctors who work with immune disorders is that a strong correlation exists between the ups and downs of these disorders and the ups and downs of emotional life. For example, a typical onset of rheumatoid arthritis in a young woman may be a flare-up in many joints of the body within hours of a severe emotional trauma.

A few years ago I saw two patients with advanced lupus (systemic lupus erythematosus or SLE, another autoimmune disease). Both were women in their thirties, one white, one black. The white woman was hospitalized with serious kidney damage and, as a result, uncontrollably high blood pressure. She also had serious toxicity from long treatment with steroids and other immunosuppressive drugs. Her prognosis was grave. The black woman was out of the hospital but also was very sick with kidney damage, high blood pressure, brain dysfunction, and drug toxicity. She was in better shape than the first patient, but her future also looked grim. The first patient underwent a religious conversion in the hospital and became a fundamentalist Christian. The second woman fell in love and subsequently married. Both went into complete remission and became symptom free.

The young science of psychoneuroimmunology is demonstrating the interconnections of mind, nervous system, and immune system. In many cases the connections are chemical, with small protein molecules called peptides being the messengers that take information from cell to cell. It is clear that the nervous, immune, and endocrine systems are in constant biochemical communication, linked by a web of peptide hormones. Wherever nerves are, the activities of the mind can travel.

Clearly, emotional states like grief and depression can interfere with immunity, just as loving can enhance it. You do not need to know any more than that to be motivated to improve your emotional health. I have already given you suggestions for action in Chapters 4, 5, 6, and 8. Do not try to stop or fight negative mental states. Instead, put energy into creating a positive state, and the negativity will tend to resolve.

SUGGESTED READING

Maximum Immunity by Michael A. Weiner, Ph.D., with Kathleen Goss (Boston: Houghton Mifflin, 1986) is a good general book on the immune system and how to fortify it.

The Healer Within: The New Medicine of Mind and Body by Steven Locke, M.D., and Douglas Colligan (New York: E. P. Dutton, 1986) focuses on the connection between the mind and the immune system. Dr. Locke, a psychiatrist, is one of the leading workers in the field of psychoneuroimmunology.

Minding the Body, Mending the Mind by Joan Borysenko, Ph.D. (Reading, Mass.: Addison-Wesley, 1987) is another good book on the same subject.

PART III

BASIC NATURAL TREATMENTS

13

SIMPLE MEASURES

YOU CAN SAVE a lot of money in doctor bills by learning to use some simple techniques of self-care. In this chapter I will describe a number of ways you can help your body heal itself, using simple, effective measures that do not require much equipment or training. I use these techniques myself and frequently recommend them to patients.

Rest is *so* simple that many people fail to think of it when they start to get sick. Your immune system requires energy to do its job. By cutting down on unnecessary expenditures of energy, you can give it a great advantage. Going to bed when you first notice a breakdown in health, canceling planned activities, and letting others take care of you is a much more sensible strategy than taking pills and going about your business. Even a twenty-four-hour rest may be enough to alter the course of an illness and put you on the road to recovery.

Fasting owes its effectiveness to a basic fact of physiology. The digestive organs are the largest and bulkiest in the body, and their routine operations consume large amounts of energy. The simple act of not eating rests this system and frees up much of that energy for the body to use in healing. Fasting means taking in nothing other than water (or water and herbal teas with no calories). Restricting yourself to liquids, fruit, or fruit juice is not fasting. These are special diets that have particular benefits but do not produce the same results as fasting.

There are two kinds of fasting, short-term and long-term, with very different consequences and uses. Short-term fasting means one to three days of taking in nothing but water. Short-term fasting alters both consciousness and physiology. It is a good home remedy for colds, flus, infectious illnesses, and toxic conditions of all kinds. If you combine it with rest and a good mental state, short-term fasting can make you feel like a new person. Many people report that even after one day of fasting their senses are sharper, their heads clearer, their bodies lighter and more energetic. Some like this feeling so much that they fast one day a week. This practice can also be beneficial as a psychospiritual discipline.

Long-term fasting continues longer than three days. *Do not attempt long-term fasting without expert supervision.* It is a drastic technique that can be dangerous. I have met people who have fasted for one to three months with good results, and I have seen long-term fasting produce complete remissions of diseases that resisted all other treatments: bronchial asthma, rheumatoid arthritis, ulcerative colitis. On occasion I recommend it, but I am not qualified to supervise it. Long-term fasting should be done only in a facility staffed by experienced health professionals.

If you want to try a short-term fast the next time you get sick, here are some points to remember:

• *Be sure to drink plenty of liquid* (water, mineral water, or herbal tea). This will help you avoid constipation and help your urinary system remove any toxic products of infection.

• *Conserve your energy.* Do not expect to maintain normal activity or your usual exercise routines.

• *Stay warm.* Your body temperature will fall when you fast. Especially if the weather is cold, do not let yourself get chilled. Dress warmly and drink some hot herbal tea. Take warm baths.

• *Do not look at food or at people who are eating.* This will only make it harder to fast.

• *Break your fast sensibly.* At the end of it, begin to eat some fresh fruit or fruit juice and light, plain foods in small amounts. If you go directly to pizza and enchiladas, you are likely to make yourself sick.

Sweating is a natural method of purification that enables the body to eliminate salt, drugs, and a variety of toxins *as long as it is supplied with adequate water.* You can do healthy sweating in a sauna or steam room. Just be sure to take along a plentiful supply of pure water and drink it often. Depending on the temperature, you can stay in the heat for ten to twenty minutes or until you are perspiring freely. I recommend sweats often, especially to people who smoke, drink, or use other drugs, suffer chemical exposures, or eat a lot of salt. Intense sweating at the very start of a viral infection may abort the illness or greatly reduce its severity.

• *Allow yourself a rest period at the end of a sweat.* You may be weak, dizzy, or unstable on your feet.

• *Continue to drink water after the sweat in order to keep urine output high.* Never let the body get dehydrated.

Steam inhalation is an excellent remedy for respiratory problems, particularly for chest congestion, bronchitis, bronchial cough, laryngitis, and sinusitis. You can rig up a steam inhalation tent in your kitchen by bringing a pot of water to boil on the stove, then standing over it with a towel over your head and the pot. (Be careful with the towel if you have an open flame.) Breathe steam through the nose for nasal and sinus problems, otherwise through the mouth with pursed lips. Another possibility is to roll a cone of stiff paper, put the wide end over the pot, and inhale steam through the narrow end. Steam vaporizers also work well.

You can increase the effectiveness of steam inhalation by adding aromatic herbs to the water. My favorites are sage and eucalyptus, either alone or in combination. Add a small handful of whole leaves or a teaspoon of the essential oils, available from herb shops. Steam mixed with sage and eucalyptus is not only soothing, it is also antibacterial, since the aromatic oils retard bacterial growth. This treatment reduces the chance of secondary infection in cases of respiratory diseases caused by viruses.

Nasal douching is the practice of rinsing the nasal passages with a saltwater solution. It is a hygienic practice of yoga as well as a marvelous treatment for sinus problems and allergic rhinitis (as in hay fever). Most people don't like the sensation of water in the nose, and some of us associate it with distress in swimming. Therefore it takes some practice to change these reactions and master the technique. Having the water at a comfortably warm temperature with just the right concentration of salt is critical.

Dissolve one quarter teaspoon of salt in one cup of warm water. This approximates the concentration of sodium in blood and tissue fluids and is soothing to mucous membranes. There are several ways to get this solution into the nose. You can pour it into your cupped hand and simply inhale the liquid through one nostril at a time while closing the other with an index finger. Or you can inhale it directly from a small cup or glass in the same way. You can tilt your head back and squirt the solution in gently with a rubber bulb syringe. Or you can pour it in slowly from a small container with a spout. (Yoga supply shops sell a ceramic device for this purpose that looks like a miniature Aladdin's lamp.)

However you do it, you want to get enough water in through your nose so that you can spit it out your mouth. Do this several times through each nostril, then gently blow your nose. Do not be discouraged if you cough, splutter, and make a mess. You will soon learn to inhale the salt water neatly and efficiently and come to like the way it feels.

People with pollen allergies should do this once or twice a day during the pollen season, as should people living in smoggy areas who experience nasal irritation from airborne pollutants. People with sinus conditions should also use a nasal douche daily, as it promotes drainage of the sinuses and speeds healing of inflamed tissues. In the case of acute sinus infection, it is important to do it even more frequently, up to four times a day. It will reduce pain and end the infection more quickly.

You may also find the nasal douche helpful in relieving the congestion and irritation of colds and flus, as long as the air passages are open enough to allow inhalation of the solution. Unlike most commercial nasal sprays, warm salt water does not cause irritation, rebound stuffiness, or drug dependence. Practice the technique while you are well so that you will be ready to use it in time of need.

Gargling is an easy way to speed healing of sore throats as well as to open congested ears and help ear infections. The idea of gargling is to keep a healing solution in contact with the tissues of the throat. The simplest gargle is a warm saline solution: one quarter teaspoon salt to one cup of warm water. Use the warmest water you can stand. The heat increases blood flow to the affected areas, and the inflamed tissues are bathed with a restorative solution. You can add goldenseal powder, an herbal disinfectant, if you like (see pp. 241–242) or goldenseal and red pepper to taste. Hydrogen peroxide makes another effective gargle when mixed half and half with hot water. It is a good disinfectant, useful in tonsillitis. Whatever mix you use, try to gargle for a few minutes at a time at least four times a day.

Hot and cold applications affect the body in simple yet powerful ways. In general, heat dilates blood vessels, increasing blood supply to an area, while cold does the opposite. You always want more blood in cases of infection. You always want less blood in cases of acute injury or of venomous bites and stings. Put hot compresses on boils, abscesses, splinters, and crampy muscles. Put cold compresses on bruises, sprains, traumatized joints and muscles, burns, bites, and stings.

Hot, wet heat is the best treatment for localized infections. Soak a towel in hot water, wring most of the water out, fold it, and apply to the affected area. Work up to as much heat as you can stand, reheating the towel whenever it starts to cool off. Do this for fifteen minutes at a time at least three or four times a day. If the infection is on the hand or foot, you can soak the part directly in a basin of hot water.

Heating pads can be useful for applying heat over larger areas and can be soothing to sore muscles. Be aware that electric heating pads may be hazardous in subtle ways. They generate powerful electrical fields that might disturb delicate biological control systems. I would be cautious about using them near the head or using them at all on a regular basis. (The same caution applies to electric blankets, which I suggest you avoid.) Hot water bottles are safe and effective for such problems as menstrual and intestinal cramps. Nonelectric heating pads are also available; you heat them in hot water, and they retain the wet heat for a long time.

An ice pack is a good way to apply cold to an injury. You can make one by wrapping ice cubes or a package of frozen peas in a towel. The faster you get it in contact with the injury, the better. (In case of burns, *immediate* immersion of the affected part in ice water is the preferred treatment.) Using an ice pack will reduce leakage of fluid into injured tissues, reduce swelling and pain, and slow the spread of any poison into the system. Try to keep ice on an acute injury for most of the first few hours, removing it occasionally to relieve any discomfort caused by the cold. Intermittent cold applications continue to be helpful for twelve to twenty-four hours after an injury; after twenty-four hours they are of little benefit.

For muscle injuries, after immediate treatment with ice, sports medicine experts often recommend alternating applications of heat and cold, ending with heat. You can try this technique to see how it works for you.

Hot and cold baths can very quickly change how you feel. Hot baths are relaxing. They increase blood flow to the surface of the body, soothe sore muscles and joints, and promote sleep. Cold baths are stimulating. They tone the muscles, circulation, and heart, increase mental alertness, and energize you. Experiment with baths of different temperatures to see how you react to them.

Healing touch is practiced in every culture. I have already talked about touch as a basic human need. For sick people the need is even greater. Many systems of touch therapy are available now, from Oriental massage techniques like acupressure to the therapeutic touch practiced by nurses. I recommend massage and touch therapy frequently. It cannot harm, and it often changes how you feel dramatically. Even if you do not have a massage therapist handy, you can apply healing touch to yourself. Just hold any part of your body that hurts. Do not be hesitant to ask friends or family to touch you in ways that will make you feel better.

I meet many people who are fascinated by the concept of detoxification. They believe that they are toxic: full of residues of junk food, drugs, and chemicals or invaded by viruses or yeasts or suffering from bad blood or accumulated waste in their intestines. These beliefs create markets for treatments and products that claim to be able to undo the damage and restore the body to a state of purity.

Ideas of pollution and purification are very powerful and universally appealing. All cultures and religions concern themselves with definitions of what is unclean and with rituals of purification. It is important to understand that these ideas may be fundamentally irrational and may generate concerns about health that have no medical reality. Most people who tell me they are toxic are not.

The body has its own self-cleaning, self-purifying systems; the best way to protect yourself from toxicity is to keep those systems in good working order. For example, the kidneys are a key component of our blood-purifying apparatus, and I have suggested ways of protecting their health by keeping them well supplied with pure water and avoiding dietary stresses like coffee, alcohol, and excessive protein. In general I favor relying on the body's own resources for detoxifying, and I urge you to guard those resources. If you stop putting toxins into your body and follow the preventive advice in this book, your own natural mechanisms of detoxification will keep your system in prime condition.

In health food stores you will see many advertisements for supplements and herbal products that claim to detoxify the system and purify the blood. None of these are necessary to good health. Detox regimens often focus on the colon. I have reviewed many systems of colon cleansing, including colonic irrigation (colonics) and the use of natural laxatives and herbal mixtures. If you eat a high-fiber diet, drink plenty of water, exercise, and move your bowels regularly, you shouldn't need any of them. (See the entry on constipation in Part IV.) The best way to care for the colon is to let its own natural physiological action keep it clean and in good working order.

There is no medical reason to irrigate the colon. Actually, the entire lining of the colon sloughs off and is regenerated every day, so it is physiologically impossible for any "encrustations" to build up on it. Some people like colonics, and some become addicted to them. There can be an element of sexual pleasure in this pattern. In addition, people can become addicted to the idea and feeling of being clean and light inside. They maintain this feeling for a short time, then slide back into habitually eating heavy food until they again become obsessed with the idea of being toxic and needing another colonic.

A better way to do internal cleansing is to go on a restricted diet for a few days, such as a "fruit fast" while taking some powdered psyllium seed husks to give the intestines plenty of bulk. Use a tablespoon of the powder stirred into a big glass of water and follow it with additional water. I have several times done a ten-day regimen that went like this: two days of nothing but fresh fruit and water, then two days of nothing but fresh fruit juice and water, then two days of fasting on water, then two days of fruit juice, and finally two days of fruit. There are dozens of different regimens of this sort, all aiming to give the digestive system a rest from its usual routine. It is not a bad idea to pick one of them that appeals to you and follow it for a week or so once a year as a general preventive measure or to use it whenever you have seriously overindulged in heavy foods or alcoholic beverages.

SUGGESTED READING

Home Remedies: Hydrotherapy, Massage, Charcoal, and Other Simple Treatments by Agatha Thrash, M.D., and Calvin Thrash, M.D. (1981, available from Thrash Publications, Route 1, Box 273, Seale, Ala. 36875) is a very complete manual describing the use of hot and cold applications for a variety of common disorders.

14

VITAMINS AND SUPPLEMENTS

MANY HEALTH FOOD STORES might better be called pill stores, given how little food they stock in relation to all the vitamins and supplements. Claims made for these products are extravagant. If they were all true, we could forget about proper diet, exercise, relaxation, and all other preventive strategies and just take pills.

Once or twice a year a new miracle supplement appears: spirulina, organic germanium, coenzyme Q, or some other natural product alleged to do any or all of the following: reduce cancer risks, enhance immunity, detoxify the system, extend life, increase resistance to stress, improve sexual functioning, promote weight loss without changing diet, give more energy and stamina, build muscles, and fight depression. It will be *very* expensive, but how can you afford not to take it?

In most cases solid research to back the claims is nonexistent, although promotional literature will often cite studies done in other countries. Usually these products are harmless (except to your pocketbook), but I think most of the benefits people report from taking them are placebo responses.

I get in the mail countless testimonials to supplements, including stories of remarkable cures of hopeless diseases in people who went on this or that powder or pill. Most medical doctors are contemptuous of testimonials to anything other than standard drugs and surgery, dismissing them as "anecdotal evidence" and therefore not worth listening to. I take a different view. To me testimonials are always interesting, but what I think they testify to is the natural healing capacities of human beings, not the power of the products.

The official view of the medical profession is that vitamins are necessary in minimal amounts to prevent deficiency diseases. Taken in excess of those doses, they do nothing, are simply excreted from the body, and in some cases can be toxic. The fact that medical education does not prepare doctors to understand or use nutritional supplements creates the basis for angry polarization when manufacturers make outrageous claims (and profits). Patients are often caught in the middle. They hear of the usefulness of some vitamin or mineral for a certain condition, but when they ask for advice, their doctors often dismiss their questions.

Even among laypeople a wide spectrum of opinion exists on the need to take supplements. Some people feel that all pills and capsules are unnatural, that we should be able to get all of our nutritional requirements from the food we eat. Others say we cannot experience optimal health or maximum longevity unless we add vitamins, minerals, and other substances to the diet.

I find myself in the middle of this divergence of views. I am not a great fan of taking pills, and I think it is desirable to get most of our nutritional needs from our diets, but I also see reasons to take certain supplements. Your diet should provide most of what you need, if it is the right diet for you, richly varied, and with mostly fresh foods. That is a big "if." Besides, many of the crop varieties grown may not be the most nutritious, and chemicals used in their production may deplete nutrients. If you use drugs like alcohol, tobacco, or caffeine, if you are under a great deal of stress, or if you are sick, your requirement for some nutrients may be greater than your diet can supply. Some nutritional supplements, in doses much higher than those recommended by the government, are useful as natural treatments for specific conditions.

Many patients who come to see me tell me they take a multivitamin and mineral supplement every day as a kind of "nutritional insurance." That is not a bad idea, as long as the formula does not contain iron (see p. 220) or other potentially toxic components. Other patients present me with long lists of supplements they take every day. Whenever possible I encourage them to cut out as many as possible, especially expensive "miracle" pills.

I would like to explain the common categories of supplements you will find in health food stores, so that you can be an informed and wary consumer.

VITAMINS

The body needs vitamins in tiny amounts for normal functioning. If it does not get them, deficiency diseases develop. (These are very rare in our society.) In addition to their basic roles in metabolism, some vitamins, taken in larger amounts, have other effects that are ignored by many nutritionists and doctors. These other actions may make them useful as treatments for particular problems.

First I want to give you some general advice about vitamins. Vitamin pills and powders can cause nausea, heartburn, and other gastric disturbances, especially when taken on an empty stomach. Always take them after a meal, with food in the stomach. If they do not agree with you in the morning, try taking them later in the day.

There is no important difference between natural and synthetic vitamins, unless the natural forms provide traces of other substances that might enhance their activity. Different brands of vitamins vary widely in cost. Buy the cheapest brands you can find that are as free as possible of fillers and additives. Very expensive, fancy vitamins are likely to be of greater benefit to the manufacturer than to you.

Vitamins fall into two general categories: those that are soluble in water and thus easily eliminated from the body (B-complex and C) and those that are fat-soluble and can accumulate in the body (A, D, E, K). The latter are potentially harmful because the body cannot eliminate any excess in the urine, but actual cases of toxicity are rare to the point of being medical curiosities. I will start with the water-soluble group.

B-complex vitamins include a number of substances needed for metabolic reactions. It is hard to become deficient in them if you eat a diet that is anywhere near balanced, but the need for them is increased by stress, use of drugs, and illness. I recommend B-complex supplements to smokers, drinkers, users of recreational drugs, people with erratic diets, people who work shifts or have stressful travel schedules, and people with chronic illnesses. Look for "B-50" or "B-100" products, which provide 50 or 100 milligrams of each of the B-vitamins. Take one a day or as the label directs.

I also recommend high doses of a few of the B-vitamins as specific treatments.

Thiamine (vitamin B-1) is selectively destroyed by alcohol. I recommend that drinkers take 100 milligrams of it once a day, especially on days when they drink.

Riboflavin (vitamin B-2) is a yellow pigment, which is what turns the urine bright yellow when you take a B-complex supplement. This is harmless, but can be upsetting if you don't know the cause. I do not know any reason to take this vitamin separately.

Niacin (nicotinic acid, vitamin B-3) produces a dramatic reaction, called the "niacin flush," when you take a sufficient dose (usually 100–200 milligrams). About ten minutes after you swallow it, a sensation of prickly heat begins on the top of the head. This quickly develops into a wave of heat and redness that spreads down the whole body from the head to the feet. I imagine it feels like the "hot flash" that women experience in menopause. After another ten minutes the skin becomes blotchy instead of solid red, and the sensation becomes more itchy and crawly. All effects disappear thirty to forty-five minutes after taking the vitamin. Some people find this reaction interesting and pleasant; others can't stand it.

The niacin flush is the result of dilation of blood vessels in the skin due to the vitamin's effect on arteries and the nerves that regulate them. It is a harmless reaction and may even be of benefit in some people with problems of blood circulation. I recommend supplemental niacin for people with Raynaud's disease (episodes of painful, blanched fingers and hands, usually on exposure to cold), smokers with leg cramps at night, and people with cold extremities. The usual dose I suggest is 100 milligrams twice a day, taken with food to moderate the flushing.

In much higher doses, niacin lowers serum cholesterol, but it can also disturb liver function. People taking 1,000 milligrams two or three times a day have had dramatic drops in cholesterol within a few weeks, but some of them have developed nausea, jaundice, and elevated liver enzymes, a toxic picture mimicking hepatitis. These symptoms go away when they stop taking niacin. A new, much safer form of vitamin B-3 is now available in health food stores. Called "flush-free" or "inositol-bound" niacin (or inositol hexanicotinate), it does not cause flushing, nausea, or liver disturbances. It is the only form I recommend for use as a cholesterol-lowering agent, and I believe it to be safer than pharmaceutical drugs used for this purpose. If you are going to try niacin to bring your cholesterol down, observe these precautions: (1) never use ordinary niacin; use only the inositol-bound form; (2) never use time-release forms of niacin; they are more likely to be toxic; (3) do not exceed 1000 milligrams three times a day; (4) have liver function tests done before the start of therapy and at intervals during it, and stop the therapy if test results are abnormal; (5) discontinue niacin if nausea or any other gastrointestinal symptoms appear; (6) monitor serum cholesterol at monthly intervals, and reduce the dose of niacin to the lowest possible level to maintain improvement.

• *Do not take high doses of niacin if you are pregnant or if you have ulcers, gout, diabetes, gallbladder disease, liver disease, or have had a recent heart attack.*

You will often see niacinamide, a closely related substance, on shelves next to niacin. Niacinamide has the same vitamin activity but does not cause flushing. However, it is ineffective for the treatment of circulatory problems or elevated cholesterol. Do not use it.

Pyridoxine (vitamin B-6) has a number of interesting effects in addition to its actions as a vitamin. High doses (100 milligrams two or three times a day) help relieve nerve compression injuries (like carpal tunnel syndrome), premenstrual syndrome (PMS), and some cases of depression and arthritis. Pyridoxine also helps protect immunity and increases the incidence of remembered dreams.

Although water-soluble vitamins are not thought of as having any toxicity, a few cases of nerve damage have occurred in people taking more than 300 milligrams of pyridoxine a day. I recommend staying below this dose and discontinuing the vitamin if any unusual numbness appears.

Cyanocobalamin (vitamin B-12) is deficient in "vegan" diets, those with no animal products at all. If you eat any dairy products, fish, or meat, you will get adequate B-12 because the body needs so little of it. Vegetarians should be aware that comfrey, miso, and fresh sauerkraut are not sources of this vitamin, as is sometimes stated.

Many doctors and patients like injections of vitamin B-12 as an occasional tonic or pick-me-up. The usual dose is one milligram, a lot for this vitamin, which the body needs in microgram amounts. No toxicity is known for B-12, and people who get shots of it often report immediate feelings of warmth, energy, and a general glow of health. These effects tend to be short-lived and are most prominent with the first injection. I regard B-12 shots as active placebos (see *Health and Healing,* chapters 19–20) and have no objection to their use, but I do not use them myself. Health food stores sell sublingual (under the tongue) and nasal forms of this vitamin.

Folic acid may help reverse mild to moderate cervical dysplasia in combination with other measures (See the entry on this condition in Part IV.). Cervical dysplasia, a precancerous condition in women, is easily diagnosed by Pap smear.

Pantothenic acid and biotin, the last members of the B-complex group of vitamins, have vital metabolic functions, but I do not know of any reason to take them separately in higher doses.

Vitamin C (ascorbic acid, ascorbate) is needed only by humans and other primates. We may have lost the ability to make our own vitamin C as the result of a genetic accident in one of our distant ancestors, a mutation that knocked out the gene responsible for synthesizing ascorbic acid. If we eat plenty of fresh fruits and vegetables, we get a lot of it, but diets lacking in these foods can be deficient, and the need for vitamin C is increased by exposure to toxins, infection, and chronic illness.

I have already written about vitamin C as an antioxidant, cancer fighter, and immune system protector (see pp. 186–187, where you will also find information about dosage and forms). I recommend taking large doses of it throughout the day as a general preventive measure. People with chronic or recurrent infections, those who are exposed to toxic chemicals (including smokers and other drug addicts and those who eat carcinogenic foods), cancer patients, and other people with serious illnesses should take even larger doses. I have never seen any adverse reactions to megadoses of this vitamin except at the limit of bowel tolerance, when flatulence and diarrhea occur. These symptoms disappear as soon as the dose is reduced.

I do not believe that vitamin C is a panacea that will cure everything from AIDS to cancer, but I do believe that we have yet to discover and appreciate all of its protective effects.

The following vitamins are fat-soluble:

Vitamin A is known traditionally for its role in the maintenance of night vision and in the normal development of skin and other epithelial tissues, but in recent years its antioxidant and anticancer effects have drawn more attention. Vitamin A toxicity does occur, both in people who eat seal and polar bear livers, which concentrate huge amounts of it, and more commonly in people who take massive doses of supplements. If you stay below 50,000 IU of vitamin A a day, you will not hurt yourself.

You can avoid the possibility of toxicity altogether by taking beta-carotene, the water-soluble precursor of vitamin A. The body can turn this into the vitamin as it needs to. Moreover, research shows that beta-carotene offers even greater protection against cancer than vitamin A itself. Therefore, I recommend only beta-carotene: 25,000 IU a day for everybody and twice that amount for people with precancerous or cancerous conditions. Natural forms (like those derived from algae) might be more effective than synthetics. There is scientific evidence that beta-carotene protects against skin cancer, cervical cancer in women at risk, and probably other forms of cancer as well.

Vitamin D, sometimes called the "sunshine vitamin," is necessary for the proper absorption and use of calcium. If the skin is exposed even minimally to ultraviolet radiation, the body can produce this vitamin from a derivative of cholesterol in the skin. Unless you are a total shut-in, or live in a basement, or in the far north during the winter, you do not need to take supplemental vitamin D, even if you are not eating the usual dietary sources of it (egg yolks, butter, fortified milk, fish livers). Growing children on vegetarian diets may need additional vitamin D, particularly during the winter. Some people with chronic diseases and disorders of calcium metabolism may also need it, but medical tests are required to confirm the need and determine the correct dose. Usually 400 IU is sufficient, and it is possible to find this dose combined with calcium. If you are healthy, eat a varied diet, and spend any time in the sun, you should not have to take supplementary vitamin D.

Vitamin E, in addition to being a powerful antioxidant, is a natural anticoagulant that offers some protection against heart attacks and thrombotic strokes. I also find it useful as a treatment for a number of female disorders, including fibrocystic breast disease, PMS, and painful or excessive menstruation. It is not toxic, even in megadoses. Applied topically, it reduces scar formation following surgery, burns, or other skin injuries. (Do not apply it until wounds have closed.) See page 185 for details on how to take this useful supplement.

Vitamin K, needed in small amounts for normal blood clotting, is present in many foods. Doctors use it to counteract overdoses of anticoagulant drugs, but there is no reason for people to take it outside of a medical setting.

MINERALS

The body needs small amounts of a number of minerals to function normally. *The best way to ensure that you get all of these micronutrients is to eat a variety of fresh vegetables.* If you do not eat many vegetables, you might want to take a daily multimineral supplement (or a multivitamin/multimineral supplement) for nutritional insurance.

As with vitamins, taking specific minerals in doses larger than needed to prevent deficiency states may have beneficial effects on some medical conditions. Dose ranges are important: if a little is good, more may *not* be better.

There is much confusion about the health benefits of mineral supplements, with many competing products, some very expensive, on the shelves of drugstores and health food stores. Promoters of these products often make extravagant and questionable claims. Medical doctors are well aware of the body's need for iron, cobalt, iodine, zinc, calcium, and selenium. We know that some other micronutrients, like copper, chromium, and manganese, are also needed by the human body, but we do not fully understand the roles they play. The metabolic functions of other substances — cadmium, strontium, nickel, silicon, molybdenum, germanium — are even more obscure. *Do not believe promotional claims made for trace elements, especially about their ability to cure diseases or the need to take them in supplement form for optimal health.*

If you decide to take a particular trace mineral — zinc, for example — and go to a pill store to get it, you will probably be completely bewildered by the variety of products offered for sale. They differ not only in dose but in composition. Do you want zinc gluconate, zinc succinate, zinc picolinate, chelated zinc, zinc in an amino acid complex, organic zinc, inorganic zinc???

I will explain these differences and then comment on several minerals that you need to know about. You need not be concerned about others if you are eating according to the dietary guidelines in this book or taking a multimineral supplement.

Most of the minerals I have mentioned are metals, which the body cannot use in their free or elemental state. It needs them in ionic, or combined, form, as found in chemical compounds. Metals react with inorganic acids to form inorganic salts. Zinc sulfate, for example, is one type of inorganic zinc. Organic salts, those formed from organic acids, include succinates, gluconates, citrates, picolinates, and fumarates. These forms may be more soluble and more easily absorbed by the body than the inorganic salts. This difference is important, because an increased need for trace minerals may be due more to failure to absorb them than to an inadequacy in the diet. Within the category of organic salts there are differences in solubility and ease of absorption. For each trace mineral one or another of these organic, combined forms may be the best way to present it to the body. For example, calcium citrate is absorbed from the intestinal tract more readily than calcium carbonate (chalk, limestone) or calcium gluconate.

Chelates are more complicated compounds in which the metal ion is held in the middle of a large organic molecule. (The word *chelate* comes from the Greek word for "claw," describing the way in which the molecule "grasps" the metal within its structure.) The iron atom in hemoglobin is naturally chelated, as are the magnesium atom in chlorophyll and most of the trace minerals in vegetables. The body may find it even easier to absorb and use chelated forms of the micronutrient metals, and many such products are available.

These are the minerals you need to know about:

Iron is necessary to make hemoglobin, the oxygen-carrying red pigment of blood. It is one of the few minerals we cannot eliminate. *Unless you are a menstruating woman or have had a significant blood loss, you should **never** take supplemental iron except on orders from a physician after appropriate blood tests have documented iron deficiency anemia.* Not only can excess iron accumulate in the body to toxic levels, it may also promote cancer and coronary heart disease.

• *If you take a multivitamin/multimineral supplement, make sure it does not contain iron unless medical tests have indicated that you need it.*

This caution is based on new information about iron that contrasts sharply with advice we heard in the past about the prevalence of iron deficiency and the wonders of iron tonics to counteract fatigue and low energy. Most of us get plenty of iron in our diets, and iron excess may be much more common than anyone thought.

The easiest source of iron for the body to assimilate is red meat, which provides two natural chelates of this element, hemoglobin and myoglobin, another red pigment responsible for the color of muscle tissue. If you do not eat meat, your best sources for iron are whole grains, dried beans, cooked greens, apricots, prunes, raisins, and food cooked in iron pots, especially if you take one of your doses of vitamin C with these foods. Vitamin C greatly facilitates absorption of iron. Vegetarians tend to have lower hemoglobin and red cell counts than meat eaters, but these values do not indicate deficiency states in the absence of symptoms such as fatigue. In fact, lower iron levels in vegetarians may help account for their lower risks of cancer and heart disease.

Sodium is another mineral you need never take in supplemental form unless you experience muscle weakness and lightheadedness as a result of heavy sweating. In some people excess sodium contributes to high blood pressure (and, as a result, increased risk of heart attack and hemorrhagic stroke) and fluid retention (increasing the workload on the heart and kidneys).

• *Make sure that any nutritional supplements you take are free of sodium.*

Potassium, the complement of sodium in the body, will be more than adequate in the diet if you eat a variety of fresh fruits and vegetables. If you have reason to think you are salt-sensitive, I recommend replacing table salt with the mixture of half sodium chloride and half potassium chloride described on page 60. The only people who need to worry about not having enough potassium are those taking prescription diuretics ("water pills"), which can cause excessive urinary loss of this element.

• *Do not take potassium supplements unless a doctor has prescribed them along with diuretics.*

• *Some people who develop muscle cramps as a result of vigorous exercise may find potassium helpful.*

Calcium helps regulate nerve and muscle function and is necessary to build strong bones. It has been much discussed recently because of concern about osteoporosis, a serious condition of weakened bones due to loss of this mineral with age and declining levels of sex hormones. Women become susceptible to osteoporosis at much younger ages than men, because men do not go through an equivalent of menopause in middle age and have high levels of sex hormones into old age. Please see pages 27 and 109 for information on osteoporosis. I will repeat here what I said in Chapter 1: *Osteoporosis is not caused by calcium deficiency in the diet, nor can it be corrected by taking calcium supplements.* Do not eat dairy products to prevent osteoporosis. Their protein content can accelerate the loss of calcium from bones.

If you do not eat dairy products, you can get calcium from cooked greens (collards especially), molasses, sesame seeds, broccoli, and tofu. If you are worried about getting enough calcium, take a supplement. A reasonable dose of supplemental calcium is 1,000–1,500 milligrams a day. Take two thirds of this at bedtime (your body will use it best then) and one third in the morning. It is good to know that supplemental calcium is not harmful, since so many people are taking it today. Calcium supplements vary tremendously in content and price, and you should be cautious in choosing one. Calcium citrate is the best form of this mineral because it it more easily assimilated than other forms and not expensive. Other choices are chelated calcium, oyster shells, and eggshells. It is O.K. to use calcium supplements containing vitamin D, as long as they do not give you more than 400 IU of the vitamin a day.

• *Do not use dolomite as a calcium source.* This mineral ore often contains lead and other toxic heavy metals. The same caution applies to bone meal.

• *Be sure to take magnesium with supplemental calcium.* Without magnesium to balance it, large doses of supplementary calcium are constipating and may be unhealthy over time.

Magnesium complements calcium in the same way that potassium complements sodium. Calcium and magnesium in balance are needed for proper conduction of electrical impulses in nerves and muscles. Taken together, calcium and magnesium are mild neuromuscular relaxants and may help promote sleep at bedtime, especially if muscle tension contributes to wakefulness. I recommend taking these two minerals together in a one-to-one ratio. For example, if you take 1,000 milligrams of calcium a day, take 1,000 milligrams of magnesium too. If this amount of magnesium causes a laxative effect, cut the dose in half. Magnesium citrate or chelated magnesium will be well absorbed, and you may be able to find them combined with calcium in some capsules or powders.

Selenium is an important antioxidant, protector of the immune system, and cancer fighter. See pages 187–188 for information on how to use it.

• *To avoid possible toxicity, never take more than 300 micrograms of selenium a day.*

Zinc in moderate doses can enhance immunity. High doses can depress immunity and should be avoided. If you cut down on foods of animal origin, as I strongly recommend, you need to take supplementary zinc, since vegetables and fruits provide little. The best vegetarian sources of zinc are legumes (dried beans, garbanzos, black-eyed peas, lentils, peas, soy products) and whole grains. If you are on a vegetarian or semivegetarian diet, I recommend that you take 30 milligrams of zinc a day. I use zinc picolinate, which is rapidly assimilated.

• *Do not exceed 100 milligrams of supplemental zinc a day.* Larger doses may have adverse effects on immunity.

Chromium helps stabilize blood sugar, may improve serum lipid profiles, and may help the body burn fat. The best form to use is "GTF chromium" in a daily dosage of 200 micrograms.

Copper balances zinc and may, in small amounts, protect against atherosclerosis. Watch for more research on this possibility. I will not recommend supplemental copper until I see more evidence of its safety and benefits.

ENZYMES

Enzymes are specialized protein molecules that catalyze, or speed up, biochemical reactions. They are involved in all aspects of metabolism, growth, and development, but there is no point in taking them as supplements. The reason is simple: enzymes that are ingested are simply broken down in the stomach and small intestine and digested like any other proteins. Enzymes injected intravenously or directly into tissues might be effective, but those taken by mouth cannot possibly be. The only exceptions to this rule are the digestive enzymes made by the stomach and pancreas, which work in the gastrointestinal tract. I sometimes prescribe capsules of these to people who have digestive problems. Do not waste your money on supplemental enzyme products, such as superoxide dismutase, catalase, glutathione peroxidase, or any other "-ases." (That suffix designates an enzyme.) Let your body make its own enzymes and don't worry about them.

The same argument applies to the nucleic acids, DNA and RNA, the molecules that carry and transfer genetic information in our cells. I can think of no possible reason to take these as supplements since your digestive system will just destroy them.

GLANDULARS

I see a great many glandular products on the shelves of health food stores: extracts of animal thymus, adrenal, pituitary, and reproductive glands to be taken as dietary supplements. *I strongly recommend against using these products.* The body's hormonal balance is maintained by a delicate and interconnected set of controls. Throwing an outside hormone into this system can make an imbalance worse. Besides, diagnoses of "adrenal insufficiency" and "thymus depletion" made by people not qualified by medical training (including nutritionists, chiropractors, massage therapists, and health food store clerks) are unlikely to be valid. You should never take hormone supplements, in either synthetic or glandular tissue form, unless a definite need has been established by appropriate medical tests. In short, avoid over-the-counter glandular supplements. At best they are unnecessary; at worst, dangerous.

AMINO ACIDS

Amino acids are the building blocks of protein molecules, relatively simple natural substances that are the first breakdown products of proteins in digestion. If you eat adequate protein, which, as I explained in Chapter 1, is much less than most people think, you will have all the amino acids you need and probably more. *There is no need to take mixtures of amino acids as nutritional supplements,* no matter what fitness instructors, bodybuilders, and athletes tell you. Read over the information on protein in Chapter 1 and remember that too much of it stresses the liver and kidneys and can irritate the immune system.

Single amino acids are another matter. If you take one amino acid *on an empty stomach,* it may build up to high levels in the blood and brain, causing useful effects. A number of individual amino acids are available in health food stores. They are not cheap, and I do not recommend taking them unless you can verify that they produce beneficial changes. Here are the ones I have experience with:

L-tryptophan is the metabolic precursor of serotonin, one of the neurotransmitters used by the brain to carry information from one part of the nervous system to another. Serotonin has general sedative effects. In theory, raising the level of L-tryptophan in the brain will cause increased production of serotonin and natural sedation. For that reason this amino acid has become popular as a natural aid to sleep.

I do not recommend using any sleeping aids, natural or not, on a regular basis. (See the entry on insomnia in Part IV.) A few years ago, doctors linked L-tryptophan to a rare disease, eosinophilic my-algia syndrome, that is very painful and can be fatal. It is likely that the problem was a contaminant in one brand of L-tryptophan from a Japanese company that changed its manufacturing process. None-theless, the Food and Drug Administration will not allow the amino acid back on the market. *If you have any old bottles of L-tryptophan on hand, throw them out.*

By the way, the "L" in L-tryptophan designates the form of the molecule. Amino acids are asymmetrical and so can exist in right-handed and left-handed forms that are mirror images of each other. Chemists call them "D" and "L." The body uses only L-forms to build its proteins.

Phenylalanine, the precursor of norepinephrine and dopamine, both excitatory neurotransmitters, has an opposite effect from tryp-tophan. L-phenylalanine can be helpful to some people who suffer from depression. D-phenylalanine works differently. It may prevent breakdown of the brain's natural narcotics and so may help some people with chronic pain. People with high blood pressure should be cautious about taking the L-form of this amino acid; it may aggravate that condition. DL-phenylalanine, also known as DLPA, is a mixture of the two forms. It is less likely to raise blood pressure and may be useful as an adjunctive treatment for depression. (See the entry on depression in Part IV.) It is the product I usually recom-mend. You will find all three forms in most health food stores.

If you do not have high blood pressure and want to experiment with phenylalanine for relief of depression or for increased energy, try taking 1,000–1,500 milligrams of DLPA on an empty stomach first thing in the morning, again with 100 milligrams of vitamin B-6, 500 milligrams of vitamin C, and a piece of fruit or glass of fruit juice. See if you notice a change in arousal, energy level, or mood.

If you do have high blood pressure, start with 100 milligrams of DLPA and raise the dose gradually over a few weeks as you monitor blood pressure.

L-tyrosine is also a precursor of norepinephrine and dopamine, even closer to them than phenylalanine is. If you do not get results with DLPA, try L-tyrosine in the same way. Be equally cautious about this substance if you have high blood pressure.

L-lysine reduces the frequency of attacks of oral herpes (cold sores, fever blisters) in some people. Take 500–1,000 milligrams a day on an empty stomach. It is more effective if you minimize consumption of seeds, nuts, peas, and chocolate.

L-arginine and **L-ornithine** supposedly increase the production of growth hormone in the pituitary, which can favor conversion of fat to muscle and development of muscle bulk. These hypothetical effects appeal to weight lifters and others caught up in the bodybuilder psychology, which I do not feel is healthy. The idea of tampering with growth hormone makes me uneasy. Besides, I cannot confirm that these amino acids do anything at all, and they are quite expensive. Arginine has an opposite effect to lysine and may activate herpes in some people.

To sum up:
• *Do not take amino acid mixtures.* They are a waste of money.
• *Take single amino acids for treatment of particular conditions. Take them only on an empty stomach and stop using them if you do not notice any beneficial effects after a reasonable trial, say two to four weeks.*

PROTEIN SUPPLEMENTS

Protein supplements are tremendously popular in our society because people fear protein deficiency and are unaware of the negative health consequences of eating much more protein than the body needs for routine maintenance and repair of tissue. *There is no reason to take protein in supplemental form, ever.*

Recently a forty-nine-year-old airline pilot consulted me after a routine blood test gave abnormal results for liver function. Specifically, his liver enzymes were greatly elevated, a pattern suggestive of an infectious disease like hepatitis or mononucleosis. Except for fatigue, he had no symptoms of those diseases, however, and tests for them were negative. This man had always been in excellent health and was an avid fitness buff, particularly committed to weight lifting and bodybuilding. I questioned him about his diet and his use of supplements and was not surprised to learn that he ingested huge amounts of protein, both in food and in blender drinks fortified with scoops of protein powder. In addition he was taking supplemental ornithine, arginine, tryptophan, and a host of other pills supposed to promote the development of muscle bulk. He assured me this was a modest regimen compared to the habits of most of his fellow bodybuilders. I ordered him to stop all supplements and switch to a low-protein, high-carbohydrate diet. I also gave him some herbal remedies to help his liver (described in the entry on liver problems in Part IV). His liver function returned to normal within two weeks.

MISCELLANEOUS SUPPLEMENTS

Yeast, in powder or flake form, has long been a popular supplement. Brewer's yeast, a by-product of beer making, tastes bitter and is not as rich in some nutrients as nutritional yeast, which is grown specifically for human consumption. Nutritional yeast is a good source of the B-complex vitamins, trace minerals, and some protein (which you do not need). It is not expensive. A heaping tablespoon of yeast will color your urine yellow (owing to its content of riboflavin) and may have enough vitamin B-3 to give you a niacin flush. If you like the taste of nutritional yeast, try sprinkling it on popcorn instead of butter, as an alternative to taking a B-complex pill. Smoked torula yeast is even tastier as a seasoning, but it is not as good a source of vitamins and minerals and probably contains some carcinogenic compounds.

Spirulina and **chlorella** are two varieties of freshwater algae, primitive plants that are cultivated for nutritional use, dried and sold as dark green powders or tablets. They are very expensive and heavily promoted as miracle supplements. What they provide is mostly protein, which you do not need, along with some vitamins and minerals. Claims made for these products are not substantiated by research.

The original source of spirulina was Lake Texcoco, a large lake just outside of Mexico City that is heavily polluted. A not very polite way of describing this supplement was dried scum from a dirty lake. I am sure that most of the early batches of spirulina were full of unhealthy contaminants. Today both spirulina and chlorella are cultivated in clean ponds, but I see no reason to take them, no matter how clean the source.

Barley grass, wheat grass, and **alfalfa** are green plants that some people believe to be full of nutritional blessings. The first two are the young shoots of sprouted grains. Alfalfa is a legume, usually grown to feed animals. Freshly squeezed wheat-grass juice is sold in some health food stores as are dried green powders and tablets of all three plants. There is no evidence to back the claims made for these products, and I do not recommend using them. Alfalfa may contain natural substances that harm the immune system.

Acidophilus is a general name for dried or liquid cultures of living bacteria that sour milk and are considered "friendly" organisms in the intestinal tract. You can buy these preparations in all health food stores. Most are milk-based, but recently some nondairy versions have appeared that use carrot juice as a base. All of them provide much higher concentrations of the desired organisms than yogurt, acidophilus milk, or other cultured milk products.

I take acidophilus with meals when I travel in underdeveloped countries. I believe it reduces the chance of getting traveler's diarrhea, the result of changes in intestinal flora. I recommend acidophilus to anyone who takes antibiotics, especially the broad spectrum ones like tetracycline and ampicillin, which wreak havoc on intestinal flora. I recommend it also to women who have frequent vaginal yeast infections. The dose is one tablespoon of the liquid culture or one to two capsules after meals unless the label directs otherwise. To treat yeast infection, you can also place the liquid culture directly in the vagina in addition to taking it by mouth.

Always check the expiration date on acidophilus products. You want to be sure the bacteria in them are alive and in good condition.

Wheat germ is a nutty-flavored, cereal-like product made from the embryo of the wheat grain. It is a natural source of vitamin E but is also high in calories and fat. Because the fat is polyunsaturated, wheat germ becomes rancid quickly. If you like it, buy it in small quantities, keep it refrigerated, and use it up fast. A derivative of wheat germ, octacosanol, is sold as an energizing supplement in capsule form. Promotional claims assert that it improves athletic stamina and performance, but few studies have been made of its effects in humans. I do not recommend using octacosanol.

Lecithin is a fatlike substance found in the cells of all living organisms. It is commonly used in the food industry as an emulsifying agent and is also widely sold as a supplement to combat atherosclerosis, improve memory, and fight Alzheimer's disease. There is no scientific evidence that it will have these effects. Lecithin is harmless but is not needed in human nutrition beyond the amounts we get in our food. I do prescribe it to patients with multiple sclerosis as a way of strengthening nerve sheaths, which are the targets of that disease.

Coenzyme Q, also called Co-Q-10, is a natural substance, present in most foods, that assists in oxidative metabolism. The supplement form is imported from Japan. Coenzymes are compounds that interact with enzymes, helping them perform their biochemical functions. (Many of the B-complex vitamins function as coenzymes in metabolic reactions.) Since they are not large protein molecules, coenzymes can survive digestion and pass into the system. Coenzyme Q may improve the utilization of oxygen at the cellular level, and patients with coronary insufficiency or diabetes may find it worth trying in doses of 30–100 milligrams a day. Some healthy users report that it increases aerobic endurance. More studies are needed to verify these effects. Coenzyme Q is harmless but not cheap.

Omega-3 fatty acids, like EPA (eicosapentaenoic acid) and DHA (docosahexaenoic acid) are the constituents of fish oils that may protect against heart attacks by thinning the blood. They also act as anti-inflammatory agents and may be worth trying if you have an autoimmune disorder or arthritis. Many versions of these substances are on the shelves of health food stores, from salmon oil to capsules of concentrated EPA. Although I frequently suggest that people eat some salmon or sardines, I do not usually recommend fish oils in capsule form, because it is not clear that adding them to the diet reproduces the benefits of eating fish. Also these supplements may be contaminated with the same pollutants that make so many kinds of fish unsafe to eat on a regular basis. If people do not want to eat salmon or sardines, I usually tell them to take flax seeds, flax oil, or hemp oil as a dietary supplement (see p. 24) rather than fish oils. Because of their effect on blood clotting, you should avoid fish oil supplements altogether if you are taking any anticoagulant drugs.

Evening primrose oil, black currant oil, and **borage oil** are natural sources of another unusual fatty acid called GLA (gamma-linolenic acid). Very hard to come by in the diet, GLA is an effective anti-inflammatory agent with none of the side effects of anti-inflammatory drugs. It also promotes healthy growth of skin, hair, and nails. I prescribe it frequently for skin conditions (including brittle nails and hair), arthritis, autoimmune disorders, and premenstrual syndrome. Do not expect immediate results; it takes six to eight weeks to see changes after adding GLA to the diet. These three products vary in the amount of GLA they supply and in cost. I usually recommend black currant oil in doses of 500 milligrams twice a day as the most economical form.

Homeopathic remedies are harmless dilutions of minerals, plant extracts, and other natural substances prepared according to the principles of homeopathic medicine. (See *Health and Healing*, chapters 1–3, for an explanation of this system of treatment.) These remedies are supposed to stimulate healing reactions by working on the body's energy field. Homeopathy is a controversial form of alternative medicine whose theories conflict with those of regular medicine, but many people find that it works for them. The art of homeopathic practice has to do with selecting just the right remedy in the right dilution out of the many thousands available. (See Appendix A for information on how to find a homeopathic practitioner.) Guidebooks are available to help patients make the selections on their own and treat themselves. If you are interested in learning how to use these remedies, two books that will help you do so are *Everybody's Guide to Homeopathic Medicines* by Stephen Cummings and Dana Ullman (Los Angeles: Tarcher, 1984) and *Homeopathic Medicine at Home* by Maesimund B. Panos, M.D., and Jane Heimlich (Los Angeles: Tarcher, 1980).

Your neighborhood health food store will certainly carry more products than I have mentioned in this chapter. In general, if you don't know what it is, you don't need it, especially if it is very expensive and said to work wonders. Concentrate on improving your diet and use supplements selectively for reasons that you understand.

15

THE HERBAL
MEDICINE CHEST

MOST PEOPLE who come to me for medical consultations leave with prescriptions for herbal remedies. For every prescription I write for a pharmaceutical drug these days, I give out forty or so recommendations for botanicals. I have practiced in this way for the past five years and in that time have not seen a single adverse reaction to any of these remedies. No physician who relies on pharmaceutical drugs can match that record of safety. In addition I have found my herbal recommendations to be effective, especially when they are part of a program of natural treatment that also includes dietary modification, proper exercise, stress reduction, and mobilization of mental resources in the service of healing.

Medical students and doctors frequently ask me how they can learn to use herbal medicine, but I have no ready answer for them. I was fortunate in being able to do my undergraduate work in botany and in having a strong background in the study of medicinal plants. Still, I did not learn what I know from books. I use books to look up information about the history, composition, effects, and possible toxicity of plants that interest me, but mostly I have learned from people who actually treat with plants — herbalists, naturopaths, American Indians, and healers. I'm afraid I do not know a substitute for going out and spending time with teachers of this sort and then experimenting on your own.

One day I may try to write a sort of *Physicians' Desk Reference* to herbal medicine, because I would like more doctors to use plants in place of the strong and dangerous chemical drugs now in fashion. In chapter 9 of *Health and Healing* I explained the differences be-

tween medicinal plants and refined or synthetic drugs. I will not
repeat that material here because I want to get right on to the
practical information. Nor is it my purpose in this chapter to write
an exhaustive guide to herbal treatment. In Part IV, under headings
for specific diseases, you will find many herbal remedies and directions on how to use them. In this chapter I give you some general
information about botanicals: what forms to use, where to get them,
what dangers to be aware of. Then I describe a number of plants
that I find to be safe, effective, and generally useful for common
conditions, plants that you may want to keep around the home as
the foundation of an herbal medicine chest.

Like vitamins and supplements, herbal medicine polarizes doctors
and industry, with patients left somewhere in the middle. The herb
industry is booming today. A great deal of its promotional efforts
are pure baloney, with unsubstantiated claims all too common. Just
as health food stores display the latest miracle supplements, so do
they glamorize miracle herbs. In response the medical profession
likes to issue dire warnings of the dangers of self-care in general
and herbal medicine in particular. Some spokesmen for the medical
profession would like us to believe that pharmaceutical drugs are
safe and herbs are not, that technology is good for us and nature
bad.

In general the herbal products you can buy in stores are not
harmful. They may be ineffective, but they are more likely to do
harm to your pocketbook than to your body. There are a few exceptions, however. One is comfrey, *Symphytum officinale,* a Eurasian
native widely grown in this country. The genus name, *Symphytum,*
comes from Greek roots meaning "to knit together," and the species
name, *officinale,* suggests the status of this plant in European medicine of the past. Comfrey has a long history of use and still enjoys a
strong reputation as a healing plant, one that helps wounds heal,
broken bones mend, and respiratory and digestive functions improve.

I meet people who attribute miraculous virtues to comfrey. They
make "green drinks" of comfrey leaves, eat bowls of the leaves as
salads, or take concentrated extracts of leaves and roots, sometimes
mixed with extracts of papaya or digestive enzymes. I have read

books and pamphlets from health food stores touting the health benefits of this plant. Some say it is a vegetarian source of vitamin B-12; it is not. All say that it is perfectly safe; it is not.

Research in the past decade shows unequivocally that comfrey contains pyrrolizidine alkaloids, compounds that are known to be toxic, which are widely distributed in plants and often are the cause of sickness and death in grazing livestock. These chemicals are particularly harmful to the liver, in which they can cause potentially fatal blockage of the hepatic veins.

Pyrrolizidine alkaloid poisoning in humans usually results from accidental contamination of grains with toxic seeds of other plants, but some cases are on record of individuals, mostly children, who succumbed to acute liver failure after drinking an herbal tea. For example, in 1977 a Mexican-American infant in Arizona died after being given a folk remedy for sore throat. The tea, purchased at a pharmacy that carried Mexican herbal remedies, turned out to be mislabeled. Instead of a harmless species of *Gnaphalium* (cudweed), the package contained an unrelated species of *Senecio*, a toxic desert plant with a high content of pyrrolizidine alkaloids.

The alkaloid content of comfrey roots is higher than that of leaves, and some commercial preparations of the plant have enough of these compounds to be harmful. One brand of comfrey-pepsin capsules — a "digestive aid" made from comfrey roots — will easily deliver enough pyrrolizidines to damage the liver of anyone who takes the recommended dose of two tablets per meal over several months. Even if catastrophic liver disease does not occur, other possible consequences of long-term comfrey use include the gradual development of cirrhosis, liver cancer, and damage to lungs and other organs.

Comfrey lovers often resist these warnings, believing them to be establishment propaganda against an innocent herb. Scientists interested in making people aware of the danger do not help their cause when they go well beyond their data to condemn all herbal teas. In fact, the chance of poisoning from comfrey tea, leaves, and juice is probably small, both because the alkaloid content of these forms is usually low and because the particular alkaloids in comfrey may be less toxic and less easily absorbed from the gut than related compounds in *Senecio* and other species. Still, given the known toxicity of this family of chemicals, it is hard to justify eating comfrey.

Topical application of the plant is another matter. It does indeed have excellent wound-healing properties, and systemic absorption of alkaloids by this route is minimal. I include comfrey in the herbal medicine chest for the treatment of wounds and sores that do not heal, and in a moment I will tell you how to use it.

The lessons I draw from all the information I have reviewed on comfrey are: (1) medicinal plants cannot be considered safe *just* because they have a long record of use in folk medicine; (2) chemical analysis of popular medicinal plants is always worthwhile; (3) even if the plant contains toxins, occasional use of dilute preparations may not be harmful; and (4) it is important to try to inform users about the real hazards of plant products in ways that will not cause them to stop listening.

If toxicity of herbal products is mostly a nonissue, the question of efficacy is a real concern. One reason that regular medicine embraced chemical drugs with such enthusiasm in the last century was that they made possible the administration of exact doses of known compounds. Herbal medicine can be terribly inexact. How can you be sure that an herbal preparation contains the right plant in the right amount or that it has preserved the desired activity of that plant?

One result of the exploding market for natural medicines has been the recent appearance of companies that are doing their best to sell quality herbal products. Still, in order to be an informed consumer, you must know some basic facts:

• *Loose herbs sold in bulk are probably worthless.* Dried plants deteriorate on exposure to air, light, and moisture. Leaves and flowers deteriorate quickly, bark and thick roots more slowly. The more finely chopped the plant parts are, the faster they lose their desirable qualities. Do not buy whole dried herbs from bins or jars in stores.

• *Encapsulated, powdered herbs are also likely to be worthless.* A major cause of deterioration of dried plants is oxidation. The greater the surface area of a plant preparation, the faster it will oxidize. When plants are ground into powders, the surface area increases tremendously.

• *Herbal products may be contaminated or adulterated.* Depending on how the plants were grown and handled before processing, they may carry residues of pesticides and molds and may be mixed with other plants, either accidentally or deliberately. The only way to avoid these problems is to buy reputable brands that advertise the purity of their ingredients. Look for herbal preparations that have been "wildcrafted" (harvested from wild stands) or cultivated organically.

Some Chinese "herbal" remedies manufactured in Hong Kong have turned out to contain powerful pharmaceutical drugs. The notorious "black pearls" taken for arthritis (*chuifong*) contained Valium and phenylbutazone, an anti-inflammatory drug now no longer used in humans because of toxicity. Buy Chinese herbal products from reputable sources (see Appendix B), and do not use any that do not list ingredients.

• *Tinctures and freeze-dried extracts of medicinal plants are the best preparations to buy.* Tinctures are alcoholic extracts of fresh or dried plants, usually containing a high percentage of grain alcohol to prevent spoilage. They are very stable and can provide the beneficial activity of plants in a concentrated, convenient form. Tinctures usually come in small medicine bottles with droppers and should be diluted in a little water before use. A typical dose is one dropperful in a quarter cup of water, taken three or four times a day with food. Shake the bottle well before filling the dropper. The amount of alcohol in one dose is not enough to affect you, but if you object to it, you may be able to find vinegar-based products from some companies. Or look for a freeze-dried preparation instead.

Freeze-drying is a method of flash evaporation at low temperature in a partial vacuum. Very potent preparations of medicinal plants are made by extracting them with chemical solvents, then freeze-drying the extracts to remove all of the solvents, and packing them into capsules. These products are concentrated and stable.

• *Discontinue use of any herbal product to which you have an adverse reaction.* Adverse reactions to botanicals are much less common than to pharmaceutical drugs, but they can occur. You may be allergic to a plant or may react to it in some unique way.

• *Do not take herbal medicines unless you need them.* Medicinal plants are dilute forms of natural drugs. They are not foods or dietary supplements, and you should not take them casually or for no good reason, any more than you would take a pharmaceutical drug casually or for no good reason.

• *Experiment with herbal remedies conscientiously.* People vary in their response to botanicals. Just because a book or person tells you an herb should work for a certain condition does not mean it will work for you. Let your own experience be your best guide and use only remedies that give you consistent results.

With that as background, I would now like to acquaint you with the herbal remedies that I keep in my own medicine chest and use frequently. They are all easy to obtain and are safe and effective when used as directed. I present them in alphabetical order.

Aloe, or *Aloe vera,* is a succulent plant from Africa widely grown as an ornamental in warm regions. Many people have discovered the healing properties of the clear gel that fills the thick leaves of this plant. It is a superior home remedy for burns, so useful that you ought to keep a potted aloe plant in your kitchen to have available in case of an accident.

There are many species of aloes, and many whose leaves are big enough to provide gel, but *Aloe vera,* the "true" aloe, has the best effect. You can buy the plants at most nurseries. They are easy to grow and will multiply for you as long as they have light and good drainage. To use the fresh plant, cut off a lower leaf near the central stalk, cut off any spines along the edge, split the leaf lengthwise, score the gel with the point of your knife, and apply it directly to the burn. It will soon soak into the skin and provide immediate, soothing relief. Use it on sunburn, thermal burns, and any areas of skin irritation or inflammation.

You can also buy aloe products in drugstores and health food stores. Its moisturizing properties make it a desirable ingredient of skin lotions and creams, but be warned that some cosmetics that boast of their aloe content have too little of it to do your skin much good. Read labels to determine the percentage of aloe gel in the formula.

Aloe vera juice, sold in all health food stores, is intended for internal use. Although many claims are made for it, the only reason I know to take it is to help heal ulcers and other irritations of the gastrointestinal tract. In high doses, aloe is an irritant laxative, so if you want it to soothe the lining of your GI tract, you must stay below the laxative dose. A reasonable amount to try is one teaspoon after meals. You can use the fresh gel, mashed up in a little fruit juice, or any commercial product that is pure. A lot of bottled aloe juice tastes nasty; shop around for a brand that is palatable.

Arnica comes from several species of the daisylike genus *Arnica*, native to high mountains of western North America. Tincture of arnica is an excellent external remedy for bruises, sprains, and sore muscles and joints. It is made by crushing whole plants and soaking them in alcohol. Both the plant and tincture have a characteristic, pleasant smell. You can buy tincture of arnica in herb stores and some drugstores.

Apply it freely to sore parts of the body, but do not use it on broken skin. Rubbed in with some massage, it is a soothing, effective liniment that reduces pain and swelling and encourages healing. Arnica products vary in strength. If the tincture causes slight skin irritation, dilute it with an equal volume of rubbing alcohol.

• *Never take tincture of arnica or arnica tea internally.* The plant is toxic when ingested. (Homeopathic arnica tablets [see p. 262] are too dilute to cause toxicity; it is all right to swallow them.)

Chamomile, one of the mainstays of European folk medicine, is the dried flowers of a low-growing plant of the daisy family. The entire plant has a pleasant, applelike smell. (The name *chamomile* comes from Greek words meaning "ground apple.") When brewed into tea, chamomile flowers release this same aroma and flavor along with a slightly bitter taste.

Chamomile tea is an excellent home remedy for upset stomachs. It relieves heartburn, indigestion, and colic and is completely harmless. In addition, it has mild relaxant and sedative properties. You can give it to infants and young children with good results, as well as to old people. Most people find the taste of the tea agreeable.

You can buy extracts of chamomile in herb stores, and ordinary tea bags of it are now available in most supermarkets. As long as they have a strong fragrance, they are fine to use. Brew the tea in a covered container to prevent loss of the volatile constituents in steam. Let the flowers steep in the hot water for ten minutes before pouring.

Comfrey in the form of a poultice for external application is a remarkably effective treatment for wounds that do not heal, such as decubitus ulcers (bedsores), diabetic ulcers, the bites of brown recluse spiders, and the terrible staph infections that affect people living on tropical beaches. All of these conditions can produce large, open, devitalized lesions that resist the strongest pharmaceutical treatments. Use the root of the plant, which you can buy dried in bulk from many herb suppliers. (This is a stable preparation.) Grind it to a powder in a blender, and mix the amount you need with water — or even better, with aloe vera gel — to make a paste. Gently pack it into the wound and cover with a bandage. Change the poultice once a day, washing out the wound with water and with hydrogen peroxide if any infection is present. You will soon notice new tissue growing in from the edges. I have seen complete healing of major skin wounds by this method.

Dong quai is a Chinese herbal remedy made from the root of *Angelica sinensis,* a large plant in the carrot family. It is often called "female ginseng," because it is a general tonic for women and the female reproductive system in much the same way that ginseng acts as a tonic for men and the male reproductive system. Dong quai is commonly available in this country in the form of encapsulated extracts. I prescribe it frequently for such female problems as irregular or difficult menstruation, PMS, menopausal symptoms, and weakness following childbirth. It is a good general remedy for women who simply do not have enough energy, whether or not they have specific gynecological problems. A usual dose is one or two capsules two to three times a day, depending on the strength of the product. Give it a two-month trial to see how it affects you.

Echinacea, obtained from the roots of several species of that genus, is a natural antibiotic and immune-system enhancer from the Native American herbal tradition. Echinacea is familiar to gardeners as purple coneflower, an ornamental plant. It grows wild throughout the plains of North America and is now extensively cultivated as a medicinal. Practitioners of natural medicine in Europe and America have long valued it. In recent years research, done mostly in Germany, has confirmed its antiviral, antibacterial, and immunity-enhancing properties.

You can buy tinctures, capsules, tablets, and extracts of echinacea in all health food and herb stores. The root produces a curious and distinctive numbing sensation when held in the mouth for a few minutes. If a commercial preparation does not do this, it is not good. Always test echinacea products by putting a bit on the tongue; return any that fail to cause numbness.

Try echinacea as a first line of treatment for common infections before resorting to conventional antibiotics. Use it for colds, flu, sore throats, and episodes of low resistance. A dropperful of tincture in water four times a day or two capsules of freeze-dried extract four times a day is the dose for adults; give children under ten half those amounts. To build immunity in the absence of infection, halve the adult dose and stay on the remedy for two weeks at a time. Echinacea loses its efficacy when taken continually; it is better to take it for two weeks at a time, alternating with two weeks off.

Eleutherococcus (Siberian ginseng) is the root of *Eleutherococcus senticosus,* a plant in the ginseng family that is different from true ginseng *(Panax).* Other names for it are spiny ginseng, eleuthero ginseng, and eleuthero. Many people in Russia, including athletes and cosmonauts, use it to increase endurance and resistance to stress, and Russian researchers have shown that it does have these properties. They call it an "adaptogen," a substance that promotes adaptation to environmental stress of all kinds. In the past such a substance was called a tonic, something that tones or stretches the system, making it more resilient, better able to bend under pressure rather than break. Traditional Chinese medicine places great value on tonic plants because it believes in strengthening natural defenses. In the West scientists pay little attention to that strategy and none at all to tonic plants.

Unlike true ginseng, eleutherococcus is not a stimulant or sexual enhancer. But like ginseng, eleuthero must be taken regularly over a period of weeks or months in order to have an effect. I recommend it to people who are run down, weak, lacking in energy and resistance, or suffering from chronic illness. Siberian ginseng products are readily available in herb and health food stores. They vary in concentration and potency, so follow the dosage recommendations of the manufacturer.

For information on true ginseng *(Panax),* see the entry on sexual deficiency in Part IV.

Garlic is a powerful natural medicine in addition to being a strong-flavored seasoning for food. In previous chapters I have referred to garlic's abilities to lower cholesterol and reduce the clotting tendency of the blood. It can also help lower high blood pressure. In addition raw garlic is a potent antibiotic, especially active against fungal infections, with antibacterial and antiviral effects as well. The best home remedy I have found for colds is to eat several cloves of raw garlic at the first onset of symptoms.

Eating raw garlic does not appeal to everyone, but garlic loses its antibiotic properties when you cook or dry it, and commercial garlic capsules do not preserve the full activity of the fresh bulb. You can make raw garlic more palatable by chopping it fine, mixing it with food, and eating it with a meal. Or cut a clove into chunks and swallow them whole like pills. If it gives you flatulence, eat less. If you eat garlic regularly and have a good attitude about it, you will not smell of it. Chewing some fresh parsley after eating garlic also minimizes the odor.

By the way, a *clove* of garlic is one of the segments that make up a head or bulb. I once told a patient with a sore throat to eat two cloves of raw garlic. He called me several days later to say that he was cured but that the treatment had been one of the hardest things he'd ever done. It turned out he thought "clove" meant the entire head.

I have in my files a recent paper from a Chinese medical journal describing the use of intravenous garlic to treat a rare and very serious fungal infection of the brain called cryptococcal meningitis. (We are seeing this more commonly now as an opportunistic infection in AIDS patients.) The Chinese researchers compared intravenous garlic to the standard pharmaceutical treatment, a very toxic antibiotic called amphotericin B. In this study the garlic worked better than the drug and caused no toxicity in any dosage.

A good home remedy for the early stage of ear infections in children is to put a few drops of warm garlic oil in the ear canal, then plug the ear loosely with a piece of cotton. To make garlic oil, crush a few cloves of garlic into some olive oil, let it sit a few days at room temperature, and strain it. Keep the oil in a container in the refrigerator and warm a bit for use as needed. Some people even suggest putting a small clove or piece of a clove of raw garlic directly into the ear, keeping it in with a plug of cotton. It will eventually dissolve.

I recommend one or two cloves of garlic a day to people who suffer from chronic or recurrent infections, frequent yeast infections, or low resistance to infection. Try it; it really works.

Gentian, from various species of *Gentiana,* is a bitter root and an excellent digestive remedy. European herbalists are very fond of "bitters" to stimulate and tone the digestive system, and they rate gentian as the best of them all. Several brands of alcoholic extracts of gentian root are available here, most with other plants added for flavor. For example, Angostura Bitters, a popular ingredient of cocktails, which you can buy in most liquor stores and supermarkets, is essentially a tincture of gentian root and has good medicinal properties.

For sluggish digestion, poor appetite, or flatulence, try taking a teaspoon of Angostura Bitters before or after meals (experiment to see which works best for you). If you do not like it straight, try diluting it with sparkling water to make a (relatively) nonalcoholic "mocktail." Gentian root is quite harmless and quite effective.

Ginger, the familiar spice, has a number of remarkable properties that recommend it for home use. It is a good treatment for nausea and motion sickness as well as a natural anti-inflammatory that is worth trying in all cases of arthritis, bursitis, and other musculoskeletal ailments. It tones the cardiovascular system and reduces platelet aggregation, as aspirin does. You can make a tea of fresh ginger by using about one half teaspoon of the grated root to eight ounces of boiling water. Cover and steep for 10 to 15 minutes, then strain, and add honey to taste if desired. You can also eat candied ginger or buy honey-based ginger syrups. Health food stores sell powdered extracts of ginger in capsules as well as alcohol extracts; both forms are convenient to use. One to two grams of powdered ginger a day is an average dose, but some people report successful treatment of inflammatory conditions with higher doses taken over several months. High doses may cause a burning sensation in the stomach; to minimize this, take ginger with food.

Goldenseal is a small woodland plant (*Hydrastis canadensis*) of eastern North America. The "root" (actually an underground stem or rhizome) is yellow inside and has a strongly bitter taste. Goldenseal is one of the most important native American medicinal plants, in such demand in recent years that it has been overharvested almost to extinction. Fortunately it is now cultivated.

When ground, goldenseal root yields a bitter, grayish yellow powder that you can buy in bulk or in capsules. These preparations are usually stable (but often adulterated with cheaper materials). Liquid extracts and tinctures are sometimes available as well.

Mostly I use goldenseal externally in the powder form. You can sprinkle it directly into a wound; it is a good disinfectant and promotes scab formation. My main use of this remedy is in the form of a rinse for irritated or inflamed mucous membranes. In one cup of warm water mix one quarter teaspoon of salt and one half teaspoon, or the contents of one capsule, of goldenseal powder. (It will not dissolve completely.) Use this as a gargle for sore throat or as a mouth rinse for such conditions as canker sores, sore tongue, tonsillitis, or infected gums (gingivitis). A little cayenne pepper is a good addition if you can tolerate it. Without the red pepper, this is also a good vaginal douche in case of vaginal irritation; let the mixture settle and strain out suspended particles before using it. An eyewash made from goldenseal is a good alternative to antibiotics for eye infections and irritations. Use sterile water in the formula above and strain out all particles. Discard if the solution becomes cloudy, indicating bacterial growth.

Taken internally, goldenseal tones the digestive system and has a reputation as a blood purifier. I sometimes recommend it to people who are debilitated, have weak digestive systems, or are susceptible to recurrent infections, but I find its internal effects less impressive than those of external application. Goldenseal is a most useful component of the herbal medicine chest.

Mullein is a common roadside weed *(Verbascum thapsus)* that produces large downy leaves and, in its second year of growth, a tall flowering spike. Indians and early settlers often smoked the leaves as a tobacco substitute and used them medicinally to treat respiratory ailments.

Tincture of mullein relieves chest congestion and dry, bronchial coughs. Take a dropperful in a little warm water every four hours. This plant has no toxicity. When you shop for mullein tincture you may also find mullein oil offered for sale. This is made by steeping the flowers in olive oil and is intended as a treatment for ear infections, much like garlic oil. Warm it slightly, instill a few drops in the ear, and plug loosely with cotton. You can add garlic for extra effectiveness.

Passionflower is a mild tranquilizer made from *Passiflora incarnata,* a climbing native of southeastern United States that also produces an edible fruit called the maypop. The whole plant is used to make tinctures and extracts, which you can find in herb stores. These are calming without being sedating and are a useful adjunct to programs of stress reduction, much safer than pharmaceutical tranquilizers. Take one dropperful of the tincture in a little warm water or two capsules of extract up to four times a day as needed.

Peppermint is another wonderful digestive remedy, especially useful for the upper GI tract, for relief of heartburn, indigestion, nausea, and the like. You can buy pure peppermint leaf tea in most supermarkets. Brew it in a covered container to avoid loss of volatile components, and drink as much of it as you like, hot or iced. I have cured numerous cases of stomach pain by simply getting people to switch from coffee to peppermint tea. If you eat too much, an after-dinner dose of peppermint helps relieve discomfort.

This herb is also soothing to the lower GI tract, but for it to reach there you should take enteric-coated capsules of peppermint oil. (See Appendix B for a source.) Enteric coating resists attack by stomach acid, so the capsules pass into the intestines intact and release their contents there. I like to give peppermint in this form to people with irritable bowel syndrome, diverticulitis, and other chronic intestinal ailments.

As with garlic, our familiarity with peppermint makes us less likely to take it seriously as a medicine, but in fact it is one of the most powerful and effective remedies for gastrointestinal complaints. It is also nontoxic.

Slippery elm, obtained from the inner bark of the red elm tree *(Ulmus rubra),* was used by Indians as a demulcent, a substance that restores the normal mucous coating on irritated tissues. You can buy slippery elm lozenges in most grocery stores. Try them for sore throats. Or buy slippery elm powder and keep it on hand for its soothing, healing properties. It makes a nutritious gruel that is a good food for infants and persons debilitated by chronic illness. It also helps heal irritated tissues of the gastrointestinal tract. Mix one teaspoon of the powder with one teaspoon of sugar and add two cups of boiling water, mixing well. Flavor with cinnamon if you like and drink one or two cups twice a day.

You can also mix slippery elm powder with water to make a poultice for burns, boils, uncomplicated wounds, and all inflamed surfaces. (Comfrey poultices, by contrast, are for complicated wounds that refuse to heal on their own.) This useful remedy is absolutely harmless and worth knowing how to use.

Tea tree oil, a recent Australian import, is extracted from the leaves of *Melaleuca alternifolia,* a native tree of New South Wales. Aborigines chewed the leaves for colds and drank a tea of them for general sickness. The oil is a powerful disinfectant and most useful herbal remedy. It is a clear liquid, strongly aromatic, with an odor similar to that of eucalyptus.

Tea tree oil is the best treatment I know for fungal infections of the skin (athlete's foot, ringworm, jock itch). It will also clear up fungal infections of the toenails or fingernails, a condition notoriously resistant to treatment, even by strong systemic antibiotics. You just paint the oil on affected areas two or three times a day.

Tea tree oil is nontoxic. Apply it full strength to boils and other localized infections. A 10 percent solution (about one and a half tablespoons to a cup of warm water) can be used to rinse and clean infected wounds with good results. The same solution makes an effective vaginal douche for treatment of both yeast and *Trichomonas* infections, but some women may find it irritating.

Tea tree oil is available in most health food and herb stores. Make sure that the label says it is pure.

Uva ursi, or bearberry, is an evergreen shrub *(Arctostaphylos uva ursi)* of northern Europe and North America. American Indians called the plant *kinnikinnik* and made a smoking mixture from the dried leaves. The leaves are a specific herbal remedy for irritation and inflammation of the urinary tract, for such conditions as nephritis, cystitis, and urethritis; they also help dissolve kidney and bladder stones. In addition they help reduce painful and heavy menstruation by gently constricting blood vessels in the lining of the uterus. Tinctures and encapsulated extracts of uva ursi are readily available and safe for short-term use. (Long-term use may irritate tissues.) The dose is one dropperful of tincture in a little water or one or two capsules three to four times a day.

Valerian is obtained from the root of a European plant, *Valeriana officinalis,* the main sedative in use in Europe and America before invention of the first barbiturate drugs in the early part of this century. The root has a distinctive, penetrating odor that cats like and some people find disagreeable. ("Like old socks" is one description I have heard.) Valerian is a safe and effective sleeping aid, more powerful than L-tryptophan (see pp. 224–225) or such other sedative herbs as hops and skullcap.

I usually recommend using the tincture form. The dose is one dropperful or up to one teaspoon in a little water at bedtime. Encapsulated freeze-dried extract may be available as well, and the dose of this would be two capsules at bedtime. Persons who are dependent on strong pharmaceutical sedatives may find valerian ineffective, but it can be an aid to weaning them off the synthetic drugs. A few people are very sensitive to valerian and may find that the recommended dose leaves them with a morning hangover. They should use less. You can also experiment with smaller doses for daytime calming if necessary.

Note that valerian, like all effective sedatives, is a depressant of the central nervous system. It is much milder than the usual sleeping pills prescribed by doctors, and I have never known it to cause addiction. Nonetheless, I recommend against using it every night to avoid any possibility of dependence or adverse effect on mood or mental functioning.

Valerian is a safe herbal remedy that really works and deserves a place in the home.

This completes my selection of botanicals for the start of your herbal medicine chest. I suggest again that you use these remedies conscientiously, keeping notes on your experiences with them, in order to find out how well they work for you and your family.

SUGGESTED READING

Herbs of Choice by Varro Tyler, Ph.D. (New York: Pharmaceutical Products Press [an imprint of Haworth Press], 1994) is an excellent general guide to botanical medicine.

Herbal Medicine by Rudolf Fritz Weiss, M.D., translated from the German by A. R. Meuss (Beaconsfield, England: Beaconsfield Publishers, 1988) is a more technical book, quite useful as a reference work. A softcover edition is distributed by Medicina Biologica, 4830 N.E. 32nd Ave., Portland, Oreg. 97211.

The American Botanical Council Bookstore, a mail-order service, has a 30-page catalog of books and other informational materials on herbal medicine: P.O. Box 201660, Austin, Texas 78720, or call 800-373-7105.

PART IV

A TREASURY OF
HOME REMEDIES
FOR COMMON
AILMENTS

You will find here detailed recommendations for managing common conditions by natural methods, including dietary adjustment, use of vitamins, supplements, and herbal remedies, and other measures discussed in earlier chapters. In some cases I suggest using allopathic medication along with these treatments. In other cases I suggest stopping allopathic medication as you start the program of natural therapy. *Never stop taking prescribed medication suddenly.* Always taper off slowly as you start to use the new treatments. For example, if you are taking a prescription drug four times a day, cut down to three times a day for a week or two, then to twice a day for another week or two, and so on. If you are taking one pill a day of some drug, cut it in half and take half the usual dose for a week or two, then half of that (a quarter of a pill) for the next week, then a quarter of a pill every other day, and so on. The more gradual the change, the easier it will be for your body to adjust to it. If symptoms get worse, do not hesitate to go back to a higher dose for a while before trying again to cut down. You might wish to discuss your intentions with the doctor who prescribed medication if he or she is open-minded.

Natural treatments usually take longer to work than strong allopathic drugs. Medicinal plants, for example, supply bioactive compounds in low concentrations by an indirect route to the bloodstream and target organs. Therefore their effects are usually more gradual and less dramatic than those of purified drugs. You may have to wait six to eight weeks to notice the benefits of herbal treatment, and the same is true of dietary change and aerobic exercise. Be patient with these recommendations, and give them adequate time to work.

The entries are in alphabetical order.

ACNE

In most people acne is more an annoyance than a calamity, although rare forms of it can cause serious disfigurement and scarring. Acne is the result of overactivity of oil glands in the skin, usually because of increased hormonal activity in adolescence. It is a very common disorder of the skin of the face, shoulders, and upper back, worse in males than in females. Infection is not the primary cause, and long-term treatment with tetracycline and other antibiotics should be avoided. Diet is also not the major determinant of acne, but it is important to avoid high-fat foods and iodine (found in shellfish and iodized salt). Clean the skin regularly with soap and water as well as with the special acne formulas containing benzoyl peroxide. This is an excellent cleansing agent and the active ingredient of many lotions and creams, both over-the-counter and prescription varieties. Do not use any skin products containing oils or dyes.

A good herbal treatment for the skin is calendula, commonly known as pot marigold. (It is not a true marigold.) Calendula is a popular ornamental plant that you can buy for your garden at most nurseries in the spring. Its bright orange flowers can be made into tinctures, lotions, and creams. Try washing your skin with tea made from the flowers, or buy ready-to-use calendula skin products at health food stores.

Most cases of acne will disappear by themselves at the end of adolescence, but if acne persists or becomes severe, it should be treated more aggressively to prevent scarring. Highly effective drugs, derivatives of vitamin A, are available. Tretinoin (Retin-A) is a topical preparation, while isoretinoin (Accutane) is for internal use. These drugs are safe when used under the supervision of a dermatologist but should not be used casually because they can be irritating and toxic.

Some very good Chinese herbal treatments for acne are available, both topical preparations and pills. I have seen them work in some cases when pharmaceutical drugs failed.

Sudden appearance of acne in adulthood may be a sign of hormonal imbalance or drug toxicity (usually from steroids). Get a medical checkup to rule out these possibilities.

ALLERGY

Allergy is misplaced immunity. Allergens like dog hair, pollen, dust, and mold cannot really hurt us, so the immune system need not react to them. Allergy is a learned response of the immune system, and anything learned can be unlearned. The goal of treatment should be to convince the immune system that it can coexist peacefully with these substances. Conventional medicine does not achieve this goal. Instead it suppresses allergic responses, perpetuating them and creating much toxicity.

Allergy has multiple roots. One is inherited, since these conditions are more frequent in children of parents with allergic histories. Another is in the mind and nervous system; emotional stress can precipitate allergic reactions, and relaxation techniques can moderate them. A person who is strongly allergic to roses may react to the sight of a plastic rose, demonstrating the involvement of mind and brain in the learned aspect of these inappropriate immune responses.

In fact, allergy straddles the mind/body border. There is no question about its physical reality, since you can die from an allergic reaction, but you can also make it vanish by changing your mental and emotional state. I have seen long-standing, severe cases disappear when people switched jobs, left a spouse, or otherwise eliminated sources of stress. One way to take advantage of the mind/body connection in allergy is to experiment with hypnotherapy. Hypnosis can lessen or completely prevent allergic reactions and can facilitate the immune system's unlearning of its pointless habits.

Another root of allergy is in the environment. Diet can greatly influence allergic responsiveness or lack of it, as can exposure to potentially irritating substances at critical times in one's development. Excessive protein may irritate the immune system and keep it in a state of overreactivity. The protein in cow's milk, specifically, is a frequent offender, and for people with a genetic predisposition to allergy it may be a hidden cause of problems. One general treatment strategy, therefore, is to follow a low-protein diet and try to eliminate milk and milk products.

The most serious kind of allergic reaction is anaphylactic shock. It can kill by suffocation, the result of swelling of the larynx and

obstruction of the airway. Anaphylactic shock can occur in response
to insect stings, ingestion of allergenic foods in sensitive individuals,
and injected or swallowed doses of medication. It is a medical emergency, but it can be treated effectively. An injection of adrenalin
(administered under medical supervision) will usually end the reaction promptly.

Medical treatments for less serious allergic reactions are much
less effective and often toxic. Antihistamines interfere with brain
activity, causing drowsiness and depression. *Never use antihistamines if you have a tendency to depression or mental dullness.* Even
when these drugs do not depress mental activity, they merely suppress allergy rather than cure it. As a result the pattern of immune
overresponsiveness is strengthened rather than weakened, meaning
that more treatment will be required in the future.

This objection applies even more to steroid drugs (cortisone and
related compounds). *Never use cortisone, prednisone, or other steroid drugs to treat allergic reactions unless they are very severe or
life-threatening. If you must take these powerful hormones, limit
your use of them to two weeks.* Steroids perpetuate allergy through
their suppressive action. They also lower immunity.

For more specific recommendations on the natural management
of allergic disorders, see the entries ASTHMA; BRONCHITIS; ECZEMA;
HAY FEVER; HIVES; ITCHING; MIGRAINE; POISON IVY, POISON OAK.

ANEMIA

Anemia must be diagnosed by examination of a blood sample. If the
number of red blood cells and amount of hemoglobin in the blood
are abnormally low, the cause must be found by further diagnostic
tests. For example, iron-deficiency anemia in adults is almost always
due to blood loss, from excessive menstrual flow, for example, or
internal bleeding into the gastrointestinal tract. The loss must be
identified and corrected. Other kinds of anemias result from increased destruction of red blood cells, which can be a manifestation
of autoimmunity. Still others result from depression of bone marrow
function by infection, cancer, or exposure to toxic chemicals and
radiation. In short, anemia is a sign of something wrong in the body,
requiring good diagnostic investigation rather than home treatment.

Common symptoms of anemia are fatigue, lethargy, and pallor. Whenever a person complains of chronic fatigue and low energy, a complete blood count (CBC) should be done. This is a very simple diagnostic procedure that will reveal anemia and suggest what other tests need to be done.

Do not attempt to treat anemia on your own without knowing its underlying cause.

ANGINA

Angina, or angina pectoris (Latin for "pain in the chest"), is a common symptom of coronary insufficiency that is distressing, disabling, and frequently predictive of heart attacks. The primary problem is narrowing of the coronary arteries by atherosclerosis so that the heart muscle does not receive enough oxygen when demands on it are high. Coronary artery spasm may also play a role. Anginal pain usually begins during exertion or after eating and subsides with rest. Conventional medicine treats it with drugs that dilate arteries (nitroglycerin, nitrites, nitrates) or reduce the workload of the heart (beta-blockers, calcium-channel blockers). These are symptomatic treatments that do not change the underlying problem, and all are strong drugs with the potential to harm. The other standard approaches are angioplasty and coronary bypass surgery, very expensive, drastic procedures that may provide temporary relief but do not halt progression of disease.

An alternative to the strong medical drugs is an herbal preparation made from the berries of a species of hawthorn tree, *Crataegus oxycantha*. Hawthorn increases coronary flow and is much less toxic than the pharmaceuticals in current use. A starting dose is one to two capsules of freeze-dried extract four times a day or one teaspoon of tincture in a little hot water four times a day. If you have to take stronger drugs, use of hawthorn may enable you to get by with smaller amounts. This plant also acts as a diuretic.

Two supplements that may be helpful are coenzyme Q (see p. 229) and L-carnitine, an amino acid that improves metabolism in heart muscle. Neither is inexpensive. The recommended dose of L-carnitine is 1,000 milligrams twice a day.

Scientific evidence exists that atherosclerosis and coronary insufficiency can be reversed by adherence to a conscientious program of lifestyle modification involving a strictly vegetarian, low-fat diet, yoga, meditation, group therapy, and moderate exercise. In the long run this approach is much more cost-effective than drugs or surgery and may offer the only hope for stopping the arterial disease that causes angina in the first place.

ANXIETY

This condition has been called the twentieth-century disease, and indeed antianxiety medications have been some of the biggest moneymakers for pharmaceutical companies in recent years. As I wrote in Chapter 6 (p. 129), these drugs are dangerous and should be avoided, as they interfere with mental function, contribute to depression, and cause an especially nasty kind of addiction.

Please read over Chapter 6 on relaxation. The breathing exercise described on pages 119–120 is the best single antianxiety measure I know. Also see the information about passionflower on page 243.

ARRHYTHMIA

Cardiac arrhythmia (irregular heartbeat, palpitation) is a general name for a variety of disorders ranging from harmless to life-threatening. The commonest arrhythmias are single "skipped beats" (actually premature contractions of the lower chambers of the heart) and runs of unusually rapid but regular beats. These can be upsetting but are mostly benign. The worrisome arrhythmias are associated with serious heart disease; they require medical treatment.

You can do a lot to encourage benign arrhythmias to happen less frequently and cause you less distress. Begin by eliminating caffeine from your life. It is one of the commonest causes and commonest aggravations of irregular heartbeat. Stop using other stimulant drugs as well (nicotine, cocaine, amphetamine, ephedrine, phenylpropanolamine, etc.). Although they are not stimulants, alcohol and marijuana can also predispose to arrhythmias and should be used with caution if at all.

Next, maintain good habits of aerobic exercise. This is the best cardiac conditioner. Neutralize the effects of anxiety and stress on the heart by practicing relaxation techniques (see Chapter 6). Bio-feedback training is a good choice, because it can quiet the sympathetic nervous system. (Arrhythmia is a common expression of excessive sympathetic tone.) Anyone with cardiac arrhythmia should practice the breathing exercise on pages 119–120 at least twice a day.

Calcium-magnesium supplements act as neuromuscular relaxants and may calm down the irritable areas of heart muscle that initiate irregular beats. You can take 1,000–2,000 milligrams of calcium (citrate or gluconate) plus an equal amount of magnesium at bedtime. Stay on these supplements indefinitely. Also experiment with coenzyme Q and L-carnitine.

If an episode of arrhythmia lasts more than a few hours or causes shortness of breath or chest pain, you should go to a physician or emergency room for an electrocardiogram and possible drug treatment to end it.

ARTHRITIS

Arthritis is inflammation of joints, a common cause of pain, disability, and deformity. Doctors speak of "hot joints" to describe the acute phase of arthritis, because the affected part is swollen, red, tender, and warm to the touch. Arthritis can result from trauma or can be a symptom of infectious disease, but most cases are either rheumatoid arthritis, an autoimmune disease affecting younger people, especially women, or osteoarthritis, a degenerative disease of older people, affecting both sexes equally. See OSTEOARTHRITIS; RHEUMATOID ARTHRITIS.

ASTHMA

An episodic constriction of the bronchial tubes, resulting in wheezing, especially on expiration, and difficulty in breathing, asthma is a common disorder of both children and adults, often mysterious and frustrating to treat. Worldwide, the incidence of asthma is increasing rapidly, almost certainly a result of worsening air pollution from cars and industry. The immediate cause of an asthmatic attack is tightening of the muscular bands that regulate the size of the bronchial tubes. These muscles are controlled by nerves, but why the nerves make them constrict inappropriately is not clear. Asthma can be primarily allergic or primarily emotional or induced by exercise or respiratory infection, or it can occur with no obvious causes, in which case doctors call it "intrinsic." Asthma can appear and disappear without warning. It can kill. The strong drugs that allopathic doctors use to treat it are often very toxic, addictive, and sadly ineffective, but a severe attack may require emergency treatment and hospitalization.

Childhood asthma with a strong allergic component that appears at very young ages often disappears spontaneously in adolescence or early adulthood. Much more serious is intrinsic asthma that first appears in middle age; it tends to be resistant to treatment.

Treatment of asthma has two aspects: management of acute attacks and long-term control or prevention. I have used several botanical remedies to manage acute asthmatic attacks. One is Chinese ephedra, *Ephedra sinica*, an ancient medicinal plant and the natural source of ephedrine, a stimulant and bronchodilating drug. You can buy dried ephedra stems (they look like the ends of a broom) from Chinese herb suppliers and some herb shops. These can be brewed into a pleasant-tasting tea that has fewer side effects than pharmaceutical ephedrine. Put a handful of crumbled stems in a glass or enamel pot with a quart of cold water. Bring to the boil, lower heat, cover, and boil gently for twenty minutes. Strain. Drink one or two cups every two to four hours as needed. Too much will cause jitteriness and insomnia. You can also find tinctures and capsules of Chinese ephedra in health food stores; use them according to dosage recommendations on the labels. (Do not use American ephedra, popularly known as Mormon tea; it has too little ephedrine to be of value.)

Another herbal treatment for an asthma attack is lobelia, or Indian tobacco *(Lobelia inflata)*. Mix three parts tincture of lobelia with one part tincture of capsicum (red pepper, cayenne pepper). Take twenty drops of the mixture in water at the start of an asthmatic attack. Repeat every thirty minutes for a total of three or four doses.

Here are some general measures for long-term control and prevention of asthma attacks:

• Eliminate milk and all milk products from the diet. Milk protein increases mucous secretion in the respiratory passages and may also contribute to the allergic component of asthma. Not only does this mean avoiding milk, yogurt, cheese, and ice cream, it also means reading labels to be sure that other food products do not contain any milk. Bread, for instance, often includes nonfat dry milk as an ingredient.

• Always drink plenty of water to keep the respiratory tract secretions fluid.

• Practice breathing exercises, such as the one on pages 119–120. Not only is this a good relaxation technique, it will help you combat the vicious cycle of panic and respiratory distress that builds up in an asthmatic attack.

• Have some manipulative work done on the chest to break up restrictive patterns in nerves and muscles that develop in chronic asthma. The best systems I know for this are osteopathic manipulation, especially from a practitioner of craniosacral technique, and Rolfing, a form of deep-tissue massage (see Appendix A).

• Experiment with radical dietary change, such as elimination of sugar, total vegetarianism, macrobiotics, or long-term fasting. Asthma will sometimes disappear in response to such a change.

• Minimize contact with respiratory irritants, such as smoke, dust, molds, and volatile chemicals. Remove sources of offending materials from your home, install a good air filtration system (see p. 85), or consider moving if the air is generally bad where you live.

• Experiment with living in other locations: in high mountains, the desert, or near the seacoast. Asthma may improve greatly with a change of climate.

• Experiment with traditional Chinese medicine and Ayurvedic medicine (the traditional healing system of India). These systems are sometimes able to offer significant help through more specific dietary adjustments and herbal treatments.

• Use standard (allopathic) medicines selectively and with caution. If you have significant asthma, you will probably have to use medical drugs some of the time. For allergic asthma, one of the safest and best drugs is inhaled cromolyn sodium (Intal). Most bronchodilating drugs are stimulants that increase sympathetic tone and anxiety. Theophylline, derived from tea, has a long history of use, but may not be as safe as doctors used to think. It can cause dramatic personality changes. Other drugs of this class can be inhaled to relieve and prevent attacks. These inhalers work, but they are often addictive, since the bronchial tubes are likely to become constricted again when one dose wears off (the same pattern occurs when these drugs are sprayed into the nose to relieve nasal congestion).

Other inhalers contain steroids. If the steroids are not absorbed into the system, they can be safe and effective. Different products vary greatly in efficacy and absorbability. At this writing the best (AeroBid Inhaler System) contains a synthetic steroid called flunisolide, which has low systemic activity. Steroid inhalers should always be used immediately following inhalation of a bronchodilator.

Oral steroids (prednisone is the commonest) are very dangerous for asthmatics, because it is too easy to become addicted to them, and toxicity from long-term steroid use is devastating. Try to avoid ever going on oral steroids. If you do have to take them, get off as soon as possible.

In general, the less medication you can take, the better. Allopathic drugs, being suppressive in nature, tend to perpetuate asthma and reduce the chance that it will disappear on its own.

ATHLETE'S FOOT

This is a fungal infection of the skin, related to ringworm and jock itch. It thrives in warm, moist, dark places, so one of the best treatments is to expose affected areas to fresh air and sunlight as much as possible and keep them clean and dry. An excellent home remedy for this problem is tea tree oil (see p. 244), which works as well as or better than pharmaceutical antifungal products. Apply a light coating to affected areas three or four times a day, and continue to apply it for two weeks after the infection disappears to make sure the fungus is eradicated.

For persistent or extensive infections by the athlete's foot fungus, doctors often prescribe an oral antibiotic called griseofulvin. It is expensive, can be toxic, has to be taken for long periods of time, especially if nails are affected, and often fails to eliminate the infection. Tea tree oil is cheap, safe, and more effective, even for diseased nails.

If you are prone to frequent fungal infections, try adding one or two cloves of raw garlic a day to your diet (see pp. 240–241). Raw garlic is a potent antifungal agent.

AUTOIMMUNITY

When the immune system mistakenly attacks the body's own tissues, a state of autoimmunity exists, resulting in diseases that can be mild or severe. The commonest autoimmune disorders are rheumatoid arthritis, glomerulonephritis, rheumatic fever, systemic lupus erythematosus (SLE), polymyositis, autoimmune thyroiditis, autoimmune hemolytic anemia, idiopathic thrombocytopenic purpura (ITP), myasthenia gravis, scleroderma, and Sjögren's syndrome. Some other diseases, such as ulcerative colitis and multiple sclerosis, may have autoimmune components.

Autoimmune reactions may be set off by infection, tissue injury, or emotional trauma in people with a genetic predisposition to them. Conventional medicine does not do a very good job with these diseases. It can manage patients through the worst crises, but its treatments are suppressive, not curative, and often fuel the autoimmune process. In addition, most of the drugs used in these disorders, especially steroids and immunosuppressives, cause terrible toxicity when they are used for more than a few weeks. (Doctors frequently put patients on them for months and years.) I have seen dramatic improvements in some autoimmune patients who stopped taking all allopathic medication and worked to improve their health in other ways.

Here are some general recommendations for autoimmunity:

• Eat a low-protein, high-carbohydrate diet of the sort recommended in Chapters 1 and 2. Eliminate milk and milk products, including commercial foods made with milk. Minimize consumption of foods of animal origin.

• Avoid polyunsaturated vegetable oils of all kinds.

• Be sure to do regular aerobic exercise. This is most important. See Chapter 5.

• Practice relaxation techniques like those described in Chapter 6. Visualization can be very effective at moderating autoimmune responses. Psychotherapy can be valuable as an aid to changing emotional states that keep the immune system off balance (see pp. 198–199). Hypnotherapy is also useful if you can find a hypnotherapist willing to take on autoimmune disease. (See Appendix A.)

• Read over Chapters 11 and 12 for information on how to protect your immune system.

• Do not stay in treatment with any practitioners who make you feel pessimistic about your condition. All autoimmune diseases tend to follow patterns of exacerbation and remission, and the potential for remission is always there. Suppressive therapies reduce the probability of lasting remission. The ups and downs of these conditions often mirror the ups and downs of emotional life, so it is worth cultivating positive mental states and working with practitioners who encourage you to experiment and try to manage your own health.

BACK PAIN, ACUTE

Sudden, severe pain in the back, often the lower back, is one of the most common, unpleasant, and disabling conditions human beings can suffer. This disaster can occur in response to lifting a heavy object, taking a misstep, or falling, but it can just as easily appear out of nowhere with no obvious cause. A viral illness may precipitate it, or an emotional trauma. The pain may come on full-blown in an instant or it may develop insidiously over a matter of hours or days out of a minor discomfort. In its most acute phase, back pain can render a person as helpless as a baby, unable to get up from a sitting or lying position unaided or to feed, wash, and dress oneself. Even the gentlest step, most cautious move, or lightest cough can set off a blinding spasm of pain that takes the breath away.

Although people whose backs hurt like this spend a great deal of money on treatments from medical doctors, osteopaths, chiropractors, physical therapists, and others, the benefits are too often not obvious. *Time is the most effective healer.* You can save both time and money if you understand the reason for the pain and know a few good remedies to hasten its departure.

In the vast majority of cases acute back pain comes from muscle spasm. The pain of a tightly contracting muscle can be unbelievably strong, as any woman in labor can testify. Many people with acute back problems think they are suffering from a slipped disc, pinched nerve, spinal subluxation (the chiropractor's bread and butter), or a torn ligament or muscle, when in fact intense muscle spasm is the sole or primary cause. Unless you also have such symptoms as urinary incontinence, tingling or numbness in the legs, or inability to move the legs and feet, there is no reason to think that the problem is anything other than muscle pain. (Consult a physician if you do have those symptoms.) Inflammation of the affected area develops rapidly: you may even feel heat coming from the site.

Spasm of back muscles is maintained by a nervous reflex through the spinal cord that sets up a vicious cycle: spasm and inflammation lead to more spasm and inflammation. Although the cycle can develop in response to injury, the ultimate cause is often in the brain, which can interfere with muscle physiology through the spinal cord. Acute back (and neck) pain are common expressions of stress and emotional stress. This is a true psychosomatic problem — not in the sense of being "all in the mind" but of demonstrating the complex interaction of mind, brain, nerves, and muscles. Frequently it is the brain's distortion of muscle function that sets us up for acute back pain by preventing muscles from responding freely to physical stresses. This may explain why the agonizing, vicious cycle of spasm and inflammation sometimes arises after what seemed like an innocent bend or twist.

An immediate first-aid measure is application of cold. An ice pack on the affected area relieves pain more effectively than any other treatment. Keep it on for fifteen to twenty minutes and repeat every hour or every two hours. The only tolerable position may be lying flat on the back with knees or legs raised; in this case put the cold compress between your back and the floor, resting your weight on it. Heat will often aggravate pain in the early stages.

Absolute rest and immobility are essential measures, at least for a day or two. If you try to go about your business — any of it — you will pay later, either with a longer recovery time or an increase of pain to the point that you will be forced to drop your daily routines and lie down.

Avoiding positions that stress the injury and spending time in those that make it feel better are also important. Do not sit. Do as little as possible of whatever brings on the pain or makes it worse.

Get help and do not be hesitant to ask for help with simple maneuvers. Try lying on your back on the floor with your buttocks near the front of a chair and legs raised at right angles with the calves resting on the seat of the chair. Or place a six- to eight-inch stack of books under your head, raise your knees, and place your feet close to the buttocks about fifteen inches apart; stay in this position ten to fifteen minutes at a time. If you can walk, a little walking between sessions of lying flat may help.

A good homeopathic remedy for acute muscle spasm is arnica montana in the 30X potency, available at most health food stores. (See p. 237 for information on homeopathic medicine.) It is useful for bruises and other trauma as well, so you might want to keep a bottle around the house in case of emergency. Take four tablets as soon as possible after the injury and repeat every hour for the first day while awake. The following day cut down to four tablets every two hours and then four tablets four times a day. You may continue this treatment for four or five days. Homeopathic tablets should be placed under the tongue and allowed to dissolve. They are most effective if you do not take anything by mouth for fifteen to thirty minutes before or after putting them under your tongue. You can also help them work by avoiding caffeine (especially coffee), mint (such as in toothpaste), and camphor (such as in many liniments and muscle rubs).

Anti-inflammatory analgesics, such as aspirin and ibuprofen (Advil, Motrin), are often useful. They all irritate the stomach, so be sure to take them with food. Acetaminophen (Tylenol) relieves pain but does not reduce inflammation.

Doctors often prescribe muscle relaxants for this condition. These drugs are expensive and often disappointingly ineffective, Some make you terrifically groggy and may work mainly by discouraging you from moving around. In some cases, combined with aspirin or ibuprofen and rest, muscle relaxants may help break the nerve-muscle reflex that is responsible for the spasm and pain.

Much cheaper and safer than these prescription drugs are topical counterirritants (Ben-Gay, Tiger Balm) that create sensations of heat and tingling when rubbed into the skin over an area of spasm. These feelings divert attention from the pain and may help the nervous system out of its unhealthy pattern. All drugstores carry counter-irritant liquids and salves. Try to find one that does not contain camphor if you are using homeopathic arnica pills.

Many people with acute back pain seek help through manipulation from chiropractors, osteopaths, or others. Well-done manipulation by a skilled practitioner may occasionally produce dramatic improvement and even cure. More often it gives only temporary relief, if any, and the added trauma of getting in and out of a car to go to a doctor's office may do more harm than the treatment helps. Beware of chiropractors who try to sell you a long and costly package of treatments for your subluxations — vertebral misalignments that show up in great numbers on X rays taken by a chiropractor. Subluxations are not the cause of acute back pain; muscle spasm is. If one or two sessions of manipulation do not bring obvious improvement, it is unlikely that thirty or forty will be any better.

One osteopathic method that may give relief is called counterstrain. The practitioner simply holds the legs and back in certain positions that can help the nervous system out of the pattern it is locked into. Most D.O.s today are not skilled practitioners of manipulation. It is good to know of one who is skilled in case you are in need (see Appendix A).

Massage, especially deep muscle work like shiatsu or acupressure, can help relieve spasm, but usually it is impossible to touch an acutely painful back until some time has passed and improvement has begun. Experiment with massage; you will know when it is the right thing to do.

Acupuncture can be helpful, too, especially if trigger points — localized areas of tenderness within the region of muscle spasm — can be identified. Have someone explore the sore part of your back by pressing on different spots with a fingertip. If certain spots cause particular pain and if the pain radiates beyond the fingertip, these may be trigger points that can be treated. Medical doctors do this by injecting the points with local anesthetics, but an equally good home remedy is to have someone massage them with a knuckle or with a round, blunt object. Or try acupuncture by a trained professional (see Appendix A). Simple needling of trigger points often gives just as good results as injecting them.

Breathing exercises are also useful, and you do not have to wait to start them. Read Chapter 4, "Air and Breath," for general information and use the exercise on page 119. Also practice taking deep, slow, conscious breaths in the form of an imaginary circle from the abdomen through the area of pain up to the nose and down again. Make the breath smooth and continuous with as little pause as possible between inhalations and exhalations. You can do these exercises in any position. Through control of the breath you can work directly on the nervous system and encourage it to relax.

Because emotions have such a great influence on nerve/muscle interactions, you should try to put yourself in a happy state of mind. Spend time with people who bring out your best moods. Watch funny movies. Don't despair. This sounds corny, but it is important.

Once the pain begins to subside, heat may speed recovery. First try alternating applications of cold and heat, ending with heat, then move on to heat alone if it feels good. Wet heat is best. If you can make it to a hot whirlpool bath, do so; it may give considerable relief. When you are able to get up and move about, you may find that a support belt around the lower back will help stabilize you and make movement easier. Drugstores carry belts in a variety of sizes and shapes.

Once muscles have learned this pattern of response, they may tend to go into it again under stress. You may be able to look back and identify a warning signal of the problem, such as an early feeling of tightness, soreness, or discomfort in the area that became the focus of acute pain. If so, you now should be able to recognize that sensation for what it is and take action to prevent another episode of spasm and inflammation. For instance, you could cut back on your activity, spend time in comfortable positions, and get some massage or manipulative therapy as soon as you become aware of the start of trouble.

An experience of acute back pain is humbling. It can also be a chance to learn how to be patient and accepting of changes in the body, how to let go of routine activity, and how to receive help from others.

If back pain strikes, always keep in mind that time is your great ally.

BACK PAIN, CHRONIC

Most chronic back pain is not due to structural injury but to unbalanced muscular contraction and inflammation resulting from an unbalanced pattern of nervous control of the musculature. One expert on chronic back pain calls this problem TMS for tension myositis syndrome (myositis means "inflammation of muscles," and tension implies that the cause is psychosomatic). He has a great record of clinical success based on nothing more than talking to patients and convincing them of the true nature of their pain. After hearing these talks, many of them report that the pain has disappeared for the first time in years, after long and expensive treatments from chiropractors, osteopaths, physical therapists, acupuncturists, orthopedists, and massage practitioners failed to provide anything more than temporary relief. For more on this subject, read *Healing Back Pain* by John Sarno, M.D. (New York: Warner Books, 1991).

I am a great believer in TMS, having seen a great many cases of chronic back pain disappear as if by magic when people fall in love or otherwise make radical changes in their emotional and mental life. This is not to say that chronic back pain is all in the mind. Obviously a lot of it is in the back in the form of real, physical distortion of muscle anatomy and physiology. The causal end of the chain of events leading to the pain is not all in the back, however. It is in the nervous system, and that system connects to the mind and the emotions.

Most people with chronic back pain go around thinking they have a bad back and that the trouble is there. In my experience all chronic back (and neck) pain should be considered TMS until proved otherwise, and most therapeutic effort should be directed at your head: specifically at changing your patterns of thinking, feeling, and handling stress that lead the nervous system into this abnormal pattern. Of course, if you have any history of back injury, that vulnerable spot will be a perfect focus for TMS.

Yoga is an excellent way to strengthen the back, balance nervous functioning, promote flexibility, and neutralize stress (see pp. 107–108). I recommend it to people who think they have bad backs along with counseling about the real nature of their pain and encouragement that tension myositis syndrome can leave without a trace once the brain stops sending the wrong messages to the muscles of the back.

BLADDER PROBLEMS

Bladder infections (cystitis) are a common, annoying problem, especially among women, whose urinary anatomy makes them much more vulnerable than men. Conventional medicine treats cystitis with courses of antibiotics and urinary anesthetics that often fail to change patterns of recurrent infection.

Common causes and aggravating factors of cystitis are addiction to coffee and other forms of caffeine, cigarette and alcohol addiction, dehydration, excessively frequent or traumatic sex, stress, and poor hygiene (such as wiping from back to front after a bowel movement instead of front to back). To end recurrent cystitis, you must eliminate bladder irritants from your life, especially coffee. Decaffeinated coffee and red pepper can also cause problems. Increase your intake of water so that you urinate more frequently. Cranberries contain a substance that makes it difficult for bacteria to adhere to the wall of the bladder. Take advantage of this property by drinking cranberry juice often, or better still, unsweetened cranberry juice concentrate (available at natural food stores) diluted with water or sparkling water.

Take vitamin C in the recommended doses (see pp. 186–187) as a general measure to deal with infection. To promote healing of the bladder, use uva ursi (see p. 244), either two capsules of freeze-dried extract three times a day or one dropperful of the tincture in a cup of warm water three times a day. Continue this treatment until symptoms disappear. Take acidophilus after meals (see p. 228) to improve the health of the digestive tract, especially during and after antibiotic treatment. Adjust your sexual behavior to minimize irritation of the urethra, and get in the habit of urinating after sexual activity. Try not to hold on to urine when you feel the urge to urinate. Of course, try to neutralize the causes of stress (see Chapter 6), which can affect your urinary system.

Interstitial cystitis, a less common and much more stubborn inflammation of the bladder, often resists medical treatment. Persons with this problem must be even more scrupulous about eliminating sources of bladder irritation. Guided imagery therapy may be helpful (see Appendix A).

Be aware that toxic chemicals eliminated in the urine may concentrate in the bladder, causing irritation and possibly increasing risks of cancer. This is another reason to avoid contact with chemicals, poisons, and strong-smelling fumes.

BODY ODOR

Most body odor is the result of bacterial breakdown of sweat. Perspiration itself is normally odorless. An easy way to reduce the amount of bacteria under the arms is to splash on rubbing alcohol. Most commercial deodorant products contain irritating or harmful ingredients, including aluminum salts and dyes. Avoid the antiperspirant varieties. You can find better products in health food stores, such as those containing extracts of green tea, which is antibacterial. Beware of "natural crystals," which contain aluminum even if they say they don't.

Stimulant drugs, including coffee and tea, contribute to body odor by increasing the activity of apocrine sweat glands, special glands in hairy parts of the body that produce strong-smelling, musky secretions. Try eliminating caffeine if body odor continues to be a problem.

BRONCHITIS

Inflammation of the lining of the bronchial tubes may result from irritation (especially in addicted smokers), allergy, or infection. The characteristic symptom is a deep, raspy, painful cough. I see the worst cases of chronic and recurrent bronchitis in cigarette addicts, and the only solution for them is to stop smoking. Worsening air pollution in cities throughout the world is certainly another common cause.

Upper respiratory viral infections sometimes move down to the chest, causing bronchitis that can last for weeks. This is also a common complication of influenza, which establishes itself in the chest to begin with. Regular doctors often jump right in with antibiotics to treat these problems, but that is not a good idea, unless there is proof or good reason to suspect that a bacterial infection is present. Bacterial bronchitis or a secondary bacterial infection following a cold or flu will generally produce a lot of phlegm and mucus, often discolored dark yellow, green, or rusty brown, along with fever. A sputum culture will confirm the diagnosis.

If bacterial infection is not present, I do not recommend taking antibiotics. The best treatments are the usual rest and fluids plus inhalation of steam containing sage or eucalyptus (see p. 205). Warm steam soothes the irritated lining of the bronchial tubes, loosens secretions, promotes healing, and, with aromatic herbs, discourages secondary bacterial growth. Use steam as often as possible while you are awake.

Unproductive bronchial coughs — those that do not cause you to bring up much phlegm — are debilitating and serve no purpose. Try to stop them with a cough suppressant. Start with tincture of mullein (see pp. 242–243). If this does not control the cough, take an OTC (over-the-counter) medication containing dextromethorphan, a safe and effective drug. If that fails to work, ask your doctor to prescribe a narcotic cough suppressant such as codeine. Narcotics are very effective for this purpose and are quite safe if used as directed for a week to ten days. They may cause drowsiness and constipation.

Productive coughs, in which phlegm is brought up, should not be suppressed because they are helping to expel products of inflammation from the bronchial system. Treat them with steam, tincture of mullein, and OTC expectorant cough medications containing guaifenesin. Prescription expectorants contain potassium iodide, which is even more effective. (A good brand is Pima Syrup.) Some individuals have allergic reactions to iodides, so use them cautiously the first time. Freshly prepared horseradish, hot mustard, and wasabi (Japanese horseradish) all help liquefy bronchial secretions. Eat as much as you can tolerate.

In allergic bronchitis try to identify the responsible allergens and minimize contact with them. Avoid exposure to respiratory irritants as much as possible, and eliminate all milk and milk products from the diet. Nonabsorbable steroid inhalers may be quite effective at controlling symptoms (see comments about them under ASTHMA).

BRUISES

To minimize swelling, pain, and bruising after a traumatic injury, always apply cold compresses to the injured area as soon as possible and keep them on for most of the first twelve hours, with occasional breaks to prevent excessive chilling. Take homeopathic arnica tablets (see p. 262) and massage tincture of arnica (see p. 237) into the bruised area.

A very effective treatment for severe bruises and hematomas is the pineapple enzyme bromelain, available in capsules at health food stores. This enzyme is absorbed from the GI tract and is able to promote healing of tissue injuries. The dose is 200 to 400 milligrams three times a day, taken on an empty stomach (at least ninety minutes before or three hours after eating). Occasionally individuals may develop an allergic rash from bromelain; discontinue it if you develop any itching.

Some people bruise much more easily than others. Vitamin C may correct this tendency by strengthening the walls of blood capillaries. Try 2,000 milligrams of vitamin C three times a day.

If you suddenly begin to bruise easily, you may have a problem with blood clotting. Go to a medical doctor for a physical examination and diagnostic blood work.

BURNS

Immediately immerse the affected part in ice water and keep it there for five to ten minutes with brief breaks. (There is a twenty-minute critical period during which this treatment is most effective.) Then apply aloe vera gel (see p. 236) or calendula tincture or lotion (see p. 250), or raw honey. Raw honey can be spectacularly effective for severe burns and is the basis of a new therapy in China that has attracted much attention from doctors in the West. It is soothing, antiseptic, and healing. Get medical help for any burn that covers a large area, results in charring of skin, or becomes infected.

BURSITIS

The bursae are the cushioning sacs that minimize friction in joints. Inflammation of a bursa, or bursitis, usually results from traumatic injury to a joint, often from repetitive use of or pressure on some part of the body. Bursitis of the shoulder is a common disaster for baseball pitchers. "Housemaid's knee" is another variety, the result of spending too much time kneeling. Conventional medicine treats bursitis with anti-inflammatory drugs, which are very rough on the stomach, and with local injections of corticosteroids, which I strongly oppose because of their harmful effect on immunity (see pp. 193–194).

The most important aspect of treating bursitis should be identifying and eliminating the cause. That may mean immobilizing and resting the affected joint to prevent further irritation and allow healing to begin. A good remedy to try is DMSO (dimethyl sulfoxide), a simple chemical made from wood pulp that penetrates the skin and promotes healing of pockets of inflammation. Use a 70 percent solution of DMSO, and paint it on the affected joint with cotton. Let it dry. DMSO may cause a sensation of warmth or stinging and may give you an odd garlicky taste in the mouth. Apply it three times a day for three days. If no improvement occurs, discontinue use. If you notice improvement, cut down to twice-a-day applications for three more days, then once a day for a final three days. Then let your body continue the healing process on its own.

DMSO is a powerful solvent that will dissolve synthetic fibers, so be careful with it. Most health food stores stock it. If you find 100 percent or 90 percent solutions of it, dilute them a bit with distilled water. (The mixture will get hot; allow it to cool before using.)

Acupuncture can provide symptomatic relief of the pain of bursitis and is much safer than anti-inflammatory drugs and injections of steroids.

For other suggestions on reducing inflammation of joints by natural methods, see OSTEOARTHRITIS.

CANDIDIASIS

Candida albicans is a kind of yeast that normally lives in the gastro-intestinal tract and vagina without causing any problems. Under certain circumstances it can reproduce wildly, causing symptomatic infections of the mouth (thrush) and vagina as well as intestinal upsets. A common cause of yeast overgrowth is antibiotic therapy, which can kill off the "friendly" bacteria that compete with candida for food and keep it in check. If you have to take broad-spectrum antibiotics, it is a good idea to take supplemental acidophilus (see p. 228) to reduce the possibility of yeast infections. Candidiasis also tends to occur in people with suppressed immunity, such as patients with cancer and AIDS and those on long-term treatment with ste-roids and other immunosuppressive drugs.

In recent years *Candida albicans* has received much notoriety in certain circles as a major cause of illness. Some holistic practitioners diagnose everyone coming through the door as having systemic yeast infections, and health food stores make a great deal of money on supplements that claim to fight yeast. I have read books and pamphlets that give the impression that everyone who has ever taken an antibiotic or steroid now is infected with candida, and that un-diagnosed yeast infections are responsible for fatigue, depression, anxiety, mood swings, behavioral problems in children, allergic reactivity, skin eruptions, and most chronic digestive problems. I have had patients who believed yeast was growing in their blood, lungs, and other vital organs and begged me to prescribe strong drugs to kill it. They shunned beer, wine, bread, vinegar, and even mushrooms in the belief that any food associated with yeast or fungus would contribute to their disease.

Most of these ideas are unsound. Diagnoses of systemic candidia-sis usually have no scientific basis, and most treatments people take for it are a waste of time and money. If you had yeast growing in your blood or vital organs, you would be in an intensive care unit, critically ill. Since candida is a normal inhabitant of the human body, no objective test can prove it to be the cause of general symp-toms. Culturing it from the throat of a depressed patient does not mean that yeast infection is the cause of the depression.

Most of the treatments prescribed for this faddish disease are harmless except to the pocketbook. One that is not is the prescription drug ketoconazole (Nizoral). It can be toxic to the liver and should not be used except on the advice of an infectious disease specialist. The more commonly used drug nystatin (Mycostatin) is usually safe because it is not absorbed from the gastrointestinal tract.

Women who have recurrent vaginal yeast infections should see the entry on that subject. Others who worry about yeast in their system would do well to eat raw garlic every day (see pp. 240–241) since it is a very effective antifungal agent. Take a course of nystatin if you wish (it must be prescribed by a doctor), and try to cut way down on sugar in the diet. Pau d'arco, an herbal remedy made from the bark of a South American jungle tree (species of *Tabebuia*, also known as palo de arco, lapacho, and taheebo) is often recommended for candidiasis, but I do not prescribe it. Much of the bark that comes into this country is contaminated with pesticides.

Candidiasis is a wonderful example of a fashionable disease. It appeals to our fears of being vulnerable to foreign invaders and satisfies a need to blame our vague and general symptoms on a specific causative agent. Ten years from now it may be out of fashion. In the meantime, if you have used antibiotics and steroids for a long time and have clear symptoms and signs of yeast infection, by all means follow the recommendations above and see what happens. If after a reasonable trial, say four to six weeks, you have not experienced dramatic improvement, consider another diagnosis.

CANKER SORES

These painful ulcerations of the mouth often come and go mysteriously. Use the goldenseal mouth rinse described on page 242 and take a B-100 B-complex vitamin supplement. Try applying tincture of propolis, available at health food stores. Propolis, the cement made by honeybees to construct their hives, has remarkable antiseptic and healing properties. Recurrent canker sores may indicate a metabolic imbalance; dietary adjustment, stress reduction, and rest often will clear it up.

CERVICAL DYSPLASIA

This is a precancerous condition of the uterine cervix, easily diagnosed by Pap smear. *Dysplasia* means that abnormal cells are found when the cervical smear is examined under the microscope. Pathologists grade dysplasia on a scale from 1 to 4, with higher numbers indicating greater degrees of abnormality. The assumption is that more advanced cervical dysplasia will eventually turn into cervical cancer. In its early stages this form of cancer is highly curable. To make sure it is caught early, all women should have a Pap smear once a year for two years. Then if these are negative, have a Pap smear once every three years. Women at high risk for cervical cancer might be wise to get tested every year. (Note: Pap smears may not be as reliable as doctors have thought in the past.) Infection with certain varieties of the human papillomavirus (HPV), which causes warts, may be responsible for most cases of dysplasia and cancer of the cervix.

Getting the news that you have cervical dysplasia can be very upsetting, especially since regular doctors rarely give you any program to follow to correct it. Dysplasias of grades 3 and 4 should be treated promptly. New forms of laser surgery are relatively simple and very effective. If you have dysplasia of grade 1 or 2, you have time to experiment and see if you can make it go away. First identify any sources of low-grade irritation in the genital tract. If you are using an IUD for contraception, have it removed and switch to a diaphragm or condoms. Get cultures and smears for possible undiagnosed infections. Low-grade vaginal infections (with such organisms as chlamydia, which may produce no symptoms) are frequent causes of dysplasia, which will clear up as soon as the underlying problem is treated.

Start taking beta-carotene right away: 50,000 IU a day. In addition, take 10 milligrams a day of folic acid, one of the B-complex vitamins. I also recommend daily vaginal douching. Use one teaspoon of white vinegar to one quart of warm water and add one teaspoon of liquid beta-carotene to this. (If you cannot find beta-carotene in liquid form, puncture several capsules and squeeze the contents in.)

After a month of the above regimen have another Pap smear done.

If it is normal, discontinue douching and cut the doses of vitamins to 25,000 IU of beta-carotene and 2 milligrams of folic acid a day; stay on these indefinitely. If the smear is still abnormal, continue the regimen for one more month and have one more smear checked before resorting to conventional treatment.

CHRONIC FATIGUE SYNDROME

This condition, also known incorrectly as "chronic Epstein-Barr virus disease" or "chronic EBV," is another faddish disease that may or may not prove to be a real clinical entity. It certainly has nothing to do with the Epstein-Barr virus, which causes infectious mononucleosis ("mono") in our part of the world and unusual cancers in Africa and Asia. Antibody tests for EBV are of no value in diagnosing the syndrome.

Typically, chronic fatigue syndrome affects young, healthy adults who feel perfectly well until they get a flulike illness from which they cannot recover. Thereafter they suffer from overwhelming fatigue and lack of energy, which often make it impossible for them to work or do anything but lie around the house. Most patients report severe disturbances of sleep and memory. Many describe unusual sensations, including tingling in parts of the body or the feeling of a motor racing inside them. Some have recurrent sore throats, fevers, and swollen glands. Yet most of them also look great, so friends and relatives often don't take their disease seriously. Chronic fatigue syndrome can last for years.

If this new syndrome really is a specific disease, it may represent chronic infection with a previously unknown virus. My feeling is that only some patients with the diagnosis actually have a chronic viral infection. Others may have many other reasons for not feeling well.

Conventional medicine has little to offer people with chronic fatigue syndrome except antidepressant drugs. Some doctors attempt treatment with injections of gamma globulin, interferon, or the antiviral drug acyclovir, but these are drastic methods likely to cause more harm than good. I advise you to stay away from them.

Here are my suggestions for people with chronic fatigue syndrome:

• Exercise regularly: twenty to thirty minutes of aerobic activity at least five days a week. This may be the last thing you feel like doing, but force yourself to do it. Keep the intensity of your activity below the level that leads to exhaustion.

• Follow the nutritional guidelines in Chapters 1 and 2, especially with regard to a low-protein, low-fat, high-carbohydrate diet.

• Take the antioxidant vitamin formula described on pages 185–188 plus a B-100 B-complex supplement.

• Eat two cloves of raw garlic a day. See pages 240–241.

• Take *Astragalus* root for its antiviral and immunity-enhancing properties (see p. 197). A good product that I use is Astra-8, a mixture of *Astragalus* with seven other Chinese herbs. The dose is three tablets twice a day; you can stay on it indefinitely. (See Appendix B for a source if you can't find this product in a health food store.)

• Avoid support groups for people with chronic fatigue syndrome. They often give you ideas for new symptoms and convey the impression that the disease will be with you for the rest of your life.

• Read *Chronic Fatigue Syndrome: The Hidden Epidemic* by Jesse A. Stoff, M.D., and Charles R. Pellegrino, Ph.D. (New York: Random House, 1988). It contains much useful information. Experiment with the homeopathic remedies described on pages 119–126.

• Ask your doctor to prescribe oxygen for home use and experiment with inhaling it for fifteen to twenty minutes once or twice a day. If it helps, continue to use it until your energy level improves enough to do without.

• Do not despair! Chronic fatigue syndrome is not a lifelong malady. Many of my patients have recovered well after one to five years of being sick. Do not expect to wake up cured one wonderful day. Do expect to have ups and downs, with the downs becoming less severe and less frequent.

COLD SORES. See HERPES.

COLDS

More OTC products are sold for relief of the common cold than for any other ailment, and I have collected and tried out innumerable home remedies for colds. Here is a summary of my research.

- To prevent colds, use vitamin C regularly (see pp. 186–187): 2,000 milligrams three times a day.
- At the first sign of a cold, eat two cloves of raw garlic (see pp. 240–241).
- Take echinacea (see pp. 238–239). This herb, like most treatments for colds, is most likely to work if you use it at the very first sign of trouble.
- Read over Chapter 13 for information on short-term fasting, gargling, and nasal douching, all of which are helpful.
- For head and chest congestion, malaise, and chills, try this powerful tea. Grate a one-inch piece of peeled gingerroot. Put it in a pot with two cups of cold water, bring to the boil, lower heat, and simmer five minutes. Add one half teaspoon cayenne pepper (or more or less to taste) and simmer one minute more. Remove from heat. Add two tablespoons of fresh lemon juice, honey to taste, and one or two cloves of mashed garlic. Let cool slightly and strain if desired. Then get under some warm covers and drink as much as you like.
- If you get more than two colds a year, your immunity may be down. Read over Chapter 12 on the immune system, and take courses of echinacea (pp. 238–239) and *Astragalus* (p. 197) in addition to daily vitamin C.

CONSTIPATION

A great many factors affect bowel function, including diet, drugs, physical activity, stress, and anxiety. Sales of laxatives run to many millions of dollars. Some of these products are safe, others are not. In my experience, more women suffer from constipation than men. Most cases of constipation will disappear following simple adjustments of lifestyle.

- Drink more water. Insufficient fluid is one of the commonest reasons for hard stools that are difficult to pass.
- Eat more fiber (see pp. 41–43). Insufficient insoluble fiber in the diet is also a leading cause of constipation. People who shift from typical diets to vegetarian or semivegetarian diets are often amazed at the welcome changes in their bowel habits.

- Use psyllium as a bulk laxative. The husks of psyllium seeds, from a species of plantain *(Plantago psyllium)*, are an excellent source of insoluble (as well as soluble) fiber and the basis of many safe commercial laxatives. You can buy powdered psyllium seed husks at health food stores without the sweeteners, dyes, and flavors that are added to drugstore products. The only caution about this wonderful remedy is that it must be used with plenty of water; otherwise the fiber will form an obstructing mass that may add to your problems. Start with one rounded tablespoon of the powder stirred well into a glass of water or diluted juice. Drink it down and follow with another full glass of water. Do this once a day for as long as you need to.
- Exercise more. Lack of exercise contributes to poor intestinal tone.
- Do not use caffeine addictively. Coffee and other forms of caffeine are strong laxatives because they stimulate nerves that increase intestinal contraction. When used addictively, these drugs prevent the bowel from following its own natural rhythms. If you are not a regular user of caffeine, a cup of strong coffee will induce a bowel movement quickly, a good treatment for *occasional* acute constipation.
- Do not use tobacco. Nicotine, being a strong stimulant, affects the bowel like caffeine. Addictive use of other stimulant drugs (cocaine, amphetamine, ephedrine, phenylpropanolamine) may also result in chronic constipation.
- Avoid constipating drugs. The commonest are opiates and derivatives of nightshades (atropine, scopolamine).
- Avoid irritant laxatives. Chemicals and herbs that irritate the bowel will induce bowel movements quickly, sometimes violently, but it is too easy to become dependent on them, and laxative dependence results in worse constipation. A common irritant chemical laxative is phenolphthalein, the active ingredient in Ex-Lax, Correctol, and Feen-A-Mint. Two common vegetable irritants are cascara sagrada ("sacred bark") from a native American tree *(Rhamnus purshiana)* and senna from the leaves and pods of a Near Eastern shrub *(Cassia acutifolia)*. Some people think that natural herbal laxatives are perfectly innocent, but these two have drastic effects that are not at all helpful over time.

• If you must use an irritant laxative, try rhubarb root (Rheum officinale). It is one of the safest and least violent, but it should be reserved for occasional use only. You can get preparations of rhubarb root in health food stores.

• Even better is an herbal mixture called Triphala, from the Ayurvedic (Indian) pharmacopoeia, now available in capsules at health food stores. It consists of three herbs and is a superior bowel regulator rather than a laxative. Follow dosage recommendations on the label.

• Avoid laxative products (like Haley's M-O and Agoral) containing mineral oil, which can interfere with absorption of fat-soluble vitamins and cause toxicity.

• Avoid saline laxatives like citrate of magnesia and milk of magnesia, which draw volumes of fluid into the intestines. They are less violent than the irritants but still too drastic to use with any frequency.

• Avoid enemas and colonics. There should be no need to use them to have regular bowel movements.

• If stools are very hard and straining is a problem, try using a stool softener containing docusate, a safe drug that comes in both prescription and OTC forms. Read labels carefully, as some products that call themselves stool softeners also contain irritant laxatives and a variety of additives. Good brands are Dialose and Colace.

• Practice relaxation techniques (see Chapter 6), especially biofeedback, breathing exercises, and yoga. Mental interference with nervous regulation of the bowels is a common cause of constipation. Women who are chronically constipated and have cold hands and feet should avoid all caffeine and take biofeedback training (see pp. 123–125); these symptoms indicate an imbalance of the autonomic nervous system.

• Doctors often teach that it is not necessary or even desirable to have a daily bowel movement. I disagree. Moving the bowels at least once a day contributes to a sense of well-being. If you are eating a sensible diet, drinking enough water, exercising, not putting harmful substances into yourself, and not letting your mind interfere with your body, you should have regular bowel movements without resorting to laxatives, natural or not.

COUGH. See BRONCHITIS.

CUTS

Freely bleeding cuts that do not require suturing need little treatment. Avoid tinctures of iodine, merthiolate, and mercurochrome, all of which irritate tissues. If disinfection is necessary, pour 3 percent hydrogen peroxide into the wound, let it foam up, repeat, and pat dry with a clean piece of gauze or cotton. Tetanus shots are not necessary for open cuts that bleed, only for deep, nonbleeding puncture wounds.

A folk remedy for deep cuts is to sprinkle goldenseal powder in them (see p. 242). This disinfects and encourages formation of a crusty scab that protects the wound from further injury.

To reduce scar formation from deep cuts, gently rub in vitamin E oil twice a day after the wound has closed. You can buy small bottles of pure vitamin E oil at health food stores, or puncture capsules of the vitamin and squeeze out the contents.

DEPRESSION

Depression is so common in our society that many people accept it as a normal aspect of the human condition. It is important to distinguish between situational depression, a normal reaction to external events, and endogenous depression, which comes from within and is unrelated to situations. You should try to work through the former kind, with help from psychotherapists or counselors, for example, rather than try to cover it up. Endogenous depression may require other kinds of treatment.

If you read pharmaceutical company advertisements in psychiatric journals, you would think depression and other forms of mental illness were easily conquered, but despite the promises, the reality is not so rosy. Antidepressant drugs are simply not as effective as psychiatrists and pharmaceutical company executives would like us to believe; they can also be toxic. The new generation of antidepressants (Prozac, Zoloft, Paxil) are more effective and less toxic, but I am deeply suspicious of marketing efforts to paint them as panaceas. Promoters of these drugs would have us believe that we cannot attain our full human potential without them. Let us see if there is still as much enthusiasm for Prozac ten or twenty years from now.

Of all the branches of medicine today, psychiatry is most mired in materialistic thinking. It believes that all mental problems result from disordered brain biochemistry, hence its total commitment to the use of drugs. It makes equal sense to me that disordered moods and thinking *cause* disordered brain biochemistry, and I am inclined to look for other ways to treat depression.

According to Buddhist psychology, depression is the necessary consequence of seeking stimulation; this view counsels us to seek balance in our emotional life instead of going for highs and complaining about the lows that always follow. Its basic prescription is for the daily practice of meditation (see pp. 125–127), and I am inclined to agree that this is the best way to get at the root of depression and change it. That requires a long-term commitment, however, since meditation does not produce fast results.

For faster, symptomatic treatment of depression I know no better method than aerobic exercise in the usual amount: thirty minutes of continuous activity at least five days a week. If you are depressed, exercise may be the very last thing you want to do, but force yourself to do it. Results will not be immediate but should be noticeable within a few weeks.

Follow the low-protein, low-fat, high-carbohydrate diet explained in Chapters 1 and 2. Also experiment with the following amino acid and vitamin formula. On arising in the morning, at least an hour before eating, take 1,500 milligrams of DL-phenylalanine (DLPA), 100 milligrams of vitamin B-6, 500 milligrams of vitamin C, and a piece of fruit or small glass of juice. (If you have high blood pressure, see the warning about DLPA on p. 225.)

Make sure you are not taking any OTC or prescribed drugs that can contribute to depression. That includes all antihistamines, tranquilizers, sleeping pills, and narcotics. Stay away from these medications if you have any tendency toward depression.

Also be very cautious about using recreational drugs if you are depressed, especially alcohol, cocaine, amphetamines, "downers," narcotics, and marijuana. These may give a temporary sense of relief, but with regular use are likely to intensify depression to dangerous levels. Addiction to coffee and other forms of caffeine can also interfere with normal moods and make depression worse.

An alternative treatment that may be worth trying in cases of depression is the prescription drug phenytoin (Dilantin), ordinarily used to control epilepsy. This is a relatively safe drug with a long history of use that may give results very fast, in twenty-four to forty-eight hours. Ask a doctor to prescribe 100 milligrams twice a day, and use this together with the other recommendations in this section. Once improvement is established, cut the dose to 50 milligrams twice a day for a week, then 50 milligrams once a day for another week, then none. For information on this unorthodox use of Dilantin, read *A Remarkable Medicine Has Been Overlooked* by Jack Dreyfus (New York: Dreyfus Medical Foundation, 1988).

One final piece of advice about depression: it is a state of high energy turned inward, negative. You will never come to terms with depression if you try to disown it or suppress it. The way to emotional freedom is to own your depressions, appreciate them, and transform them. You will then be able to use all the energy they contain.

DIABETES

Diabetes mellitus (sugar diabetes) is an inherited disorder of metabolism that comes in two distinct forms: type I (juvenile-onset) and type II (adult-onset). The former begins in childhood or adolescence, is more severe, requires regular injections of insulin to prevent death, and is an autoimmune disorder. The latter affects older adults, is less severe, not autoimmune in origin, and often can be controlled by maintaining normal weight and eating sensibly or by taking oral medication.

It is beyond the scope of this book to go into detail about ways to manage diabetes without relying exclusively on pharmaceutical drugs. I will note that most schools of traditional medicine have methods to regulate blood sugar and help people with this disease, which has been recognized as a disease since antiquity.

Insulin-dependent diabetics are unlikely to be able to get off insulin completely and should never attempt to do so, although they may be able to reduce their insulin requirement through natural therapies and lifestyle modification.

The goal of juvenile-onset diabetics should be to reduce their insulin requirement to a minimum while maintaining the best possible health, especially of the cardiovascular system, through attention to diet, exercise, and stress reduction. The goal of adult-onset diabetics should be to avoid insulin and other prescribed medication altogether, keeping the disease in control by adhering to a healthy lifestyle.

A surprising number of plants used in traditional medicine throughout the world show hypoglycemic activity — that is, they lower elevated blood sugar. One that is common in Europe and North America is blueberry *(Vaccinium myrtillus)*. Blueberry-leaf tea is a mild, safe regulator of blood sugar if taken over a long period of time. Drink one cup in the morning and one in the evening for at least three months. You can find blueberry-leaf tea in health food stores, sometimes along with more concentrated tinctures and extracts.

Stronger hypoglycemic herbs are often available from practitioners of traditional medical systems. For example, Ayurvedic practitioners in India use a plant called gurmar ("sugar destroyer"), which is *Gymnema sylvestre*. Extracts of it are now available in health food stores in this country. It is safe and effective and worth experimenting with.

Some research reports indicate that coenzyme Q (Co-Q-10, see p. 229) can stabilize blood sugar. Try taking 100–200 milligrams a day for at least three months.

Aerobic exercise seems to be the single most important way that adult-onset diabetics can control their disease, even more important than diet. Thirty minutes of daily aerobic activity may prevent onset of the disease in those at risk and may cause complete disappearance of symptoms in those who have it.

Stress can affect the course of diabetes dramatically, and through suggestion you may be able to lower your insulin requirements. Experiment with hypnotherapy and with other relaxation methods described in Chapter 6.

It is easy to think that diabetes, especially the juvenile-onset form, is an unmitigated curse, but it is helpful to look at it in a less negative way. There is a surprising amount of diabetes in the world, surprising for a genetically controlled disorder that can make people so ill and shorten life considerably. One way to account for the persistence of the responsible genes is to consider how they might have been advantageous in the past. In fact, in populations living near starvation or living through cycles of feast and famine, which would probably include many of our ancestors, diabetics might be better off than nondiabetics. They have a different sort of metabolism, one that becomes a disadvantage only when food is present in abundance all of the time.

If this view is correct, as I believe it to be, then diabetes is not a disease or curse in itself but rather an alternative genetic constitution that becomes a disease *only in relationship to lifestyle and environment*. One suggestion that follows from this line of thinking is that perhaps lifestyle and environment can be manipulated in ways that encourage the disease to recede. Our present medical treatments do nothing of the sort. They simply control one manifestation of diabetes (dangerously high blood sugar) without going to the root of the problem. I have no alternative program to suggest, except to encourage diabetic patients to experiment actively with diet, with the frequency and size of meals, and with all aspects of lifestyle to see if they can lower the amount of insulin they require. This means taking on a lot of responsibility for your own health, but, after all, that is why you are reading this book.

DIARRHEA

A number of safe, effective remedies exist for this common and distressing complaint. One of the best is Kaopectate, a suspension of an absorbent clay. I recommend using the concentrated tablets, which are free of additives. This preparation is not a drug and works simply by absorbing and binding irritating material in the gut.

Another possibility is Pepto-Bismol, a preparation of bismuth subsalicylate. It is effective but contains synthetic red dyes and saccharin, and salicylates can cause allergic reactions in sensitive individuals.

A good natural remedy is carob powder, available at health food stores. Start with one tablespoon, mixed with some applesauce and honey to make it palatable. Take it on an empty stomach with acidophilus (see p. 228). Carob is very soothing to irritated intestines.

A good herbal remedy for diarrhea is blackberry root bark *(Rubus macropetalus)*. It contains tannins, which have a desirable astringent action on the intestinal lining. Boil the root bark in water for twenty minutes, strain, and drink a cup every two to four hours till the diarrhea ends. You may be able to find tinctures of this useful plant in herb stores, or you can make your own if you live in an area where blackberries grow. Take a teaspoon of tincture in water every two to four hours.

If diarrhea is accompanied by painful cramps, the best treatment is opium, an old-fashioned remedy that is blessedly effective and quite safe if used in proper dosage for a short period of time. The best preparation is deodorized tincture of opium (DTO), a concentrated extract. Take ten to fifteen drops in a little water every three or four hours as needed. Alternatively, use camphorated tincture of opium, or paregoric, a less concentrated preparation, one teaspoon in water at the same frequency. Both forms are prescription drugs, and both can be used with Kaopectate or Pepto-Bismol. Do not take opium preparations for more than forty-eight hours, and do not use them for noncramping diarrhea.

I recommend against using Lomotil, Donnatal, belladonna, or other derivatives of nightshade plants to quiet an overactive gut. These drugs are more toxic than opium and have unpleasant effects on mind and body.

Diarrhea can lead to dehydration unless you replace lost fluids. Drink plenty of clear liquids: noncaffeinated teas, broth, juice. Add frequent small, soft feedings as tolerated. Avoid milk and milk products, raw vegetables and fruits, bran, whole-grain cereals, sugary foods, spices, caffeine, and alcohol.

Acute diarrhea with fever and blood or mucus in the stool may indicate infection with bacteria or parasites, especially if you are in an area of the world with poor sanitation. Have stool cultures and examinations to check on these possibilities and take appropriate medical drugs if specific organisms are identified.

Chronic diarrhea has many causes. Two of the commonest are addiction to coffee (and other forms of caffeine) and emotional stress. Recurrent episodes of diarrhea along with intestinal gas, bloating, pain, and constipation often lead people into fruitless encounters with gastroenterologists who, after a great many diagnostic tests, call the problem "irritable bowel syndrome" and have little to suggest to correct it. See the separate entry on this vague term, and see also ULCERATIVE COLITIS, a different and more serious disease with chronic diarrhea as a major symptom.

DIVERTICULITIS

In this common condition, abnormal pouches (diverticula) in the wall of the colon become inflamed, leading to episodes of cramping, lower-abdominal pain, and constipation, or constipation alternating with diarrhea. I believe diverticulitis to be a disease of lifestyle, because I do not see it in people who eat healthy diets, who avoid coffee and cigarettes, who exercise, and who know how to prevent stress from deranging their digestive systems.

Simple remedies for uncomplicated cases of diverticulitis begin with high-fiber diets. Add extra fiber in the form of wheat bran or psyllium (see p. 277), being careful to take plenty of water with these bulking agents. Stool softeners may be helpful (see p. 278). Avoid eating raw vegetables until the acute problem subsides; they can be irritating to an inflamed colon. Take aloe vera gel after meals (see p. 236), staying below the dose that causes any laxative effect. Two other excellent herbal remedies are oil of peppermint in enteric-coated capsules (see p. 243) and slippery elm powder prepared as a gruel (see pp. 243–244).

It is essential to eliminate all caffeine from the diet, avoid tobacco, and practice techniques of stress reduction.

If diverticulitis is complicated by infection or if it causes intestinal obstruction, treatment with antibiotics and surgery may be necessary.

EAR INFECTIONS

In young children middle-ear infections (otitis media) are so common as to be accepted as a normal part of growing up. They are also the bread and butter of allopathic pediatricians, who treat them

with frequent courses of antibiotics and decongestants and sometimes with surgery.

I have described the use of an osteopathic technique called craniosacral manipulation to end recurrent ear infections in children (see
p. 87). I cannot recommend this treatment too highly (see Appendix A).

In addition I suggest eliminating all milk and milk products
from the diet for at least three months to see if any benefits result.
That means avoiding all dairy products as well as breads and other
foods containing milk in any form. Soy, rice, and nut milks are all
right.

External ear infections (otitis externa) are more common in older
persons. They are easily treated by putting garlic or garlic oil
(pp. 240–241) or mullein oil (p. 243) into the ear canal. Warm the
oils slightly, put some into the affected ear with a medicine dropper,
and plug loosely with cotton. Sometimes this treatment, combined
with oral doses of echinacea (pp. 238–239), will also end a middle-
ear infection, if you get on it at the very start.

Children who are old enough to gargle should be encouraged to
do so frequently when they first notice the pain of an ear infection.
Warm saline solution works fine (see p. 206); it promotes healing
by bringing more blood to the Eustachian tube, which connects the
ear with the throat.

ECZEMA

Also known as atopic dermatitis, eczema is an allergic skin condition, common in infants, children, and young adults, that produces
itchy, thickened, red areas on various parts of the body. It tends to
come and go and often travels with other allergic conditions such as
asthma.

Dermatologists treat eczema with topical steroids. I do not, since
I believe this kind of treatment is suppressive, not curative, and
strengthens the disease process. Steroids also have a weakening influence on the immune system.

I have had good success with eczema with the following regimen:
• Eliminate milk and all milk products from the diet.

• Take 500 milligrams of black currant oil twice a day (see p. 230). Give children under twelve half that dose. This takes six to eight weeks to produce the desired effect.
• Try visualization or hypnotherapy to take advantage of the mind/body connection in allergic skin disorders.
• In Japan, doctors have achieved spectacular success with severe eczema by the use of hot spring therapy. Patients are required to soak each day in hot spring water (delivered to homes in large bottles) and participate in individual and group counseling. No medications are used.
• Try aloe vera gel (p. 236) and calendula lotion or cream (p. 250) on irritated skin.

EPILEPSY

Epilepsy, or seizure disorder, results from an irritable focus of electrical activity in the brain that periodically disrupts normal brain function. You can be born with such a focus or develop one. Seizures can be very dramatic, as in grand mal epilepsy, or barely noticeable, causing nothing more than momentary lapses of awareness. *Anyone who has a first-time seizure should go to a neurologist for diagnostic evaluation.*

Regular medicine treats seizure disorders with drugs and, rarely, surgery. The drugs control some kinds of seizures very well and others not so well. A new generation of antiepileptic drugs, just released, may be much more effective than those of the past. Even when the drugs work, patients often dislike taking them because all are depressants and sedatives that affect moods and energy levels. Most doctors have no suggestions for patients who want to try to treat their seizures in other ways and cut down on medication.

I do have suggestions for these patients, but I always caution them about the dangers of stopping anticonvulsant drugs. Even normal people will have seizures if you put them on these drugs for a time, then cut them off suddenly. Therefore *you must never stop taking antiepileptic drugs suddenly. Always cut the dose gradually and not until you begin using other measures to reduce the chance of seizures. If a seizure occurs, go back up to the prescribed dose.*

Since the challenge in treating seizure disorders is to reduce the excitability of the brain, the first thing to do is to eliminate all stimulants from your life, including tobacco, coffee, tea, cola, chocolate, and other drugs (see pp. 116–117, 135–147).

• Use tincture of valerian (p. 245) as a natural, mild depressant. Take one dropperful in a little water three or four times a day.

• Take a calcium-magnesium supplement to decrease nervous irritability: 1,000 milligrams of each at bedtime and 500 milligrams of each twelve hours later. (Citrates, gluconates, or chelated forms are best.)

• Practice the breathing exercise on pages 119–120.

• Experiment with brain-wave biofeedback (see pp. 123–125) if you can find a therapist who is set up to do it. You want to learn to produce slower brain waves: more alpha and theta rhythm.

Once you have made some of these changes — *not before* — begin cutting down your dosage of anticonvulsant medication. This process should be gradual: give yourself several weeks at each new level before cutting further. Remember, the goal is not to eliminate the drugs totally (although I have seen occasional patients succeed at that) but to reduce them to a level you can live with, so that you can enjoy normal alertness and still not have seizures.

EPSTEIN-BARR VIRUS DISEASE (EBV). See CHRONIC FATIGUE SYNDROME.

EYE PROBLEMS

The best treatment for dry, red eyes is to wash them with sterile normal saline solution, which you can get at any drugstore. Not all OTC eye drops are safe to use. Stay away from those containing tetrahydrozoline, a drug that clears up redness by causing little blood vessels to constrict. Rebound dilation follows, as with nose sprays, and will get you into an addictive cycle with the drops. For irritated, sore eyelids, try using cool compresses soaked in calendula lotion (see p. 250) or cool, wet tea bags.

Eyestrain is a not uncommon cause of frontal headaches. If you have such headaches, make sure you are wearing the right corrective lenses.

I wish I could tell you that you could throw away your glasses by doing eye exercises, yoga, and special breathing techniques, but my experiences with vision training have not left me optimistic. Eye exercises like the Bates method require a lot of practice over long periods of time, and the rewards are usually modest at best.

I recommend caution about the relatively new surgical procedure of radial keratotomy to improve vision. This is a simple operation in which a series of cuts are made in the cornea to allow it to assume a new shape. Immediate results may be good, but long-term ones may not be. A newer, better technique using lasers instead of knives will soon be available.

Two common, serious causes of visual impairment in older people are cataract and macular degeneration. You can reduce risks of the former by protecting your eyes from ultraviolet light. Wear sunglasses or get UV-protective coatings on other glasses. Taking the antioxidant formula (pp. 185–188) will reduce the risk of macular degeneration.

If you work with computers and have to watch a video display terminal for long periods, protect your vision by periodically looking away from the screen at some distant object.

FEMALE PROBLEMS. See BLADDER PROBLEMS, CERVICAL DYSPLASIA; FIBROCYSTIC BREAST DISEASE; MENOPAUSE; PREMENSTRUAL SYNDROME; UTERINE FIBROIDS; VAGINAL YEAST INFECTIONS.

FIBROCYSTIC BREAST DISEASE

This condition produces benign breast lumps that fluctuate in size, usually in phase with the menstrual cycle, and that sometimes become painfully inflamed. These lumps do not become cancerous, but breast cancer occurs more frequently in women with this condition, and early detection of it is more difficult. Many cases of fibrocystic breast disease will disappear or improve markedly if you take the following actions:
• Eliminate all sources of caffeine from the diet, including chocolate.
• Take vitamin E, 400 IU two or three times a day (see p. 186).

• Minimize consumption of foods containing estrogens: meats, poultry, eggs, and dairy products, unless these are certified to have been produced without the usual hormones. Less important are some vegetable sources of estrogenic activity: carrots, parsley, thyme, licorice, and sarsaparilla.
• Follow a low-fat diet and get regular aerobic exercise.

Remember also that fibrocystic breast disease will naturally tend to disappear at menopause unless you take estrogen replacement.

FLATULENCE

Pay attention to which foods or which combinations of foods cause flatulence, and try to modify eating patterns. For some people, eating fruit with starches causes flatulence. For many, foods like beans, cabbage, and cherries do it. A new product called Beano, available in health food and drugstores, is a plant-derived enzyme that helps the digestive system break down substances in foods that contribute to gas. You put a few drops on the first bite of the offending food; the treatment is somewhat effective.

A number of herbs, called carminatives, help expel gas from the intestinal tract. One of the most effective and easiest to get is fennel seed, which you can buy in the spice section of any supermarket. Try chewing a half-teaspoon of fennel seeds at the end of a meal or any time you feel distended from gas.

FLUID RETENTION

Some women retain fluid before the start of their menstrual periods, causing abdominal bloating and swelling of the fingers. This is an uncomfortable but benign effect of hormonal change that causes great psychological distress to women who have distorted body images and obsessive fears of getting fat. Some get in the unhealthy habit of taking OTC or prescribed diuretic drugs, which are likely to be harder on the system than retained fluid.

You can mitigate the problem of fluid retention by eating sensibly, restricting sodium intake in the premenstrual phase, and exercising. Regular black tea is a safe, natural diuretic that will work for you if you are not a regular user of caffeine. Two other herbal diuretics that I recommend frequently are cornsilk tea and freeze-dried dandelion leaf. Both are mild and nontoxic. You can get cornsilk tea in health food stores or make it yourself if you have access to fresh corn by steeping the silks in boiling water for ten minutes. Drink one cup two to four times a day. See Appendix B for a source of freeze-dried dandelion leaf. The dose here is one or two capsules two to four times a day. Hawthorn berries (p. 253) are a stronger diuretic. Take these remedies only when symptoms are present.

Please do not take pharmaceutical diuretics unless you have a real medical need for them (such as hypertension or heart failure).

GALLBLADDER DISEASE

Gallstones and resultant inflammation of the gallbladder are more common in women than men. Most gallstones are composed of cholesterol. They are unlikely to form in people who eat low-fat, mostly vegetarian diets. Removing the gallbladder has been a favorite activity of surgeons for many years. It is possible to live with gallstones if they do not cause symptoms, but attacks of gallbladder pain are serious, requiring surgery or other allopathic treatment. A new method of breaking up gallstones with sound waves is just becoming available; it promises to be safer and simpler than surgical removal of the gallbladder. If you must have your gallbladder removed, insist on the new technique of laparoscopic surgery, which is much less traumatic than standard abdominal surgery.

GOUT

This painful condition of joints, usually in the big toes, results from deposition of urate crystals in the joints. Damage to kidneys can also occur. Gout results from an inherited metabolic disorder, mostly affecting men, in which high concentrations of uric acid circulate in the blood. Uric acid is a breakdown product of protein metabolism, particularly of a class of proteins called purines, which are found in organ meats, sardines, anchovies, and lentils. It is possible to go through life with elevated uric acid and never experience symptoms of gout. Good drug treatments exist for acute attacks of gouty arthritis and for reduction of serum uric acid between attacks, but a few simple measures may enable you to minimize or avoid the use of drugs.

- Follow the dietary guidelines in Chapters 1 and 2.
- Never take protein supplements.
- Eliminate coffee and all other sources of caffeine from the diet. Caffeine and related drugs can raise uric acid levels.
- Always drink plenty of water to keep urine output high. This will help flush uric acid out of the system and prevent deposition of urate crystals in the urinary tract.
- Minimize consumption of alcohol. It promotes dehydration and irritates the urinary tract.
- Maintain normal weight; obesity correlates with symptoms in gout.

GUM DISEASE

Gingivitis — inflammation of the gums — with resultant recession of gum tissue and damage to teeth is a common condition of middle-aged people that often necessitates painful, costly surgical treatment. Most gum disease can be prevented by eating a good diet, not smoking, and practicing good oral hygiene.

- Get in the habit of using dental floss at least once a day. Use *unwaxed* dental floss if possible, and get it under the gum line to scrape the tooth surface. Have a dental hygienist teach you how to use it.
- Whenever you have a chance, massage the gums with your fingertips. Also stimulate gums by running the end of a round wooden toothpick under the gum line.
- If gums are sore, mix hydrogen peroxide and baking soda to a paste and work this mixture into and under them with a toothbrush. Leave it on for a few minutes, then rinse.
- Use the goldenseal mouth rinse described on page 242.
- Have your teeth and gums cleaned by a dental hygienist twice a year; get treatment for any pockets of infection that are discovered.
- Take coenzyme Q, 60–100 milligrams a day.

HAIR PROBLEMS

For dry, brittle, thinning hair, try adding black currant oil to your diet (see p. 230), 500 milligrams twice a day. You will see changes in six to eight weeks. Once improvement occurs, cut the dose in half and stay on this supplement indefinitely.

HAY FEVER

This common, annoying ailment, also known as allergic rhinitis and seasonal pollen allergy, makes life miserable for many people at certain times of the year. Like all allergy (see pp. 251–252), it is an example of misplaced immunity, since pollen cannot harm us.

In my opinion, conventional treatments for hay fever are not very good. Having had an intense ragweed allergy for most of my early life, I have tried them all. Desensitization shots are expensive, painful, and not without risk. (I once had an allergic shock reaction to one that could have been fatal.) Moreover, the percentage of patients who experience satisfactory relief of symptoms after years of shots is disappointingly low.

Antihistamines are the mainstays of hay fever treatment. They will often reduce itching in the eyes, ears, and throat, dry up a runny nose, and reduce sneezing attacks, but their actions on the brain also make you drowsy and depressed. I consider antihistamines toxic drugs with adverse effects on consciousness, and I would go to great lengths to avoid them. In the past few years new antihistamines have appeared that are not absorbed into the brain. The first of these on the market was the prescription drug terfenadine (Seldane). These products do not cause drowsiness and depression, but they do not work for everyone, and they are expensive.

An objection to all antihistamines, whether they enter the brain or not, is the suppressive nature of their action. They do not change the allergic process, merely block its expression. Suppressive treatment can perpetuate disease by frustrating it. All allergies have the potential to disappear if you make changes in your lifestyle and mental state. Regular use of suppressive therapies reduces that possibility.

Steroid drugs are even more powerful suppressors of allergic reactions than antihistamines. Doctors often prescribe steroid nasal inhalers (Beconase and Vancenase, for example) for hay fever sufferers. The drugs in them are not supposed to be easily absorbed into the system. These can be strikingly effective in relieving symptoms, but some of the steroids are bound to get into the rest of the body, and these hormones weaken our immune systems. A much safer prescription drug is cromolyn sodium (Nasalcrom Nasal Solution).

A safe, natural alternative to prescription drugs is the stinging nettle plant *(Urtica dioica)*. It relieves hay fever symptoms quickly in most people, has no toxicity, and is even a valuable source of iron and trace minerals. Stinging nettles are common plants throughout the world, well known to anyone who has brushed against them on walks in the country. Fresh plants have stinging hairs that inject irritant chemicals under the skin with spectacularly unpleasant results. When dried or cooked, nettles lose their sting and are much prized by wild food enthusiasts as a source of pleasant tea and cooked greens. You can buy stinging nettle tea in most health food stores.

For hay fever the best form to use is a freeze-dried extract of the leaves, sold in capsules (see Appendix B for the source). The dose is one or two capsules every two to four hours as needed to control symptoms. I have taught many patients to get off antihistamines and on to stinging nettles with good results. Laboratory studies have documented the effectiveness of this helpful plant.

Another natural product that helps manage hay fever is quercetin, a bioflavonoid obtained from buckwheat and citrus fruits. Quercetin appears to stabilize the membranes of cells that release histamine, the mediator of pollen reactions. Its action is preventive rather than symptomatic. The best way to use quercetin is to start taking it a week or two before the expected onset of the pollen season, continuing till the end.

Many quercetin products are sold through health food stores. Some contain the pure substance; others combine it with vitamin C and other bioflavonoids like rutin and hesperidin, which may or may not enhance its effectiveness. Pure quercetin powder is yellow, insoluble in water, and messy to take. It is easier to use in the form of a coated tablet. The recommended dose is 400 milligrams twice a day between meals. Take this regularly through the allergy season.

I often teach hay fever sufferers to practice nasal douching (see pp. 205–206) with a warm saline solution. This rinses pollen grains off nasal tissues and soothes irritated mucous membranes. Of course, general measures for quieting allergies are also helpful, especially decreasing dietary protein and minimizing or eliminating consumption of milk and milk products.

If all else fails, you can move to another part of the world and leave offending pollens behind. This will often give you one to three years of freedom from hay fever until new sensitivities develop.

I have met a few people who claim to have lost pollen allergies by eating local bee pollen over several months. This must be done with caution, since you may have a violent reaction to eating pollen if you are strongly allergic. The pollen must be from local bees (get it from a beekeeper or a health food store), and you should start consuming it well before the onset of the hay fever season. Start with a tiny crumb and work up slowly to a teaspoon a day. Decrease the amount or stop altogether if you experience itching in the throat.

HEADACHE

In no other condition is it so important to make a correct diagnosis, since different kinds of headaches require very different treatments. I do this by taking time to ask patients about all the details of their headaches: how often they occur, what time of day, what part of the head is involved, whether pain is throbbing or steady, what makes it better and worse, what other symptoms accompany it, and so on. Many people who develop headaches fear they have brain tumors, but if you were to list causes of headache in order of probability, brain tumor would be near the bottom.

Right at the top of the list would be muscle tension. Tension headaches usually begin in the afternoon or early evening and produce steady pain that comes up the neck and back of the head. The muscles of the neck and shoulders may be sore and will feel tight to a trained body worker. Tension headache is a very common stress-related disorder, and the best way to get rid of it is to practice relaxation techniques (see Chapter 6). Biofeedback training aimed at reducing muscle tension in the shoulders, neck, and scalp may be helpful. Massage can be a godsend to tension headache sufferers; I recommend shiatsu and Trager work especially, but even a garden-variety neck and shoulder rub can do wonders. Eliminate caffeine from your life; it increases muscle tension as well as anxiety. Practice the breathing exercise on pages 119–120. Taking aspirin or other pain relievers on a regular basis is not the way to deal with this malady.

Musculoskeletal problems in the upper back and neck can produce headaches that resemble tension headaches. Try osteopathic manipulation from a doctor trained in craniosacral technique (see Appendix A). Also follow the recommendations in OSTEOARTHRITIS.

Steady headache pain that occurs in the forehead or around the eyes often comes from eyestrain or pressure in the sinuses. Have your eyes checked if you have not done so in a while. For what to do about sinus headaches, see SINUS PROBLEMS.

Very high blood pressure can produce headache that typically occurs in the back of the head and is present on waking. If you have frequent or persistent headaches you should make sure your blood pressure is not elevated. See HYPERTENSION for how to deal with this problem.

Throbbing headache arises from an imbalance in the arteries of the head and so is called "vascular." The commonest type of vascular headache is migraine. "Migraine" is not simply a name for a bad headache. It is a particular disorder with many variant forms. See MIGRAINE.

A rarer type of vascular headache is the cluster headache, so called because it occurs in clusters over several days or weeks. It may come at the same time of day every day for two weeks, then disappear for months. The pain of cluster headache is severe, typically one-sided, and has distinctive associated symptoms, such as redness and tearing of the eye on the affected side, runny nose or nasal stuffiness, and visible swelling of blood vessels on the affected side of the head. The prescription drug ergotamine is effective for aborting and preventing attacks. Follow the recommendations for migraine as well.

Vascular headache is also the chief sympton of caffeine withdrawal as well as a common symptom of caffeine addiction (see pp.

142–143). Anyone prone to vascular headaches should avoid using this drug on a regular basis.

If you have headaches that appear suddenly and persist or increase in severity, you should go to a physician for diagnostic evaluation.

HEARTBURN

This condition is a clear sign that you are offending your stomach: by eating too much, by eating too often, by eating the wrong foods, by consuming irritating substances and drugs, by letting anxiety and stress interfere with digestion. Consuming antacids like after-dinner mints is not the solution. If you clean up your diet, you should never suffer from heartburn or have to buy antacids again. Your stomach is your friend. Be nicer to it.

Here are a few guidelines:
• Change your eating habits. Follow the recommendations in Chapters 1 and 2. Pay attention to the kinds of food that make your stomach unhappy and stop eating them.
• Stop drinking alcohol. Or cut way down and be sure to have food in your stomach when you indulge.
• Stop smoking. Tobacco irritates the stomach too.
• Stop drinking coffee and decaffeinated coffee. They are strong stomach irritants. Other forms of caffeine are not as bad.
• Drink peppermint tea frequently (see p. 243). It is an excellent stomach soother (but may exacerbate esophageal reflux by relaxing the sphincter at the junction of the esophagus and stomach). Chamomile tea is an alternative (see p. 237).
• Practice the breathing exercise on pages 119–120 along with other relaxation techniques (Chapter 6).
• If you have to use an antacid, read labels carefully. Avoid those containing aluminum. Calcium carbonate (Tums) and magnesium hydroxide (milk of magnesia) are all right. Do not use sodium bicarbonate (baking soda, bicarb); you do not want to eat extra sodium.

HEMORRHOIDS

Almost everyone at some time or another is bothered by hemorrhoids. They are distended veins around the anus that can become inflamed, causing itching, pain, and rectal bleeding (usually seen as bright red streaks on toilet paper). Common causes of hemorrhoids are pregnancy (these go away after delivery), prolonged sitting, constipation that results in straining at stool, and irritants in the diet. See CONSTIPATION for advice on how to manage that problem. The most obvious dietary irritants are coffee and decaffeinated coffee, alcohol, red pepper, mustard, and other strong spices. Avoid them if you are prone to hemorrhoids. Stay away from tobacco too.

• A good natural treatment for symptomatic hemorrhoids is the sitz bath. Sit in a bathtub filled with enough warm water to cover the anal area for fifteen minutes several times a day.

• Apply aloe vera gel (see p. 236) to the area frequently; it feels good and promotes healing. In addition, take one teaspoon of liquid aloe vera after meals.

• Instead of dry toilet paper, use compresses of witch hazel to clean the anal area after bowel movements. You can get witch hazel at any drugstore. Just moisten sheets of toilet paper with it.

• Many OTC products are sold for symptomatic relief of hemorrhoids. Avoid those containing benzocaine or other topical anesthetics. Preparation H is safe; it is an unlikely but effective combination of a yeast culture and shark liver extract.

HERPES

The herpes simplex virus (HSV) causes cold sores (fever blisters) on the lips and in the mouth and genital herpes on the genitals. It can also appear on the buttocks, thighs, or abdomen. I had one patient who got it on her thumb. The hallmark of HSV infection is a blister or cluster of blisters that often feels tingly and itchy at first, becoming sore later, eventually crusting over and disappearing. A first episode of herpes may produce fever, malaise, and enlargement of local lymph nodes; recurrences are usually milder but may begin with a brief period of general malaise. Once you get infected, the virus is with you for life. It lives in nerve cells where the immune system cannot find it, becoming activated from time to time. Common activators of herpes outbreaks are colds and other viral infections, fatigue, sun exposure, physical irritation of the skin, and emotional stress. Some people are bothered by outbreaks once a year or less; others may get them every few weeks.

• You can reduce the frequency and severity of oral herpes attacks by taking L-lysine as a daily supplement (see p. 226). This does not usually work for genital herpes, unfortunately.

• A simple treatment for oral herpes is to put a drop of ether (diethyl ether) on the lesion. This promotes crusting and speeds healing. Pharmacists will sell you small quantities of ether for this purpose.

• I regret to say that I have not found any effective home remedies for genital herpes, though I have tried out many suggestions. The prescription drug acyclovir (Zovirax) will shorten episodes and suppress the virus. It is very expensive and not curative.

• Try visualizations and mental affirmations to let the herpes virus know that it is welcome in your body only if it stays in its dormant state.

HIATAL HERNIA

This kind of hernia is a protrusion of a portion of the stomach through the muscular ring at the junction of the esophagus and stomach. In most cases it produces no symptoms, but, depending on diet and other factors, the herniated portion of the stomach can become irritated or cause acid to reflux into the lower portion of the esophagus. The result is upper gastrointestinal distress (heartburn, belching, distension, difficulty in swallowing, regurgitation). You should be able to make these symptoms go away.

• Follow the recommendations for HEARTBURN.

• Do not lie down or go to bed within two to three hours of eating a meal.

• Try eating smaller amounts more frequently.

• If you are bothered at night, try raising the head of your bed by six to eight inches with blocks of wood.

HIVES

One of the more dramatic manifestations of allergy, hives can cause terrific mental and physical discomfort. Usually a response to something ingested (a food or drug), most cases of hives are self-limited.

Occasionally hives persist for weeks or months, resisting efforts to find a cause and not responding to medical treatments.

It is worth trying to find the reason for an outbreak of hives so that you can avoid that cause in the future. If you reacted to a particular drug or food, you will not want to put that substance into your body again. Sometimes hives result from contact with allergens, such as residues of detergents and dry cleaning chemicals on clothes. If you are cursed with chronic hives and cannot trace them to anything you ate, you may have to eliminate all possible allergens from your home.

Bear in mind that emotional upsets can be the primary trigger of hives, sometimes of giant hives and angioneurotic edema, a disfiguring and annoyingly itchy swelling of the lips. The mind is deeply involved in this variety of allergy, a connection you should work with if the condition persists.

Antihistamines will often relieve acute episodes. They are less successful with chronic hives and, because they are a suppressive treatment, may contribute to persistence of the disorder. Do not let anyone talk you into taking prednisone or other steroids. Try using stinging nettles and quercetin instead, according to the directions in HAY FEVER. For topical treatment use cornstarch or colloidal oatmeal added to bath water. A good oatmeal product for this purpose is Aveeno Bath Treatment, available at drugstores.

I strongly recommend hypnotherapy as a way of dealing with chronic or recurrent hives. The systems responsible for this reaction in the skin have intimate connections to consciousness and are responsive to suggestion. Also try homeopathic treatment (see Appendix A).

If you fail to get relief, you may have to look carefully at your lifestyle to find the cause of the imbalance. You could be allergic to your spouse, your home, or your job.

Let me give you one final word of consolation: it is much better to have disease on the surface of the body than in the interior. Hives are a great hardship, but they will not injure your vital organs. Remind yourself frequently that surface problems can disappear without a trace if you figure out the adjustments they are asking you to make.

HYPERTENSION (HIGH BLOOD PRESSURE)

Much of the information in Part I is relevant to the prevention and treatment of hypertension. Read Chapters 6 and 9 especially.

Most cases of high blood pressure are called "essential hypertension" because doctors do not understand the cause. Probably the cause lies in the brain and the sympathetic nervous system, which prepares the body for emergencies, for "fight or flight" responses. In an emergency the most critical function is maintenance of circulation to the brain. When the sympathetic nervous system is activated, it shunts more blood to the brain by constricting peripheral arteries, raising arterial blood pressure. In essential hypertension the nervous system seems to be reacting to an imaginary threat that never goes away. Sympathetic tone is constantly too high, arteries are constantly constricted, and blood pressure remains elevated to levels that can eventually damage the heart and arteries, kidneys, and other organs.

Because the sympathetic nervous system deals with fear and uses adrenalin and nonadrenalin as its chemical messengers, it is not surprising that anxiety is a factor in essential hypertension. One of the clearest demonstrations of this is the artificial elevation that often occurs when a doctor or nurse reads a patient's blood pressure — the so-called white coat syndrome. Doctors inadvertently aggravate hypertension when they contribute to patients' anxiety about it.

The first piece of advice I will give you on this subject is to verify for yourself that your blood pressure is elevated by learning to take it yourself in your own home when you feel secure and relaxed. You can buy, from medical supply stores or mail-order catalogs, easy-to-use blood pressure monitors that give digital readouts. You may well find that the values your doctor gets in his office are much higher than your norm, in which case you can feel more confident about managing the problem on your own without medication.

There is good reason to try to treat hypertension without medication, because most of the medications are toxic. Diuretics, intended to decrease fluid volume in the circulatory system by stepping up urinary excretion of sodium and water, may increase the risk of heart attack. Most other hypertensive drugs work by interfering with nerves that regulate arteries, blocking their constricting influence. Not only do these cause many uncomfortable side effects (including impotence in men), they do not get at the root of the problem and may perpetuate it. The brain is not stupid. It has many ways of monitoring the results of its actions. When it finds that the message it sends through the sympathetic nerves is being blocked, it will try even harder to get it through.

The bottom number of a blood pressure reading, called the diastolic pressure, is the measurement during the relaxed phase of the heart's pumping cycle. It is the more important one in determining health risks. If it is consistently 100 or above, you must do something to get it down to 80 or below. Do so by following the recommendations I am about to give you. Give them a reasonable trial — say, two months of conscientious work. After that, if you have not been able to bring your pressure down, you will have to consider taking medication as a last resort.

• Discontinue use of all stimulant drugs, including coffee and tobacco.

• Lose weight if you are more than five pounds above your ideal weight. Follow the dietary guidelines in Chapters 1 and 2.

• Get on a regular program of aerobic exercise, according to the guidelines in Chapter 5.

• Practice relaxation techniques (Chapter 6). Start using the breathing exercise on pages 119–120. Take biofeedback training to lower blood pressure, then practice the technique on your own.

• Decrease your intake of sodium and increase your intake of potassium. See pages 220 and 221 for information on these minerals.

• Take supplemental calcium and magnesium: 1,000 milligrams of each at bedtime and 500 milligrams of each twelve hours later. You can stay on these supplements indefinitely.

• If you have to take antihypertensive medication, do not feel that you will have to take it for the rest of your life. Continue to practice all of the suggestions in this section and periodically try to reduce your dosage. Never stop the drugs suddenly. Always make gradual cuts in dosage, and see, by monitoring it yourself, if you can maintain satisfactory pressure.

HYPOGLYCEMIA

This term means low blood sugar. It is another faddish and questionable disease, one that now seems to be going out of fashion, as candidiasis and chronic fatigue syndrome have become more popular. Rare individuals have highly unstable blood sugar and episodes of dizziness, weakness, sweating, and fainting as a result. A major reason why this condition is rare is that maintenance of blood sugar is critical to normal brain function, since the brain lives on glucose as its only fuel. The body does not take chances with variables affecting the equilibrium of the brain and so has many fail-safe mechanisms to ensure a constant blood sugar regardless of what we eat.

Until the newer fad diseases appeared, many people who complained of fatigue, low energy, weakness, and depression were diagnosed as hypoglycemics, especially after undergoing glucose tolerance tests. This procedure begins with having the patient drink a large volume of sugar water. Then blood samples are taken at set intervals over the next few hours for blood sugar determinations. In my opinion this test is worthless because it distorts normal physiology and gives many false positives. Even if hypoglycemia can be documented, it is likely to be a symptom of an underlying nervous imbalance rather than a primary disease.

Health practitioners who like to diagnose hypoglycemia usually recommend dietary changes that are quite unhealthy: minimizing consumption of carbohydrate and eating mostly protein, for example. They also urge people to take all sorts of vitamins and supplements that are unlikely to be of any value.

If you think you have unstable blood sugar, follow the recommendations I have given you about diet (Chapters 1 and 2), exercise (Chapter 5), and relaxation (Chapter 6). Minimize the sugar in your diet, but by all means eat plenty of starches and keep protein consumption low. Avoid caffeine and alcohol. Supplemental chromium is supposed to help stabilize blood sugar. Try 200 micrograms a day of the GTF (or niacin-bound) form, which is most easily assimilated, and stay on it for at least two months.

Do not blame depression, fatigue, lack of sexual energy, or lack of enthusiasm for life on low blood sugar. Look for the real causes of these states and work on changing your lifestyle to correct them.

IMPOTENCE

Male impotence — inability to have penile erections sufficient for intercourse — is much more likely to have a psychological cause than a physical one. There is a very simple way to distinguish psychological impotence from physical impotence: the postage-stamp test. Glue a strip of postage stamps around the shaft of the penis before you go to bed. If the strip is intact in the morning, you have not had any erections during sleep, meaning something is wrong with the mechanics of the system. See a urologist for further diagnostic work. Drugs are a common cause of this sort of impotence, especially tobacco (which interferes with blood circulation to the genitals), cocaine and other stimulants, alcohol and other depressants, and antihypertensive and psychiatric medication.

If, as is more likely, the ring of stamps is broken, nothing is wrong with your penis. Instead the problem has to do with interaction of your mind and penis. This calls for counseling or therapy with a psychotherapist or sex therapist.

Men spend lots of money on products that claim to boost male potency, few of which actually work. The only drug currently listed in the *Physicians' Desk Reference* as a sexual booster is yohimbine, derived from the bark of an African tree *(Pausinystalia yohimbe)* and long rumored to be an aphrodisiac. Yohimbine is a stimulant that sometimes appears as a street drug. Users report distinctive and pleasurable tingling sensations along the spine and in the genitals. Manufacturers say it increases erections in men. Currently it is a prescription drug, available under the brand names Yocon, Yohimex, and Aphrodyne. Yohimbe bark and extracts are sometimes offered for sale in health food stores.

Yohimbine is relatively safe, with minor side effects in recommended dosage, but little scientific research exists to back up the claims made for it. The drug does increase sexual arousal and performance in male rats. Whether it acts the same in male humans is unclear. It does not appear to increase human sexual desire but may boost erectile and ejaculatory ability, which would make it worth trying in cases of physical impotence. (A doctor must prescribe it.)

Of all the categories of products recommended to increase male potency, hormones have the strongest biological effects. Both male and female sex hormones are manufactured in the adrenal glands of every body, both male and female, as well as in the ovaries and testes. The body makes them by complicated reactions from cholesterol. The "sterol" part of that word refers to a distinctive molecular structure that occurs in many hormones and drugs — steroids.

Male sex hormones are also called anabolic steroids because they stimulate anabolism, the building-up phase of metabolism. Under their influence protein synthesis increases in bone, muscle, and skin, leading to increased bone density, muscle mass, and skin tone, all desirable effects. These hormones are also androgens; that is, they stimulate the development of male sexual characteristics: facial and body hair, male distribution of fat and muscle, deep voice, and so on. If not enough androgens are circulating in the system, men lose libido, erections, and, eventually, some of their sex characteristics as well.

Testosterone is our principal androgen. Long recognized as regulating sexual function in men, it now appears to have widespread behavioral effects in both sexes. Recent research makes testosterone look very attractive as a sexual booster, but oddly enough, women may benefit from it more than men. Getting the dose right is critical, as is selecting the right way of introducing it into the system.

Unless men are deficient in testosterone, taking extra is not going to do much. It can be a miracle cure for men who have suffered injuries to their testes or who were born with insufficient testosterone or who have little free testosterone in their blood as the result of aging. Even in these cases the manner of giving it is very important, since the body has a daily cyclic rhythm of testosterone production that is not matched by taking it in pill or injectable form.

A few years ago a group in England tried out a testosterone cream to be rubbed on the skin of the abdomen. But the female sex partners of men using the treatment started growing beards, ending that line of research. Today the most promising method also administers this hormone through the skin but in a much more sophisticated manner. A testosterone patch is about to come on the market. It is applied to the scrotum and delivers the hormone in amounts and rhythms that closely mimic the natural state. You have to keep your scrotum shaved and apply a new patch every day. This product is intended as a treatment for sexual dysfunction with a physical basis, not for normal men who want to have more and bigger erections. Potential users include elderly men whose bones have become weak (from osteoporosis) as a result of low levels of free testosterone.

No doubt many nondysfunctional men will continue to experiment with testosterone preparations, but there is really no evidence of any beneficial effect on sexual desire or performance. Besides, unusually high levels of androgens may hurt men physically or emotionally, causing a higher risk of heart attacks, for example, or increased aggressiveness.

The function of testosterone in women is not known — they produce about one tenth the amount men do — but it appears that giving women additional small amounts can dramatically increase libido. For women who lack sexual interest and desire, the treatment can be life-changing. Although good scientific studies support these observations, most women and most physicians remain unaware of the beneficial effect of testosterone on female sexuality.

INFECTIONS

Frequent or recurrent infections may indicate weakened immunity. Read Chapter 12 for information on how to protect your immune system. To keep from getting infections:

• Take vitamin C, 2,000 milligrams three times a day (see pp. 186–187).
• Eat some raw garlic every day (see pp. 240–241).
• Take echinacea (pp. 238–239), *Astragalus* (pp. 197 and 275), and immunity-boosting mushrooms (shiitake, enokidake) (p. 198).
• Try tincture of propolis (p. 272), both topically and internally.

You will find advice on how to treat acute infections in Chapter 13.

INFLAMMATION

Inflammation is a normal response of the body to injury and infection and a major component of healing. The redness, warmth, swelling, and pain that characterize inflammatory reactions are all evidence that the immune, circulatory, and hormonal systems are actively working to boost the efficiency of the body's defenses and speed the repair of damaged tissue. Inflammation creates illness when it continues beyond its normal limits or serves no purpose. It is often an unwelcome feature of autoimmunity, for example, and a major component of musculoskeletal disease.

Medical doctors treat inflammation with anti-inflammatory drugs, which can injure the stomach, and with corticosteroids, which are suppressive and toxic. There are natural alternatives.

Inflammation is regulated by a group of hormones called prostaglandins. Some prostaglandins intensify the inflammatory response while others reduce it. Aspirin, ibuprofen, and other nonsteroidal anti-inflammatory drugs work on the prostaglandin system. You can also affect this system by diet, specifically by the kinds of fats you do and don't eat, since the body makes prostaglandins from fatty acids.

Many polyunsaturated vegetable oils favor the synthesis of stimulatory prostaglandins; they should be excluded from the diet if you suffer from any kind of chronic inflammatory disease. Also eliminate sources of *trans*-fatty acids, such as margarine and partially hydrogenated vegetable oils. Gamma-linolenic acid, found in black currant oil (see p. 230), favors the synthesis of inhibitory prostaglandins and should be added to the diet. The omega-3 fatty acids in sardines and other oily fish (p. 229) and in linseed oil (p. 24) also increase inhibitory prostaglandins. You may have to wait six to eight weeks to notice the results of these dietary changes, but they will occur and will not be accompanied by any toxicity.

If you need faster symptomatic relief, use aspirin and ibuprofen judiciously. Be sure to have food in your stomach when you take them, and discontinue use if you develop stomach pain or other untoward symptoms. An herbal alternative to these drugs is ginger (see p. 241).

Applications of heat and cold may be of benefit in some cases of inflammation (see Chapter 13). Also try homeopathic treatment (see Appendix A). In addition, since the immune system is the central player in this process, the mind can influence it in the right direction. Try hypnotherapy and visualization to take advantage of this connection.

INSOMNIA

Read Chapter 6 in its entirety. A great deal of insomnia is the result of stress, anxiety, depression, and the use of stimulant drugs.
• Eliminate all stimulants from your life (see pp. 116–117).
• Maintain good habits of aerobic exercise. Experiment with the time of day that you exercise. You may find that exercising at a particular time will help you sleep at night.
• Take a warm bath before bedtime to relax tense muscles.
• If muscle tension is causing sleeplessness, try taking preparations of hops *(Humulus lupulus)* before bedtime. In addition to its use in beer, hops has a long history of use in medicine as a sedative/relaxant. (It is also the only close botanical relative of marijuana.) Try two capsules of a freeze-dried extract of hops (see Appendix B for a source).
• Also try taking calcium and magnesium as neuromuscular relaxants: 1,000 milligrams of each at bedtime (the gluconate and citrate forms are easily absorbed).
• Try eating a portion of starch, such as a plain baked potato or piece of bread, thirty minutes before bedtime. This may increase production of the brain's own sedative neurotransmitters.
• Use the breathing exercises on pages 119–120 when trying to fall asleep.
• Try the herbal sedative valerian (see p. 245).

IRRITABLE BOWEL SYNDROME

A common disorder of lifestyle, this syndrome is ultimately rooted in nervous interference with the natural operations of the lower digestive tract. Symptoms are variable and change over time. They may include diarrhea, constipation, gas, abdominal distension and pain, and intolerance to certain foods. It is easy to get rid of irritable bowel syndrome by making adjustments of lifestyle. Do not get involved with gastroenterologists, elaborate diagnostic workups, or pharmaceutical drugs until you have exhausted the remedies listed here.
• Eliminate the following drugs from your life: coffee and decaffeinated coffee, all other caffeine sources, tobacco, and all other stimulants (see pp. 137–147).

- Eliminate milk and milk products from the diet.
- Avoid products sweetened with sorbitol (such as sugarless chewing gum).
- Eat a high-fiber diet (see pp. 41–43), adding psyllium as needed to have regular bowel movements (see p. 277).
- Take one or two enteric-coated capsules of peppermint oil three times daily between meals (see Appendix B for a source).
- Take a milk-free brand of acidophilus culture with meals (see p. 228).
- Experiment with using gentian root before or after meals (see p. 241).
- Experiment with carob powder (see pp. 283–284).
- Practice the breathing exercise on pages 119–120.
- Take relaxation or stress-reduction training. Biofeedback, yoga, and meditation would all be helpful.

ITCHING

Itching is a mysterious phenomenon. Although it can be a symptom of allergy and of rare metabolic disorders (like the one resulting from liver obstruction), many cases appear to have no physical causes. Doctors frequently prescribe antihistamines for itching, but these drugs are dangerous (see pp. 293–294), as are topical steroids (see pp. 193–194).

If itching is generalized, try taking stinging nettle capsules (p. 294) and soaking in baths containing cornstarch and colloidal oatmeal (Aveeno Bath Treatment). Also try homeopathic treatment (see Appendix A).

If itching is localized, try applying counterirritant ointments or creams like Ben-Gay from the drugstore or the famous Chinese herbal remedy Tiger Balm, which you can get at many health food stores.

Itching eyes are a common allergic symptom. Use calendula lotion compresses (p. 250) and take stinging nettle capsules (p. 294).

Anal itching is a special case. If not due to hemorrhoids (pp. 297–298), it is likely to be caused by irritants in the diet, especially mustard and red pepper. Eliminate these. Apply witch hazel topically.

KIDNEY PROBLEMS

Kidney disease may be congenital (polycystic kidney), autoimmune-related with an inherited component (glomerulonephritis), the result of infection (pyelonephritis), injury, or hypertension. Since the body has a redundancy of kidney tissue, damage to these organs must be advanced before kidney failure becomes apparent, so what doctors diagnose as early kidney failure may in fact represent a late stage of kidney disease. Left untreated, kidney failure will be fatal, and the treatments for it — dialysis and kidney transplantation — are far from easy or pleasant. When patients are already in frank kidney failure, conventional doctors warn them to avoid eating protein and other habits that put stress on whatever functional kidney tissue remains. If patients had this information much earlier, they might be able to avoid the drastic interventions.

Here are the most common kidney stressors: tobacco smoking, which cuts down blood flow to the organs; high blood pressure; dehydration; alcohol, caffeine, and other stimulant drugs; jarring motion, as in running or horseback riding; and a high-protein diet. The metabolism of protein puts a huge workload on the kidneys. If you know that you have abnormal kidneys or have had any kidney disease in the past, the two most important things you can do to protect yourself are to follow a very low-protein diet and never allow yourself to become dehydrated.

LIVER PROBLEMS

Acute and chronic hepatitis and alcoholic liver disease are the problems I see most frequently in my practice. Regardless of the cause, liver ailments have a common treatment. Since this organ has great regenerative potential, the goal of therapy should be to eliminate as many stresses on the liver as possible, while encouraging it to heal. If your liver function is abnormal for any reason (usually indicated by elevated liver enzymes in blood test), you should follow these recommendations:

• Eat a very low-protein, low-fat diet. Avoid concentrated protein foods at any given meal. You can have lots of starches, vegetables, and fruits.

- Strictly avoid alcohol and tobacco.
- Try to avoid *all* drugs, whether prescribed or over-the-counter, legal or illegal. Most drugs are metabolized by the liver.
- Avoid all protein and amino acid supplements.
- Avoid exposure to chemical fumes and vapors (gasoline, solvents, etc.).
- Drink plenty of water and get plenty of rest.
- Take steam baths or saunas frequently, being careful to drink plenty of pure water when you do. Sweating helps the body eliminate toxins and takes some of the workload off the liver.
- Drink dandelion-root tea as often as you like. You can find it in health food stores, and it is good for the liver.
- Take extracts of the seeds of milk thistle *(Silybum marianum)*. This herbal remedy is nontoxic, and European research shows that it stimulates regeneration of liver cells and protects them from toxic injury. Most health food stores stock this product under the names milk thistle, silybum, or silymarin. Take two capsules two or three times a day until liver function returns to normal.
- Together with milk thistle, take schizandra berries, the fruits of a Chinese medicinal plant *(Schisandra chinenis;* see Appendix B for a source). The dried berries look like red peppercorns and have a fruity, peppery taste. You can either eat them whole or, better, make them into a tea. Add two teaspoons of berries to a quart of cold water, bring to the boil, cover, lower heat, and simmer twenty to thirty minutes. Strain and drink throughout the day. Or look for capsules of this herb. Schizandra berries promote healing of the liver, especially with hepatitis and other inflammatory conditions.

LUPUS (SYSTEMIC LUPUS ERYTHEMATOSUS, SLE)

One of the major autoimmune diseases, affecting young women mostly, lupus can be mild or life-threatening. It frequently causes arthritis that behaves like rheumatoid arthritis, skin eruptions, and kidney disease that can result in hypertension. The drugs that allopathic doctors use to treat lupus are suppressive and highly toxic. They may be necessary for brief periods of crisis, but it is important to hold them in reserve for times of need and to get off of them as soon as possible. If you take them regularly, you will reduce the chance of having the lupus go naturally into remission. Here are the recommendations I give patients with this disease:

• Eat a very low protein diet, with lots of starches and fresh fruits and vegetables. Avoid milk and all milk products.

• Avoid all polyunsaturated oils. Use only extra virgin olive oil and cold-pressed canola oil.

• Eat sardines packed in sardine oil three times a week (p. 46) or take supplemental linseed oil (p. 24).

• Take black currant oil, 500 milligrams twice a day (p. 230).

• If arthritis is a problem, take an herb called feverfew *(Tanacetum parthenium)*. Use only freeze-dried feverfew leaves (available at most health food stores) and take one capsule twice a day. This has an anti-inflammatory effect, helpful in cases of autoimmune arthritis. Use it as long as symptoms persist.

• Drink plenty of water.

• Get plenty of rest.

• Do aerobic exercise regularly. Swim if arthritis is a problem.

• Do not stay in treatment with any medical doctors who make you feel hopeless about your condition. Lupus, like all autoimmune diseases, has a high potential to go into remission. The suggestions of practitioners, for good or ill, can be powerful influences on your state of health.

• Experiment with traditional Chinese medicine, Ayurvedic medicine, Native American medicine, and other forms of unorthodox medicine, including healers.

• Use the breathing exercise on pages 119–120 and work with other techniques of relaxation and stress reduction.

• Use visualization and hypnotherapy to increase the likelihood of remission.

• Read *Lupus Novice: Towards Self Healing* by Laura Chester (Barrytown, N.Y.: Station Hill Press, 1987) for the story of one woman's adventures with this disease and her encounters with regular and alternative medicine.

MALE PROBLEMS. See IMPOTENCE; PROSTATE TROUBLE.

MEMORY LOSS

In taking a medical history, I ask a question that seems to surprise some patients: "How is your memory?" A majority answer by saying, "Not as good as it used to be," or "Terrible." In an age when Alzheimer's disease gets so much publicity, anxiety about memory loss is very common. In my experience this fear is more of a problem than memory loss itself, since the vast majority of people who think they are losing memory are not.

The secret of memory is attention. If your attention is not in the right place when something goes by that you want to remember, you will not remember it no matter how good your memory is. The secret of attention is motivation. In fact, many of us are not really as interested in remembering as we think we are. It may be that motivation changes as we age, more than memory itself.

Try not to worry about your memory. The chances are good that nothing is wrong with it. If you follow the lifestyle suggestions in this book, take the antioxidant formula on pages 185–188, and keep your mind active, your memory should serve you well into old age.

If you are still concerned, I have one remedy to suggest, an herbal preparation made from the leaves of the ginkgo tree *(Ginkgo biloba)*. Ginkgo is the ancient and once rare Chinese tree now planted on many city streets throughout the world. Female trees provide edible nuts used in Chinese cuisine. Recently extracts of ginkgo leaves have attracted much attention from researchers because of their ability to increase blood flow to the brain. You can buy capsules of these extracts in most health food stores, although different brands vary considerably in their content of active ingredients (ginkgolides). For memory enhancement try taking two capsules twice a day for a two-month trial. Ginkgo is nontoxic.

MENOPAUSE

This condition is not a disease, despite the ads of pharmaceutical companies and the treatment philosophy of most gynecologists. Many women sail through the change of life with minimal discomfort, and I see many vital postmenopausal women who have never taken replacement hormones.

Mental attitude has a lot to do with how you experience menopause. If you see it as a tragic end to youth and sexuality, it will cause you great distress and leave you susceptible to the persuasions of those who will try to sell you eternal youth in the form of pills. If you see it as a natural transition to the next phase of life, you can accept it with serenity and without the help of the medical profession.

Doctors often rationalize their promotion of hormone replacement therapy as scientific treatment for uncomfortable symptoms. Declining estrogen levels at menopause do create two practical problems for some women: hot flashes and vaginal dryness, but you do not have to take estrogen replacement to deal with them.

Hot flashes are harmless but annoying. I recommend an herbal formula to control them. Get tinctures or capsules of the following three herbs at a health food store: dong quai (see p. 238); chaste tree *(Vitex agnus-castus),* a regulator of the female reproductive system; and damiana *(Turnera diffusa),* a plant native to Texas and northern Mexico with a reputation as a tonic and female aphrodisiac. Take two capsules of each of these herbs once a day at noon or one dropperful of each of the tinctures mixed in a cup of warm water once a day at noon. This formula is safe and effective. Continue it until you do not experience any more hot flashes, then cut the dose gradually and try to stop altogether. Eventually the hot flashes will disappear for good. Note also that diets high in soy foods may prevent hot flashes by virtue of the phytoestrogens contained in soybeans.

Vaginal dryness (atrophic vaginitis) can make sexual intercourse difficult, but it does not mean that your sex life is at an end. Try Replens Vaginal Lotion, an excellent over-the-counter product, and get in the habit of using lubricant jellies before sex. If these fail to help, your doctor can prescribe a topical estrogen cream and instruct you in its use. Used occasionally, this will restore normal vaginal tissue, and although some of the estrogen cream will be systemically absorbed, it will be a fraction of what you would get with estrogen replacement.

I am in a small minority of physicians today who oppose hormone replacement therapy for all women at menopause. I have no objection to estrogen for women who undergo premature menopause because they have lost their ovaries or for women who have specific medical needs for it, but I think the current wave of enthusiasm for this hormone blinds us to its possible hazards, especially of increased cancer risks (see pp. 172–173).

MIGRAINE

Classic migraine is a one-sided, severe, throbbing headache, often preceded by some sort of "aura" (visual disturbances are common), and accompanied by nausea and vomiting. This disorder has so many variants, however, that talk of a classic type may confuse people and make diagnosis more difficult. In women, migraine almost always disappears during pregnancy, a good diagnostic feature of this headache.

Migraine is most unpleasant for patients, often putting them out of action for days at a time, as well as frustrating for doctors, who often find that it resists their best efforts at treatment. Allopathic doctors dose migraine sufferers with a great many strong drugs, some of which do more harm than good.

The vascular instability that is the immediate cause of this headache is influenced by many factors. Allergy often plays a role, since in many sufferers specific foods trigger attacks. Hormonal fluctuations are a factor, at least in women. Not only does pregnancy block migraines, birth control pills can make them happen. Stress is clearly involved, too, as is heredity. It may be impossible to disentangle all the elements that lead to migraine in an individual case.

My recommendations for bringing migraine under control are as follows:

• Eliminate coffee and decaffeinated coffee from your life, as well as all other sources of caffeine. Make sure you are not taking any OTC or prescription drugs that contain it. Once you are off caffeine, you can use coffee as a treatment for migraine. Drink one or two cups of strong coffee at the first sign of an attack, then lie down in a dark, quiet room.

• Eliminate other common dietary triggers of migraine: chocolate, wine (red is usually more of an offender than white, but both can do it), all strong-flavored cheeses (cottage cheese and cream cheese are all right), fermented foods (including soy sauce and miso), sardines, anchovies, and pickled herring.

• Take feverfew herb, one or two capsules a day. Make sure the product you buy specifies that the leaves are *freeze-dried* or that it is a standardized extract. This remedy reduces the frequency of migraine attacks in many people. You can stay on it indefinitely.

• Take a course of biofeedback training (see pp. 123–125), with the specific goal of learning to raise the temperature of your hands. Once you master this technique, it will be a tool you can use to abort a headache at the start of an attack.

• Use allopathic medication sparingly and cautiously. Experiment with the prescription drug ergotamine to abort migraine attacks. It is a powerful constrictor of arteries that must be used at the very first sign of a headache to be effective. An under-the-tongue form is available, or use the suppository form if nausea is a problem. Your doctor will tell you how to use this drug.

• Do not take the prescription drug Fiorinal on a regular basis. Doctors hand it out like candy to migraine sufferers without warning them that it contains an addictive downer (butalbital, a barbiturate) and caffeine in addition to aspirin.

• Do not take prednisone or other steroids to prevent migraines. The dangers of steroids outweigh any benefits.

• If you continue to have attacks, try to change the way you think about the headaches. Migraine is like an electrical storm in the head, violent and disruptive but leading to a calm, clear state at the end. It is not so bad to let yourself have a headache once in a while. Take coffee and aspirin or ergotamine, lie down in a dark room, and be with your headache. It is a good excuse to drop your usual routines and go inward, letting accumulated stress dissipate. As you come to accept migraine in this way and see it as serving a purpose in your life, you may not have to have it so frequently.

MOOD SWINGS

Mood swings are a symptom of imbalance, a lack of centeredness in life. They are more likely to have nonphysical than physical causes, but you should experiment with some dietary variables in addition to working on the mental level.

• Eliminate all forms of caffeine as well as other stimulant drugs (see pp. 116–117) from your life. While you are at it, you would do best to avoid all mood-altering drugs, whether illegal or legal, over-the-counter or prescribed.

• Experiment with cutting down on or eliminating sugar. Some people find that it is a major cause of unstable moods. Eat fruit instead of sugary desserts.

• Exercise aerobically according to the guidelines in Chapter 5.

• Take a B-50 or B-100 B-complex vitamin supplement every day.

• Practice the breathing exercise on pages 119–120.

• Begin a meditation practice (see pp. 125–127). As a seed of balance and centeredness in your experiential life, daily meditation is the ultimate solution to mood swings.

Severe oscillation of moods between wild elation and despair is the hallmark of manic-depressive psychosis, also known as bipolar disorder, a major mental illness that usually requires psychiatric evaluation and drug treatment.

MOTION SICKNESS

Many people report that ginger prevents and treats motion sickness. You can drink fresh ginger tea, eat slices of candied ginger, or take the powdered spice in capsules (two to four, as needed) if you do not like its strong flavor. Try ginger immediately before you travel if you are susceptible to this malady, or eat it at the first sign of discomfort. Some people report that eating food allays motion sickness, and most people find that deep breathing helps.

The usual allopathic preventive is OTC antihistamines (Dramamine, Bonine), which strongly interfere with consciousness. An alternative is a prescription device, the scopolamine patch (Transderm Scop) that you wear behind the ear. It delivers steady, tiny doses of this drug through the skin. Scopolamine is a nightshade derivative that is quite toxic by most routes of administration, but in this form side effects other than dry mouth are rare, and I prefer it to antihistamines.

A nondrug treatment is a special wrist band with a peg that presses on an acupuncture point just below the palm. Many people report that wearing the band controls nausea.

MULTIPLE SCLEROSIS

This is one of the most baffling of all diseases because we understand so little of its causes and the factors that influence its course and outcome. The immediate problem is localized inflammatory damage to the sheaths surrounding nerve fibers, resulting in interference with the conduction of nerve impulses and disturbance of body functions. Typical symptoms are loss of vision, motor strength, coordination, and bowel and bladder control.

Although the immune system is certainly the agent of the nerve damage, multiple sclerosis does not look like a simple matter of autoimmunity. Researchers have long suspected viral involvement, suggesting, for example, that the measles virus may somehow trigger the immune reaction. That does not explain why multiple sclerosis is most common in northern latitudes and rare near the equator. Medical science also cannot explain why the disease takes so many different forms. Some people have transient symptoms at the onset and are never bothered again for the rest of their lives. Others experience alternating cycles of intense disturbance and remission. Still others go rapidly downhill to disability and death.

Conventional medicine now has a specific treatment for one form of MS — beta-interferon — but this drug is scarce and expensive, produces side effects, and is far from a sure thing. In most cases, medicine has little or nothing to offer victims of this disease once the diagnosis is made. It may even do harm by giving patients a sense of hopelessness and incurability. I consider multiple sclerosis a fascinating and challenging condition to work with because it is so variable, because it has significant potential to stabilize or go into remission, and because lifestyle modification and stress reduction can strongly affect its course. When I see new patients with this diagnosis, I give them long lists of suggestions to experiment with.

• Do not stay in treatment with doctors who make you feel you cannot get better. That kind of negative suggestion can have disastrous effects on your health.

- Stay away from caffeine, alcohol, and tobacco. All of them can complicate your problems by their effects on the nervous system and on the gastrointestinal and urinary tracts.
- Follow the dietary guidelines in Chapters 1 and 2. Eat very little protein. Avoid milk and all milk products.
- If constipation is a problem, take acidophilus culture (see p. 228) and psyllium (p. 277). Read CONSTIPATION.
- Avoid all polyunsaturated oils. Use only extra virgin olive oil and cold-pressed canola oil.
- Take black currant oil, 500 milligrams twice a day (see p. 230).
- Eat sardines at least three times a week (p. 46) or take supplemental linseed oil (p. 24) as sources of omega-3 fatty acids.
- Take the antioxidant vitamin formula (pp. 185–188) and a B-100 B-complex vitamin supplement daily.
- Take a multimineral supplement once a day.
- Take soy lecithin granules, 5 grams a day (see p. 229). Keep this product in the refrigerator.
- Take coenzyme Q (Co-Q-10), 30 milligrams two or three times a day (see p. 229).
- Be sure to exercise regularly. Pick aerobic activities that you can manage, and do not push yourself to the point of exhaustion.
- Use visualization, meditation, and hypnotherapy to redirect your mental energies in positive directions.
- Find out about possible benefits of apitherapy — bee-sting treatment. Honeybee venom contains a number of powerful anti-inflammatory compounds that may help induce remission in auto-immunity. One of them, apamin, is under investigation in France as a possible new treatment for MS. Purified bee venom is available for injection, but many apitherapists prefer to apply living bees to the body. In experienced hands the procedure is quite safe. The best way to find out about this therapy is to consult a local bee-keeper.
- Try a variety of healing methods to see if they improve your condition: acupuncture, physical therapy, manipulation, yoga, and so on, but beware of questionable practitioners selling "cures."
- Get to know some people who have multiple sclerosis and are doing well with it. They can inspire you to take more responsibility for your own health.

MUSCLE CRAMPS

Two very common causes of night cramps in leg muscles are tobacco and inactivity. The solutions to these problems are obvious.
• A good remedy for night cramps is a calcium/magnesium supplement at bedtime, 1,000 milligrams of each (gluconate or citrate forms are best). You can take this indefinitely.
• Also try the B-vitamin niacin (see pp. 214–215) along with calcium/magnesium.
• A hot bath before bedtime increases blood flow to the muscles and may also help.

NAIL PROBLEMS

For weak, brittle nails try black currant oil, 500 milligrams twice a day (see p. 230). You will see results in two months. Taking gelatin as a supplement is of no value.

You will find advice about fungal infections of nails in ATHLETE'S FOOT.

NERVE DAMAGE

Nerves in the central nervous system (brain and spinal cord) are supposed to be irreplaceable, which is why strokes and traumatic injuries to the brain and spinal cord can be so devastating. One treatment worth trying in such cases is the prescription drug Hydergine, derived from ergot, a natural fungus. It is nontoxic and may stimulate some regeneration of nerve function. One drawback is its expense, since you will have to take high doses for months or years; cheaper generic forms are available. Try 5 milligrams three times a day for at least three months. Sublingual (under-the-tongue) tablets are more effective than oral ones, but new liquid capsules may be even better. Extracts of the leaves of the ginkgo tree increase cerebral blood flow (see p. 313) and are also worth trying in cases of brain injury.

Peripheral nerve injury often results from compression, as in carpal tunnel syndrome, in which pressure from ligaments in the wrist affects the function of nerves going to the hand. Before you resort to surgery for this condition, try taking vitamin B-6, 100 milligrams three times a day (see p. 215).

Acupuncture can also stimulate healing of peripheral nerve injuries.

OSTEOARTHRITIS

This condition is primarily the result of not using the body correctly, either not exercising it enough or using it in wrong ways. You can prevent this degenerative disease of joints by following the guidelines for general health in Part I, especially the advice about exercise in Chapter 5. Osteoarthritis is a common cause of aches, pains, and inability to move, especially in older people who complain of "rheumatism." Regular doctors mostly hand out anti-inflammatory drugs for this condition, but there are many other strategies to try:
• Read INFLAMMATION and follow the dietary suggestions there.
• Take vitamin B-6, 100 milligrams twice a day.
• Experiment with niacinamide, a variant of vitamin B-3. Start with 500 milligrams twice a day, increasing by 500 milligrams at three-week intervals if necessary, to a maximum daily dose of 2,000 milligrams.
• Take ginger regularly (see p. 241), for its anti-inflammatory effect.
• Experiment with the Ayurvedic herb *Boswellia* or with boswellin, the extract made from it. This is available at health food stores; use the dosage recommended on the product.
• Soak in hot water, hot mineral baths, or hot whirlpool baths as often as possible.
• Use ice packs on acutely inflamed, "hot" joints; they may provide great relief.
• Swim for your aerobic exercise. If you are not a good swimmer, try water aerobics or just get in the water and move. Avoid cold water.
• Try acupuncture for pain relief (see Appendix A).
• Experiment with homeopathy, traditional Chinese medicine, folk remedies, osteopathic manipulation, and different forms of massage, such as Trager work (see Appendix A).

• Use visualization and meditation to try to affect your condition with your mind.

• Do not let anyone inject cortisone into your joints. This treatment is suppressive and harms your immunity.

• Experiment with a TENS (transcutaneous electrical nerve stimulator) unit. This device delivers pulses of electricity through the skin and can be dramatically effective in relieving chronic arthritis pain. Ask your doctor or physical therapist about getting one.

OSTEOPOROSIS

See pages 27, 109, and 221–222 for information on this common disease of bones. Osteoporosis might be under tight genetic control, and a genetic test may soon be available to screen for those at risk. Women become susceptible earlier in life than men, because their sex hormones decline at around age fifty, while men maintain high levels through their seventies. Bone-density measurements can determine if the disease is present and how much bone has been lost. Once osteoporosis has developed, the best treatment is calcitonin, a hormone from the parathyroid glands of salmon, which regulates calcium balance. Avoid the pharmaceutical drug etidronate (Didronel).

POISON IVY, POISON OAK

These plants produce an intense contact dermatitis in susceptible individuals (about half of the population). Allergy to poison ivy or oak can suddenly come and suddenly go.

The best defense against this uncomfortable and disfiguring reaction is to learn to recognize the plant and avoid contact with it. If you do touch the plant, you have about twenty to thirty minutes in which you can wash the oil off with soap and water. After that it is absorbed into the skin. The reaction usually begins thirty-six to forty-eight hours later and can last for weeks. An excellent over-the-counter product, Tecnu lotion, will remove the oil from the skin up to twenty-four hours after contact. If you are highly allergic to poison ivy/oak, you should keep this product handy and take it with you on outdoor trips.

• The best treatment for poison ivy or oak dermatitis is to run hot water on the affected áreas, as hot as you can stand. This will seem counterintuitive, as heat increases the itching and cold soothes it, but trust me. Under hot water the itching will briefly become very intense, then will stop for several hours, as if the nerves responsible for conveying the sensation to the brain become overloaded and quit. As soon as itching starts again, go back to the hot water. If you do this conscientiously, the whole reaction will complete itself quickly, and your skin will return to normal much faster than it would otherwise.

• If you wish, use calamine lotion as a topical treatment.

• Do not take oral prednisone for poison ivy or oak unless the case is so severe that you become systemically ill (fever, difficulty in urinating, etc.). Do not use topical steroids either.

PREMENSTRUAL SYNDROME (PMS)

PMS is a controversial subject, since many (male) doctors maintain that it is an imaginary condition. Their opinion notwithstanding, it is obvious that many women suffer terribly before the onset of their periods with such symptoms as mood swings, depression, irritability, bloating, headaches, joint pain, and more. Some of them also are disabled by very painful cramps during their periods. It is possible to eliminate or greatly reduce the severity of PMS by making the following changes:

• Eliminate caffeine from your life, including chocolate, which some women crave intensely in the premenstrual phase.

• Do regular aerobic exercise according to the guidelines in Chapter 5.

• Avoid all polyunsaturated vegetable oils.

• Take black currant oil, 500 milligrams twice a day (see p. 230).

• Take dong quai herb, two capsules twice a day (see p. 238). An alternative is chaste tree herb *(Vitex)* in the same dosage.

• For painful menstrual cramps, try raspberry-leaf tea, which you can get at a health food store. Drink as much as you like — it is nontoxic. Also try calcium/magnesium supplements, 1,000 milligrams of each as needed. A stronger herbal remedy is crampbark or viburnum *(Viburnum opulus),* from a European bush. Take one dropperful of the tincture in a little warm water as needed. Many women report satisfactory relief of menstrual cramps with ibuprofen (Motrin, Advil). Be sure to have food in your stomach when you take it. A hot water bottle on the abdomen is also helpful.

• Use the breathing exercise on pages 119–120 and practice other relaxation techniques (Chapter 6).

PROSTATE TROUBLE

The prostate gland is a walnut-size organ surrounding the urethra at the neck of the bladder in men. Its secretions are one component of semen. Prostatitis, or inflammation of the gland, is a common ailment of young men who get urinary tract infections. Unfortunately this condition easily becomes chronic and is difficult to treat. Older men are subject to a different sort of problem, enlargement of the gland, which can interfere with urination.

Prostatitis causes pain on ejaculation and urination, urinary frequency, and sometimes urethral discharge; chronic prostatitis can be a cause of low backache. This condition resists treatment because the gland has a poor blood supply, making it hard for the immune system to defend it against infection and making it hard for antibiotics to reach the site. Regular doctors can do little except give antibiotics; too often the condition recurs whenever the drugs are stopped. You can get over prostatitis if you follow these suggestions:

• Eliminate all prostatic irritants from your life. The most important ones are coffee and decaffeinated coffee, other caffeine sources, alcohol, tobacco, and red pepper.

• Drink more water! Dehydration is one of the great stresses on the prostate. Keep your urinary output high and never let yourself get dehydrated.

• Avoid jarring motion to the perineal (seat) area, as can happen from riding a horse, motorcycle, or bicycle. Also avoid prolonged sitting.

• Take zinc picolinate, 60 milligrams once a day. Once symptoms subside, cut the dose in half and continue on this supplement indefinitely.

• Take vitamin C, 2,000 milligrams three times a day (see pp. 186–187).

- Adjust your frequency of ejaculation. Both too much and too little encourage prostatitis.
- Try warm sitz baths (see p. 298).
- Prostatic massage is helpful. Have a partner do it for you or do it yourself by inserting a finger in the rectum and gently pressing on the gland (it will be tender). This helps drain the gland and increases blood flow to it.
- Use antibiotics if you have acute symptoms but do not stay on them for more than two weeks. Antibiotics alone will not solve the problem.

Most men over the age of fifty develop benign prostatic hypertrophy (BPH), an enlargement of the gland that may be due to accumulation of testosterone in it. This condition can be asymptomatic or it can cause a number of urinary problems: increased frequency, decreased force of urination, and nighttime awakening to empty the bladder. If these symptoms become severe, doctors will urge surgery to remove all or part of the gland.

It is worth trying to manage symptomatic BPH by natural methods before resorting to surgery:

- Avoid the prostatic irritants listed above.
- Take zinc picolinate, 30 milligrams daily.
- Use an herbal remedy made from the berries of the saw palmetto *(Serenoa repens)*, a small palm tree native to the coastal region of southeastern United States. You will find saw palmetto products in health food stores, but the best form to use for BPH is a standardized extract, 160 milligrams twice a day (see Appendix B for a source). This remedy protects the prostate from the irritating effects of testosterone and, by promoting shrinkage of the gland, improves urinary function (a mechanism similar to that of the much more expensive pharmaceutical drug finasteride [Proscar]). Saw palmetto is nontoxic, and you can stay on it indefinitely. You may also combine it with another herb that benefits the prostate, *Pygeum africanum*.
- Add soy foods to the diet. The phytoestrogens in soybeans may greatly reduce the risks of both BPH and prostate cancer.
- Men fifty and older should get a PSA blood test, useful as a screen for prostate cancer.

PSORIASIS

In this mysterious disease, cause unknown, areas of skin grow too fast, resulting in thickened, red, scaly patches that are itchy and unsightly. The scalp, knees, and elbows are common sites of involvement, but the disease can spread over large areas and produce an associated arthritis that is difficult to treat. Psoriasis may have a genetic or biochemical basis, but as with most chronic skin ailments, severity varies over time, and the ups and downs often correlate with stress levels and mental outlook. Conventional treatments are toxic and not very satisfactory.

I recommend the following course of action:
• Spend time in the sun and consider moving to a desert climate. Sunlight is of great benefit in psoriasis.
• Follow the dietary and other guidelines in Part I.
• Take the antioxidant vitamin formula on pages 185–188.
• Experiment with seeds of milk thistle (*Silybum marianum;* see p. 311). You can find extracts of the seeds in health food stores, sometimes under the name silymarin. They are nontoxic, have a beneficial effect on the liver, and may help some people with psoriasis. Take two capsules twice a day for at least three months.
• Practice stress reduction techniques (Chapter 6), and experiment with hypnotherapy to promote healing of lesions. The skin is very responsive to hypnotic suggestion.

RHEUMATOID ARTHRITIS

One of the common autoimmune diseases, rheumatoid arthritis is more easily influenced by lifestyle changes than osteoarthritis. Read AUTOIMMUNITY and INFLAMMATION. Also try these suggestions:
• Take feverfew herb, one or two capsules twice a day (see p. 312).
• Make the following dietary experiments, one at a time, trying each for two months to see what you notice: (1) eliminate milk and all milk products, (2) eliminate all sugar except natural fruits, (3) eliminate all citrus fruits, (4) eliminate all nightshade vegetables (tomatoes, potatoes, eggplant, peppers, paprika, chili). At the end of each trial period restore the eliminated items to your diet. You

may find that one or more has an influence on your arthritis. Knowing this will give you more control over it.

• Use swimming as your primary form of aerobic exercise.
• Use aspirin and other anti-inflammatory drugs for symptomatic treatment.
• Experiment with the anti-inflammatory herbs ginger (see p. 241) and *Boswellia* (see p. 321).
• Try to avoid taking strong prescription drugs: gold salts, steroids (prednisone), penicillamine, or immunosuppressives (Cytoxan). Patients who use those therapies are less likely to respond to nontoxic natural treatments or go into long remissions.
• Study the information in Chapter 6 and commit yourself to a program of mind/body work. Meditation, yoga, visualization, and hypnotherapy can all be very helpful to you.
• Experiment with traditional Chinese medicine, Ayurvedic medicine, homeopathy, Native American medicine, folk remedies, and healers (see Appendix A). Also experiment with long-term fasting, but only under supervision (see pp. 203–204); it can induce long-lasting remissions.
• Consult a beekeeper to find out about apitherapy (see p. 319).

SEXUAL DEFICIENCY

Many people, mostly older men, complain of not having enough sexual energy. Read IMPOTENCE for a discussion of psychological versus physical causes and the role of sex hormones. Of the many sexual tonics on the market, ginseng has the longest history and greatest reputation. Much prized in the Far East as the ultimate sexual restorative for men, ginseng was long ignored by medical researchers in the West. Once they began to study its chemistry and pharmacology, they found that it does indeed have many biological effects.

Two species of ginseng are prominent in commerce: Oriental ginseng *(Panax ginseng)* and American ginseng *(Panax quinquefolium)*. Both are full of compounds (ginsenosides) that work on the pituitary-adrenal axis, increasing resistance to stress and affecting metabolism, skin and muscle tone, and hormonal balance. Oriental ginseng is more of a stimulant and can raise blood pressure in some people. If you have high blood pressure, use it with caution if at all, or use only the American species.

The quality of ginseng on the market varies enormously, with better, older roots selling for very high prices. If you want to experiment with this famous tonic plant, you must shop around for high-quality material and be prepared to pay for it. Also you must take ginseng regularly over a period of months to notice its effects. You can buy whole dried roots and boil them into teas or use more convenient extracts in the form of liquids and capsules. Follow dosage recommendations on the products.

Chinese men advise against wasting ginseng in your youth. Save it for old age, they say, then see what it can do for you.

Recently, an Ayurvedic herb for sexual deficiency in men has become available here: *Withania somnifera,* known by its Indian name, ashwaganda ("smells like a horse"). It comes in capsules; follow dosage recommendations on the product.

SINUS PROBLEMS

Sinusitis, both acute and chronic, causes great misery. The worst cases I see are in cigarette addicts, but people who suffer from upper respiratory allergies may also develop bad sinus problems (pain, headache, congestion, postnasal drip, obstructed breathing, and so forth). Regular doctors treat sinusitis with a lot of drugs (antibiotics, antihistamines, decongestants, and steroids) and sometimes with surgery. I will certainly prescribe penicillin for an episode of acute sinusitis, but I try not to keep patients on antibiotics for long periods, and I do not use the other kinds of drugs. Instead I urge sinus sufferers to take a number of actions:

• Read INFECTIONS.
• Eliminate milk and all milk products from the diet, including prepared foods that list milk as an ingredient. An overwhelming majority of patients report dramatic improvement in sinus conditions after two months of this dietary change.
• Do not smoke. Do not spend time around smokers or in smoky environments. Consider moving if you live in a smoggy area. Equip your home with air filters (see p. 85).

• Practice nasal douching regularly (see pp. 205–206) and use this technique as a treatment for acute sinus infections also.
• At the start of sinus trouble, put hot wet towels over the whole upper face. Work up to as much heat as you can stand and keep applying them for fifteen minutes. Do this three or four times a day. It is an excellent home treatment for sinus congestion and sinusitis, since it promotes drainage and increases blood flow to the area.
• Read ALLERGY if your problem is mainly allergic. Try using capsules of stinging nettle (see p. 294) to relieve allergic symptoms.

SPRAINS

Apply ice to the injured area as soon as possible (see pp. 207–208). Take homeopathic arnica (p. 262). Use DMSO (p. 270) or tincture of arnica (p. 237) or both as a topical application. Protect the sprain from further injury (by using an elastic bandage, for example). After twenty-four hours try alternating applications of heat and cold.

STOMACH UPSETS

The best home remedies are peppermint tea (p. 243) and chamomile tea (p. 237). Read HEARTBURN.

TEMPOROMANDIBULAR JOINT (TMJ) SYNDROME

Another fashionable and questionable disease, TMJ syndrome is now a big moneymaker for some dentists, chiropractors, and holistic practitioners. Ear and jaw pain combined with difficulty in opening and closing the mouth usually results from a vicious cycle of muscle spasm and inflammation around the articulation of the temporal bone of the skull and the mandible (lower jaw) — the same sort of problem that accounts for most acute back pain (see BACK PAIN, ACUTE). Why this site should be so vulnerable is not clear, but it is often involved in osteoarthritis as well.

Do not undertake long and costly treatments for TMJ syndrome or, especially, surgery until you try out simple remedies. Since mus-

cle tension is the underlying cause, relaxation techniques can be most valuable.
• Take a course of biofeedback training (pp. 123–125) focused on relaxation of muscles of the head and face.
• Practice the breathing exercise on pages 119–120 along with visualization exercises (pp. 122–123).
• Experiment with guided imagery therapy (see Appendix A).
• Have some cranial work done by an osteopath trained in craniosacral technique (see Appendix A). One session may be enough; the practitioner can tell you whether you need any more.
• Try acupuncture for symptomatic relief.
• Use calcium and magnesium (citrates or gluconates) as muscle relaxants: 1,000 milligrams of each at bedtime and 500 milligrams of each twelve hours later. Continue these supplements as long as symptoms persist.

THYROID PROBLEMS

The thyroid gland controls so many aspects of metabolism that disturbance of its function can produce symptoms in almost every system of the body. Medical doctors have put far too many young women on supplemental thyroid hormone. Some women have been taking thyroid for most of their lives because they were chubby and depressed in adolescence and young adulthood and placed their trust in doctors. Since thyroid pills suppress the gland's natural production of hormone, it is now very difficult for them to stop taking the pills, even though they may never have needed treatment in the first place. In fairness to doctors, I must say that the patient is often at fault here, too, since many women use an underactive thyroid as an excuse for being out of shape mentally and physically.

Overactivity of the thyroid gland causes weight loss, insomnia, hand tremors (shakes), palpitations, heat intolerance, and digestive disturbances. It is less common than underactivity of the gland and usually requires conventional (allopathic) treatment with drugs or surgery.

Unfortunately, thyroid function tests are not reliable, sometimes indicating that people are in normal thyroid balance when they are not.

• If you are taking thyroid replacement (Synthroid is the usual prescribed brand) and feel you do not need it, never attempt to stop it suddenly. You can experiment with cutting down the dose very gradually, giving yourself a few weeks at each new level to see how you feel.

• Practice the yoga posture called the shoulder stand. Learn it from a yoga teacher or a book and try to work up to doing it twenty minutes at a time, at least once a day. It stimulates the thyroid and will be even more effective if you combine it with a visualization of your gland waking up from a long period of inactivity.

• Take tablets of Norwegian kelp (available in health food stores), up to twelve a day.

• If you develop any of the following symptoms, increase your dose of thyroid: mental and physical sluggishness, increased cold sensitivity, weight gain, joint stiffness, increased menstrual flow, digestive problems. Remember that it takes a while to feel the effects of dose changes.

• If you feel you are not getting enough thyroid, increase the dose in gradual steps. Cut back if you develop any of these symptoms: insomnia, jitteriness, hand tremors (shakes), palpitations, intolerance for warmth, digestive problems.

• If you are or ever have been on thyroid replacement or have had any history of thyroid dysfunction, be sure to tell any doctor you consult about it, no matter what your present symptoms are.

TONSILLITIS

Not long ago recurrent tonsillitis was always justification for tonsillectomy. Doctors were taught that the tonsils had no function and were just useless organs waiting to get infected. Today we know that tonsils (and adenoids) are important components of the immune system, and tonsillectomies, fortunately, are performed much less frequently.

Read over INFECTIONS. At the first sign of tonsillitis begin gargling with hydrogen peroxide, mixed half and half with hot water. Do this at least four times a day; it is a good disinfectant. Take a course of echinacea (pp. 238–239) and eat raw garlic (pp. 240–241). Do not take antibiotics unless a throat culture demonstrates a bacterial infection.

ULCER (PEPTIC ULCER; DUODENAL OR GASTRIC ULCER)

An ulcer used to be considered one of the classic stress-related disorders, but in recent years medical doctors have tried to downplay its connections to the mind and have looked instead for purely physical causes — in particular, infection by an organism called *Helicobacter pylori*. Simple tests can reveal the presence of these bacteria, which can be eliminated by a course of antibiotics. Anyone with chronic gastritis or ulcer should be tested and treated if the tests are positive. I still believe mental factors to be important in these conditions, because they can determine the susceptibility or resistance of tissues to bacterial attack. (Many people infected with *H. pylori* suffer no damage.)

Ulcers usually form in the beginning of the duodenum (the first section of the small intestine), just below the outlet of the stomach. More rarely they occur in the lining of the stomach itself. In either case the tissue becomes vulnerable to damage by stomach acid. The diagnosis of ulcer is confirmed by X ray and by direct viewing of the lesion through an instrument (gastroscopy). Ulcers can come and go. When active they cause pain, which is relieved by eating, and a variety of other unpleasant symptoms in the upper digestive system.

Conventional medical treatments include many drugs: antacids, protective coatings, antispasmodics, and especially new compounds that suppress the production of acid in the stomach. Two of the most popular of these new drugs are cimetidine (Tagamet) and ranitidine (Zantac). They are highly effective in the short run but do not get to the root of the problem (tissue susceptibility). Being suppressive, they may perpetuate the disease instead of undoing it. Too often doctors dismiss patients with prescriptions for these drugs without teaching them how to modify their lifestyle to minimize the chance of future recurrence.

If you are prone to ulcers, you must take the following actions:
• Strictly avoid all coffee, decaffeinated coffee, other sources of caffeine, alcohol, and tobacco.
• Strictly avoid all aspirin and other salicylates and all nonsteroidal anti-inflammatory drugs. If you need a pain reliever, use acetaminophen (Tylenol). Do not take any steroids.
• Drink peppermint tea frequently. It soothes the lining of the digestive tract.
• Avoid milk and milk products. Doctors used to recommend them to coat the stomach, but it has been found that they increase acid secretion.
• Eat smaller amounts of food more frequently. Do not let your stomach go empty for long periods.
• Use a natural product called deglycyrrhizinated licorice (DGL) to protect the lining of the stomach and duodenum. Licorice has excellent soothing and healing properties in cases of ulcer, but whole licorice contains a fraction (glycyrrhizin) that can raise blood pressure. This is removed to make DGL extract (see Appendix B for sources). The dose is two tablets of DGL extract chewed slowly before meals or between meals, or one half teaspoon of the powder swallowed at the same times. You can stay on this remedy as long as symptoms are present.
• Try taking aloe vera juice, one teaspoon after meals (see pp. 236–237). It helps heal ulcers.
• Experiment with cayenne pepper. This may sound absurd, but in fact spicy foods do not aggravate ulcers, and red pepper specifically can help them. It has a good local anesthetic effect and also brings blood to the surface of the tissue. Try sips of red pepper tea (one quarter teaspoon of cayenne pepper steeped in a cup of hot water) or a small capsule of the powder if the taste is too strong.
• Read Chapter 6 again and make serious efforts to neutralize stress in your life. Practice the breathing exercise on pages 119–120. Take a course of biofeedback training. Use visualization and hypnotherapy to help heal your ulcer. Concentrate on making the lining of your digestive tract strong and healthy.
• If necessary, change your job, your living situation, your relationships — whatever in your life is causing you most stress.

ULCERATIVE COLITIS

Another of the classic stress-related disorders, this one is also now being regarded more as a purely physical disease. Medical students no longer learn that the mind plays a major role in it, and medical researchers have written that they cannot understand why it occurs more frequently in ex-smokers of cigarettes but not in current smokers. (The reason is obvious to me: smoking burns up a lot of nervous energy. When that outlet is closed, increased nervousness can produce many symptoms, including disturbances of digestion.)

In ulcerative colitis, inflammation damages the lining of the colon, causing bloody diarrhea, pain, and a great many complications that often require drastic treatments. Autoimmunity plays a role in this disease, but the factors that trigger it are not all known. Medical doctors treat ulcerative colitis with strong drugs, including long-term steroids; if these fail to control it, all or part of the colon is removed. In Crohn's disease, a closely related problem, inflammation damages the whole wall of the colon, not just the superficial lining. Crohn's disease can involve the small intestine as well and is even more resistant to treatment.

These ailments follow alternating cycles of exacerbation and remission. The goal of treatment should not be to suppress the inflammatory process but to encourage remission. I have seen many patients do very well once they changed their lifestyle. One woman who had severe ulcerative colitis for years went into complete remission when she went on a macrobiotic diet.

Here are the suggestions I give to people with ulcerative colitis and Crohn's disease:

• Strictly avoid coffee, decaffeinated coffee, all other sources of caffeine, and all stimulant drugs.

• Avoid milk and all milk products.

• Avoid products sweetened with sorbitol.

• Follow the general advice under AUTOIMMUNITY.

• Follow the dietary guidelines in Chapters 1 and 2, but be aware that raw fruits and vegetables may be irritating during an active phase of colitis.

• Take slippery elm in the form of a gruel (see pp. 243–244).

• Take aloe vera juice, one teaspoon after meals, or less if that dose is laxative (see pp. 236–237).
• Practice the breathing exercise on pages 119–120.
• Take a course of biofeedback training (pp. 123–125). Experiment also with hypnotherapy and other relaxation methods described in Chapter 6.
• Use psychotherapy to work on emotional conflicts.
• Experiment with traditional Chinese medicine, Ayurvedic medicine, radical dietary change, and long-term fasting under supervision (pp. 203–204).

URINARY PROBLEMS

The most common urinary problem in women is cystitis (see BLADDER PROBLEMS). Urinary frequency and urgency in both sexes is a common symptom of caffeine addiction, especially addiction to coffee. Nocturia (having to get up at night to empty the bladder) is more common in men. Although this problem might be due to enlargement of the prostate (see PROSTATE TROUBLE), coffee is often the culprit here, too, and eliminating it will bring great improvement. Other forms of caffeine and other stimulant drugs can cause the same symptoms.

If you are prone to urinary problems, it is important to avoid alcohol, tobacco, and caffeine. Drink more water and never let yourself get dehydrated.

UTERINE FIBROIDS

Fibroid tumors are benign muscle tumors that cause enlargement and distortion of the uterus in premenopausal women. They may make menstrual periods painful and heavy, leading to anemia in some cases.

Many gynecologists use the mere presence of fibroids as an excuse to remove the uterus (hysterectomy), but surgery is not indicated unless the tumors are creating significant problems. You can live with very large fibroids as long as they are not causing you pain and excessive bleeding. They do not turn malignant.

Fibroids are dependent on estrogen for their growth. If you can live with them till menopause, they will shrink down and not be heard from again, as long as you do not go on estrogen replacement therapy. Even if you are years away from menopause, you can take actions to lower your estrogen levels and slow the growth of fibroids:

• Eat a low-fat diet.
• Avoid estrogenic foods (see pp. 289–290), but note that soy foods may have a protective effect.
• Increase aerobic exercise.
• Take vitamin E, 400 IU twice a day.
• If painful periods are a problem, take blue cohosh herb *(Caulophyllum thalictroides)*, two capsules twice a day for a month. If this seems to help, continue the treatment for another month, then cut the dose in half and gradually reduce it to nothing.
• If menstrual bleeding is heavy, have a complete blood count done to be sure you are not anemic.
• Use visualization exercises to try to decrease the size of the fibroids.
• Resist hysterectomy. Remember that time is on your side. If surgery is necessary, investigate new techniques of laser surgery that permit excision of the tumors rather than removal of the whole uterus.

VAGINAL YEAST INFECTIONS

Symptomatic vaginal infections are often caused by yeast. If you get them frequently and are not on antibiotics, you may have a metabolic imbalance. Try cutting way down on sugar and adding raw garlic to the diet (see pp. 240–241). Take acidophilus culture after meals (see p. 228). For topical treatment, insert one tablespoon of liquid acidophilus culture directly into the vagina with a rubber bulb syringe, or douche with a solution of tea tree oil (see p. 244), which is at least as effective as the usual prescription remedy (nystatin vaginal suppositories).

VARICOSE VEINS

An inherited weakness in the structure of veins, much more common in women than in men, predisposes a person to varicosities when veins are subjected to increased pressure over time. The best preventive measures are avoidance of prolonged standing, frequent elevation of legs when seated, and conscientious use of elastic support stockings if standing is necessary. Conventional medical and surgical treatments are very invasive and often not successful. A promising alternative is topical application of an extract of horsechestnut (*Aesculus hippocastanum*), sometimes sold under the name escin. This herbal remedy is much better known in Europe than in America, but creams containing it are becoming available here. (European doctors also prescribe escin internally, but because of potential toxicity I recommend it only for topical use.)

APPENDIX A

FINDING PRACTITIONERS

Acupuncture and Chinese Medicine

The practice of acupuncture in the United States is in great confusion at the moment, since people with very different training and degrees do it, and state laws regulating it vary widely. There is sharp division between M.D.s who use acupuncture and non-M.D.s who claim to be better trained in the philosophy and techniques of Oriental medicine beyond just sticking needles in people.

If you want to find out about professional standards and licensing requirements for acupuncturists, contact:

> National Commission on the Certification of Acupuncture
> 1424 16th Street N.W., Suite 501
> Washington, D.C. 20036
> 202-232-1404

You can obtain referrals of practitioners from another group that shares the same office:

> American Association of Acupuncture and Oriental Medicine
> 1424 16th Street N.W., Suite 501
> Washington, D.C. 20036
> 202-265-2287

The professional organization for M.D.s who practice acupuncture is:

> American Academy of Medical Acupuncture
> 5820 Wilshire Boulevard, Suite 500
> Los Angeles, Calif. 90036
> 213-937-5514

Ayurvedic Medicine

The traditional healing system of India classifies people into different body types requiring different treatments and emphasizes dietary
adjustment, massage, and herbal prescriptions from the vast Indian
repertory of medicinal plants. Ayurvedic clinics and practitioners
are appearing in the United States. For information, contact

> Maharishi Ayurveda Health Center for Stress Management
>   and Behavioral Medicine
> P.O. Box 344
> Lancaster, Mass. 01523
> 508-365-4549

or look for independent Ayurvedic practitioners, who might be
much less expensive.

Biofeedback

Biofeedback therapists usually list themselves in the yellow pages of
the telephone directory. Or contact:

> Biofeedback Certification Institute of America
> 10200 West 44th Avenue, Suite 304
> Wheat Ridge, Colo. 80033
> 303-420-2902

Feldenkrais Work

This is a system of postures, movements, and body work designed
to retrain the nervous system to interact with muscles in new ways.
It is an excellent technique of rehabilitation for people who have
suffered injuries and strokes and a good therapy for those with
chronic pain. It is also very useful in cases of developmental retardation. You can obtain a directory of practitioners from:

> The Feldenkrais Guild
> P.O. Box 489
> Albany, Oreg. 97321
> 1-800-775-2118

Guided Imagery Therapy

This new organization maintains a database of health professionals who use guided imagery in their work:

> Academy for Guided Imagery
> P.O. Box 2070
> Mill Valley, Calif. 94942
> 415-389-9324

Holistic Medicine

Members of the American Holistic Medical Association are M.D.s and D.O.s (osteopaths) who subscribe to the general belief that human beings are more than just physical bodies and that good treatment must address the whole person. Holistic doctors may use alternative or complementary techniques in addition to or in place of regular practices, and there is wide variation in what they do. The AHMA can provide you with names of member physicians in your area and tell you what methods they use.

> American Holistic Medical Association
> 4101 Lake Boone Trail, Suite 201
> Raleigh, North Carolina 27607
> 919-787-5146

Homeopathic Medicine

A great variety of people practice homeopathic medicine: M.D.s, naturopaths, chiropractors, and lay practitioners with no formal degrees. The best source of information about this system is:

> Homeopathic Educational Services
> 2124 Kittredge Street
> Berkeley, Calif. 94704
> 510-649-0294

They publish and distribute books, tapes, and medicine kits for home use.

The following organizations have referral services and can provide you with names of homeopathic practitioners:

National Center for Homeopathy
801 North Fairfax Street, Suite 306
Alexandria, Va. 22314
703-548-7790

International Foundation for Homeopathy
2366 Eastlake Avenue East #301
Seattle, Wash. 98102
206-324-8230

Hypnotherapy

Check the yellow pages of the telephone directory under "Hypnotists." If you want to work with an M.D. who is a hypnotherapist and can't find one in the phone book, contact:

American Society of Clinical Hypnosis
2250 East Devon Avenue, Suite 336
Des Plaines, Ill. 60018
708-297-3317

Naturopathic Medicine

Three sorts of naturopaths (N.D.s) are in practice today. A few very old ones are the last of the group that founded this system of natural treatment in the early years of this century. If you can find one of them, you will be pleased, because they are good practitioners with much experience. Many middle-aged naturopaths are really chiropractors who took mail-order courses in naturopathy and awarded themselves N.D. degrees. They are not nearly as well trained as the younger naturopaths produced by two schools: the National College of Naturopathic Medicine in Portland, Oregon, and the John Bastyr College of Naturopathic Medicine in Seattle. (A new school, the Southwest College of Naturopathic Medicine, has just opened in Phoenix.) The graduates of those schools are well educated and trained, and I refer patients to them. Naturopaths are currently licensed in fewer than a quarter of the states in this country (mostly in the west), but the profession now seems to be growing in stature and may win the legal right to practice in other states. You can locate practitioners nearest you by contacting:

American Association of Naturopathic Physicians
2366 Eastlake Avenue East, #322
Seattle, Wash. 98102
206-323-7610

Osteopathic Manipulation, Cranial Therapy

Most osteopaths (D.O.s) today are indistinguishable from M.D.s. They give drugs and do surgery — a far cry from osteopaths of previous generations. A minority of them use manipulation as a main modality of treatment. They belong to a professional organization called the American Academy of Osteopathy, which will provide you with names of practitioners nearest you.

American Academy of Osteopathy
3500 DePauw Boulevard, Suite 1080
Indianapolis, Ind. 46268
317-879-1881

Of these manipulating osteopaths, an even smaller percentage have taken training in cranial therapy. You can find those through:

Cranial Academy
3500 DePauw Boulevard, Suite 1080
Indianapolis, Ind. 46268
317-879-0713

Rolfing

Rolfing is a system of deep-tissue massage that works especially on the connective tissue (fascia) that attaches muscles to bones. It can also release emotional stresses that have been stored in the musculature. You can locate practitioners through:

Rolf Institute
205 Canyon Boulevard
Boulder, Colo. 80306
303-449-5903

Trager Work

This gentle massage system, useful as a relaxation technique as well as for rehabilitation and the relief of chronic pain, is practiced by trainees of the Trager Institute. For the names of practitioners nearest you, contact:

The Trager Institute
33 Millwood
Mill Valley, Calif. 94941
415-388-2688

FINDING SUPPLIES

Chinese Medicinal Herbs

Herbs such as schizandra berries for the liver, *Polyporus umbellatus* mushrooms, and *Astragalus* root for immune-system enhancement, as well as crude Chinese ephedra and dong quai roots can all be ordered from:

Nuherbs Company
3820 Penniman Avenue
Oakland, Calif. 94619
1-800-233-4307

The manufacturer of Astra-8, the herbal combination for immune-system enhancement, and other Chinese herbal formulas is:

Health Concerns
8001 Capwell Drive
Oakland, Calif. 94621
1-800-233-9355

Excellent Chinese herbal tonics and information about them are available from:

The Tea Garden Herbal Emporium
903 Colorado Boulevard, Suite 200
Santa Monica, Calif. 90405
310-450-0188

Freeze-Dried Herbal Extracts

The only supplier I know of freeze-dried stinging nettles, dandelion leaves, and hawthorn berries is the Eclectic Institute. This company also makes good herbal tinctures.

Eclectic Institute
14385 S.E. Lusted Road
Sandy, Oreg. 97055
1-800-332-4372

Herbal Pharmaceutical Products

Products such as enteric-coated peppermint oil capsules, deglycyrrhizinated licorice (DGL) extract, saw palmetto extract, and preparations of ginkgo and Chinese ephedra are made by:

Phyto-Pharmica
P.O. Box 1745
Green Bay, Wis. 54305
1-800-553-2370
414-435-4200 (in Wisconsin)

This company sells only to health professionals, so you will have
to have a doctor place an order for you.

Organic Produce

The Organic Network by Jean Winter is a directory of organic
growers. The national directory costs $15; directories for most
states are available at $2 each. Write to:

Eden Acres, Inc.
12100 Lima Center Road
Clinton, Mich. 49236
517-456-4288

Vitamin C

The best form of this vitamin I have found is called C-salts, an effervescent powder that is nonacidic and sodium free. It is made by:

Wholesale Nutrition
P.O. Box 3345
Saratoga, Calif. 95070-9942
1-800-325-2664

Vitamins and Supplements

It is a challenge to find sources of quality products at less than exorbitant prices. Two mail-order houses carry many brands and publish comprehensive catalogs:

L & H Vitamins
37-10 Crescent Street
Long Island City, N.Y. 11101
1-800-221-1152

The Vitamin Shoppe
4700 Westside Avenue
North Bergen, N.J. 07047
1-800-223-1216

Another company that makes good vitamin and mineral preparations is:

Bronson Pharmaceuticals
1945 Craig Road
P.O. Box 46903
St. Louis, Mo. 63146-6903
1-800-235-3200

ACKNOWLEDGMENTS

Of the people who helped me write this book, I must first acknowledge the many patients who were willing to try unusual and sometimes experimental remedies and report back to me on the results.

Several persons read the manuscript and gave me helpful suggestions, primarily my friend and colleague Dr. Steven Rayle. Other readers were Sabine Kremp, Sue Fleishman, and Kim Cliffton, and Dr. Joseph Alpert.

Practitioners who gave me information that went into the book include Deborah Morris, Nancy Aton, N.D., David Jaffrey, Theresa Cisler, D.O., Dean Ornish, M.D., Robyn Power, Francis Brinker, N.D., and Michael Moore.

Thanks to Nancy Kaye Lunney of Esalen Institute, who prompted me to begin giving workshops on nutrition. The information I organized for them became Chapters 1 and 2.

I have had the help of a good editor, Signe Warner Watson of Houghton Mifflin.

Thanks also to Peg Anderson, Lynn Nesbit, Harriet Larkin, Victoria Tolmach, Brian Becker, Mike Meyer, Cliff Berrien, the Alchemy Rhythm Band of Tucson, Arizona, Pete Craig, and, especially, to Sabine.

INDEX